Challenges in Medical Ethics:

the South African context

Editors:

Chris Jones
Mariana Kruger
Juri van den Heever
Anton van Niekerk

SUN PRESS

Challenges in Medical Ethics: the South African context

Published by African Sun Media under the SUN PReSS imprint
Place of publication: Stellenbosch, South Africa

First edition 2022

ISBN 978-1-991201-94-2
ISBN 978-1-991201-95-9 (e-book)
https://doi.org/10.52779/9781991201959

Set in Adobe Caslon Pro 11/14

Cover design by African Sun Media Create
Typesetting and production by African Sun Media

SUN PReSS is an imprint of African Sun Media. Scholarly, professional and reference works are published under this imprint in print and electronic formats.

This publication can be ordered from:
orders@africansunmedia.co.za
Takealot: bit.ly/2monsfl
Google Books: bit.ly/2k1Uilm
africansunmedia.store.it.si *(e-books)*
Amazon Kindle: amzn.to/2ktL.pkL

Visit africansunmedia.co.za for more information.

Contents

Acknowledgements

The editors wish to thank all the co-authors for making the time in their busy schedules to reflect on the crucial issues addressed in this book. Making this publication a reality was indeed a team effort.

A lot of hard work has been done by the staff members of African Sun Media. Thank you for believing in this book project right from the start, and for improving the text.

Much appreciation goes to the reviewers. Thank you for the time spent on evaluating the manuscript, and for valuable comments.

A word of sincere appreciation to the Unit for Bioethics, based in the Centre for Applied Ethics at Stellenbosch University, for its financial contribution towards this book project.

The Editors

Research Justification

This double-blind peer reviewed book academically reflects on important and relevant challenges in medical ethics within the South African context such as the law and bioethics; Universal Health Coverage, National Health Insurance, and a sustainable workforce; reproductive health and the termination of pregnancy in contemporary South Africa; gender in sport, with Caster Semenya as a case in point; ethics of transplantation; ethical issues in the HIV-positive to positive transplant setting; the South African legal response to organ trafficking and transplant tourism in international perspective; the ethics of mental health service delivery in a multicultural setting; a more globally inclusive and relevant neuroethics; significantly increased longevity; end-of-life choices; how to treat private and sensitive medical and genetic data; cyberspace-related risk aspects in the medical ecosystem; and how biotechnology will transform human health, with reference to the peril and promise of genetic engineering. It is mainly written from a qualitative and conceptual methodological research perspective, including autobiographical and participatory views.

In the respective 14 chapters, the authors present their research systematically and intersectionally, rooted in proper theoretical analysis and reasoning. It is a scholarly book aimed at peers, scholars, and researchers, providing arguments for open discussion of the perspectives on the different challenges in medical ethics, mainly in the South African context.

We can confirm that all the chapters of this collected work are based on original research and that no part of the book was plagiarised from another publication or published elsewhere. It disseminates original research and new developments within these specific fields of study.

The Editors

Preface

This is a book about a number of serious challenges that bioethicists have to deal with in our time, particularly in the South African context. The term 'bioethics' will, in what follows, be used interchangeably with the term 'medical ethics'. By bioethics/medical ethics we mean the outcome of systematic reflection on moral problems that arise in health care and the life sciences generally, as well as the institutional practices that provoke or are influenced by such reflection (e.g., the institutionalised generation of abortion laws in Parliament).

Bioethics ironically represents both the oldest and one of the newest 'sciences' widely practiced at the current-day university. As an instance of intellectual endeavour, it originally draws on the work (particularly the oath) of the ancient Greek physician, Hippocrates. The Hippocratic tradition, however, never developed into a systematic body of scholarship. The latter only occurred in the course of the 20th century, mainly as a result of the rapid development in current-day medical science and technology. At the same time, the 20th century brought, in a very notable manner, the realisation that, in spite of the unprecedented strides made by medical sciences in our times (e.g., the successful treatment of ischemic heart disease, various cancers, transplantation technologies and the like), health care professionals are not only prone to do good, but can indeed sometimes indulge in ethically questionable practices. In this respect, one hardly needs to be reminded of more than the abominable 'medical experiments' on (particularly disabled) human subjects by Nationalist Socialist 'doctors' (like Joseph Mengele) during World War II, or, alternatively, the infamous Tuskegee medical 'research trials' in the USA in the early part of the 20th century.

These (and many other) events launched bioethics as not only a prevailing, but indeed an extremely necessary intellectual endeavour. From an almost non-existent 'science' at the beginning of the 20th century, bioethics has since been growing with unprecedented strides and established itself as a major field of study across the world.

This book is an acknowledgement of the relevance and actuality of this development of bioethics, not only internationally, but particularly in South Africa. The saga surrounding the death of Steve Biko in the late 1970s amply testifies how bioethical issues also permeate the South African socio-political context.

This book is not only an inter- and multidisciplinary composition of contributors, but also a very good reflection of the interdisciplinary approach that is, in our time, universally required for bioethical work. The contributions also testify to diversity in background.

In chapter one, Anita Kleinsmidt looks at the relationship between law and bioethics. She considers how societies came to adopt laws as their governing systems and specifically describes sources of law and how laws are made in South Africa. There is a brief description of the increasing use of the criminal law in medical negligence matters and also the current pressing problem of unaffordable insurance for obstetricians due to massive civil claims in their discipline. South Africa has a culture of human rights necessitating a discussion on the nature of rights and opposition to rights as a concept. Finally, at the intersection of medical ethics and law, there is a selection of cases from the South African courts summarising judgments involving ethical concepts such as confidentiality, medical professionalism, the doctor-patient relationship, abortion, surrogate pregnancies, and physician-assisted suicide.

Mariana Kruger, in chapter two, reasons that everybody has the right to health. According to the World Health Organization (WHO), this is achievable through universal access to health coverage (UHC). Countries should provide access to quality health services which addresses the need of the population with priority setting regarding health care interventions for the improvement of general health. Usually these decisions focus on safety, efficacy, and cost-effectiveness, but health care decision-makers should also address issues such as equity, fairness, financial protection, and impact on the national budget. South Africa is in the process of implementing UHC through the establishment of National Health Insurance, which is crucial to address the inequity of health care provision during the apartheid era. There are four key interventions planned, namely the transformation of the health care service provision with a sustainable health care workforce, a complete overhaul of the health care system, administration and management changes, and provision of a comprehensive health care package for all South Africans.

In chapter three, Carike Noeth provides a brief overview of recent historical legislation regarding the termination of pregnancy in South Africa, focusing on the Abortion and Sterilization Act of 1975 and the Choice on Termination of Pregnancy Act 92 of 1996. This is followed by a discussion of the reasons why the termination of pregnancy is regarded as an ethical dilemma in the 21st century, such as politics, technology, paternal rights, and religious conviction. The complexities and challenges of the termination of pregnancy are then discussed to determine where the shortfalls are regarding the Choice on Termination of Pregnancy Act 92 of 1996. By determining the challenges, it is argued that different role-players are key to accepting ethical responsibility when it comes to reproductive health in South Africa to ensure that policies, laws, and regulations are implemented practically. This includes the acceptance of the ethical responsibility to ensure the implementation of rights as set out by South African laws to promote the furtherance of gender equality, women's rights, and the right to reproductive health care.

In chapter four, Juri van den Heever and Chris Jones point out how sex and gender have been contentious issues, historically and up to the present time, in various walks of life, none perhaps more so than in international athletics. They examine the origins and historical development of sex and gender discrimination from the perspective of hunter-gatherer societies to the present, referring to the influences of agricultural practices, religion, and legal systems. Advances in biological disciplines such as neurobiology, embryology, and genetics have revealed, and made public, a wide range of detailed insights about the physical realities of human sexuality and gender choices that can no longer be ignored. It is suggested that administrative bodies, such as the International Association of Athletics Federations, now World Athletics, and indeed the public in general, avail themselves of this information, thereby fostering a more balanced view of issues pertaining to sex and gender. Finally, they suggest a tentative option which may allow World Athletics an escape route from the impasse they currently find themselves in regarding sex and gender discrimination.

Willie Koen, in chapter five, writes about the ethics of transplantation and refers to the different factors that must be considered regarding cadaver organ transplantation. He also focuses on living donor organ transplantation, where the organs are harvested from a live donor opposed to cadaver organs. The author further writes about the allocation of cadaver organs in transplantation, the transplant waiting list, artificial mechanical circulation, stem cell transplantation, Xeno transplantation, and non-lifesaving organ transplantation such as penile, facial, and uterus transplantations. He concludes that the field of transplantation is fraught with ethical challenges. However, these challenges can be addressed by the fundamental question of 'risk versus benefit' by following the first part of the Hippocratic oath of the medical profession namely "do no harm", and by adhering to the four main principles of medical ethics: respect for autonomy, beneficence, non-maleficence, and justice.

Elmi Muller, in chapter six, describes the decision-making process around the use of HIV-positive donors for HIV-positive patients with renal failure for the purpose of kidney transplantation. It highlights the very specific South African health care environment in which this decision was made when the programme was started in 2008. It also discusses some of the ethical considerations surrounding these transplants. It is important to note the landscape for HIV-positive patients in South Africa at the time – there were no treatment options available for HIV-positive patients with renal failure. The author writes the chapter from a personal perspective: both as the transplant surgeon who planned and executed the procedures, as well as the person who followed up with these patients over the long term. The chapter uses Alain Badiou's essay on the understanding of evil as a starting point to think about some of the decisions that had to be made. It also reports on the clinical risks that had to be considered for a medical procedure where there was no evidence-based treatment guidelines available. In clinical medicine, evidence-based practice is considered best medical practice. This chapter considers how difficult decisions can be if there is no evidence available in a context where patients and their health care providers are faced with their own mortality.

In chapter seven, Rosaan Krüger outlines the South African legal framework in response to organ trafficking and transplant tourism with reference to the international legal standard set out in binding and non-binding instruments. It does so by comparing the legal framework in place at the time of the organ trafficking scandal in South Africa in the early 2000s, which involved the Netcare group, with the framework currently in place in terms of the National Health Act and its regulations and the Prevention and Combating of Trafficking in Persons Act. The current legal framework adheres to the international standard by reflecting the principles of non-commercialism and altruism in donation but fails to address the issue of organs supply for transplantation adequately.

In chapter eight, Hanru Niemand investigates to what extent the political dilemmas of multiculturalism translate to obligations, particularly in mental health service delivery. He discusses some of these obligations, all of which can be summarised under the heading of cultural competence. He also discusses different types of cultural competence in terms of (1) the obligations on larger structures, including policymakers, educators and selectors to create structures for cultural equality; and (2) the obligations of practitioners and theorists to practice an approach characterised by (a) an awareness of the cultural conditioning involved in their existing models and (b) a willingness to understand models with different cultural origins as if from the inside, and not as so-called neutral observers. In this regard, he pays special attention to criticisms aimed at the scientific method as practiced by mainstream psychology. He also introduces the distinction between simple and complex multicultural problems. He concludes that the progressive equality to be striven for, particularly by larger structures, represents a solution to simple (but practically difficult to achieve) multicultural problems. In contrast, the freedom from bias that is to be achieved, particularly by practitioners and theorists, is a logical impossibility. For this, he suggests a process model of justification, whereby the obligation that rests with practitioners and theorists lies in their attitude, that is, in the process in which they approach these matters.

Andrea Palk, in chapter nine, engages with neuroethics as an interdisciplinary field, encompassing the full array of ethical, legal, and social implications of our study, understanding and deepening knowledge of the human brain, including our ability to increasingly alter or enhance our brains. While the field is broad in scope, it has largely been shaped by the input of researchers situated in high-income countries, with less participation from low-resourced contexts. Participation of African scientists and ethicists, in particular, has been lacking in the field. In light of these observations, she takes as her point of departure a need to critically engage with neuroethics, with the aim of working towards a field that is more globally informed and inclusive of a range of concerns and perspectives. Given that neuroethics is not well established in Africa, in the first half of the chapter, she provides an overview of the traditional conceptualisation of the field as concerned with the 'ethics of neuroscience' and the 'neuroscience of ethics', with examples of typical areas of discussion. She then considers four suggestions for developing the field in African contexts, thus working towards increasing its global relevance. Her suggestions include: building neuroethics capacity through the growth of neuroscience research collaborations across the African continent; exploring congruence with the global mental health movement to engage in neuroethics activism to address brain and mental health research and treatment priorities in Africa; drawing on the strong tradition of empirical ethics research on the continent to establish an evidence-base comprising the perspectives of underrepresented populations on established neuroethics concerns; and finally, engaging with the underlying moral framework of neuroethics by drawing on African moral frameworks. While developing neuroethics in Africa will benefit those who are impacted by its reach in African contexts, the field itself also stands to benefit insofar as it is recognised that any field or area of focus is improved by including a plurality of perspectives, concerns, and input.

In chapter ten, Anton van Niekerk investigates (bio-)ethical issues related to indefinite life expectations and significantly prolonged longevity. It is shown that Yuval Noah Harari regards increased longevity and life expectation as the central scientific, medical, and technological agenda of the 21st century. The contribution of Aubrey de Grey, who advocates the indefinite prolonging of life, is submitted to critical scrutiny. Attention is paid to the causes of death, and particularly to the question as to whether old age ought to be interpreted as a disease. A key argument in the chapter is the prudence of preferring better health than a longer life as one matures. The danger of immeasurable boredom associated with indefinitely prolonged life is argued. The chapter is concluded with arguments about the organic nature of human life and the fact that human life is essentially a narrative quest. These concerns do not support the idea of significantly prolonged human life.

In chapter eleven, Willem Landman reasons that for some, dying is peaceful and dignified. For others, it is suffused with fear, suffering, and loss of autonomy and dignity. We need not die while suffering physically and mentally, with loss of control over one's body. Morally and legally, we have choices that can mitigate what would otherwise be an even worse death. There are four categories of end-of-life choices: end-of-life pain management that hastens death; refusal of and refraining from life-sustaining treatment; advance directives; and assisted dying – referring to assisted suicide and voluntary euthanasia. The first three are, and should be fully recognised as, standard medical practices, but they present several problems relating to their exact legal status and unanswered questions about how they should function in practice. This calls for legislative clarity.

The fourth is more controversial. Rendering assistance with dying – in the forms of assisting with suicide and practising voluntary euthanasia – constitutes the common-law crime of murder. Significantly, though, assisted dying presents a formidable and untenable tension between our common law and rights recognised and protected by the Bill of Rights in our Constitution such as the rights to autonomy, dignity, and bodily integrity, including control over one's body. The crucial public-policy question is how to get the embedded right to assisted dying recognised. In a 2016 ruling, the Supreme Court of Appeal (SCA) made it clear that our common law will "no doubt evolve" when the court is presented with a "full argument and time to reflect". The court would then declare an "incompatibility" between the common law and the Constitution "to enable parliament to remedy the deficiency". In the final analysis, moral responsibility for decriminalising assisted dying rests with our dysfunctional Parliament. The prior challenge is for a dying person, with access to the necessary monetary means, to bring an application to our courts, and remaining alive while the case proceeds through successive court processes.

Himla Soodyall and Jerome Singh, in chapter twelve, write that public trust and confidence in researchers and medical professionals are essential when engaging with research subjects and patients. Coupled with this, there have been a range of ethical challenges related to consent; privacy; ownership of samples; data sharing; re-identification of previously de-identified participant information; access to electronic health records; the collection, storage, and secondary use of biospecimens; and issues related to incidental findings that have been raised in the context of sensitivities to medical and genetic data. While research subjects and patients are mostly happy to consent as participants for research, they still have many concerns about confidentiality of data, particularly in the era of data-sharing and electronic access to information. Patients are also part of families and sometimes their medical information impacts on other family members. Disclosure of such information often poses challenges around privacy and confidentiality, while in other instances family members have shown gratitude for such engagement. Advances in genomic and other diagnostic technologies have vastly improved on diagnosis, treatment, and delivery of health care. Such capabilities have raised concerns about how to deal with incidental findings and whether to disclose this information to patients or not. In this chapter, they address some of the ethical issues outlined above when dealing with sensitive medical and genetic data.

Basie von Solms, in chapter thirteen, argues that new developments in technology have, over the ages, always been core drivers in the dramatic improvement in all areas of health care. Such developments include the availability of newer and more effective drugs as well as the possibility to implant a stent and a pacemaker in the body to address a problem which, only a few years earlier, may have needed a massive invasive operation. Technology developments, operating in what we today experience as 'cyberspace', have already become massive new drivers in improving health care, and will continue to do so at a dizzying pace in coming years. Such technological developments have, among others, led to the implementation of the internet of medical things (IoMT) where numerous sensors and devices are used in the medical ecosystem. However, as has always been the case with any new technology, there are always risks which must be managed as comprehensively as possible to prevent the new technology from causing negative consequences. The IoMT is specifically prone to such risks, which can even threaten the lives of patients. Medical ethics has an essential role in the IoMT as well as in the whole medical ecosystem. This relationship between cyberspace, cybersecurity, and medical ethics in the medical ecosystem is also addressed. This chapter gives an overview of how cyberspace has already impacted the medical ecosystem, and what are some of the important risks which must be identified and managed.

In chapter fourteen, Susan Hall argues that technological advancement often gives rise to novel ethical problems. This is as true with respect to the development and application of biotechnology in the context of health care as elsewhere. The best known and probably most contentious possible application of biotechnology in the context of health care is genetic engineering. While genetic engineering holds great potential for the treatment of disease and disability, to many the prospect of the development and use of interventions which aim to manipulate our genetic makeup evokes discomfort or repugnance, particularly when such interventions aim not only to treat but also to enhance. In this chapter, the author outlines the bioethical debate surrounding genetic engineering. She considers two groups of arguments against the development and use of gene editing technologies which focus on (1) the inherent nature of genetic modification itself and its relationship to human nature, and (2) the likely consequences of gene editing, and she explores possible lines of defence against these challenges. Finally, she briefly puts forward the case that both genetic therapy and some forms of genetic enhancement hold great potential for the transformation of human health, and, in the case of enhancement, human well-being more generally. We should therefore be cautious of rejecting these technologies out of hand.

The Editors

1

Law and Bioethics

Anita Kleinsmidt

"In civilized life, law floats in a sea of ethics" (Warren, 1962)

Keywords: conduct; confidentiality; dual loyalties; euthanasia; informed consent; intersection between law ethics; medical ethics; medical law; professional conduct; surrogacy

---

1.1 WHAT IS LAW AND WHAT IS ETHICS?

Although the answers may seem obvious, let us consider the questions of what law is, what ethics is, and which of the two takes precedence.

Laws consist of rules and guidelines which are enforced through social institutions to govern behaviour. Laws are made based on the moral values of a particular society. Laws represent the minimum standards of human behaviour expected in a society. Legal systems include penalties such as fines and imprisonment for breaches of the law, i.e., infringements of the law usually result in punishments of some kind. If, however, we agree with the normative content of a law, we would obey it even if there were no penalties. The same goes for disagreement with a law in the sense that we sometimes disobey laws when we disagree with them, even if there are penalties. This is aside from circumstances where we may disobey a law through necessity or if we believe that we can escape the consequences. We may ignore the costs of disobedience if a law is greatly at odds with our personal views on what is right (*SA History Online*, 2019).[1]

An ethical position results from a considered analysis or intellectual inquiry of whether an action is good or bad, inherently or in terms of its impact on others.

---

1   South Africa has a long history of protest against unjust laws, often with fatal consequences for protestors.

Ethics and morality are often used interchangeably – morality describes the viewpoints held by a group or individual that certain behaviour is right or wrong. Ethics is often associated with professional practice, e.g., in health care, it has resulted in policies, guidelines, and codes of conduct (Hare, 2019).

The question then arises: where does law come from and why do societies have laws? Natural law theorists believe that natural law arises from nature, irrespective of the society under consideration. Thus, natural law may or may not be present in the legal rules of a society, but exists nonetheless, independently of whether it was incorporated into written legal rules. The concept of natural law was discussed by Aristotle in ancient Greece (384-322 BCE). Some concepts that were 'natural' to the ancient Greeks would be unacceptable or unnatural to us today, e.g., slavery and the subordination of women to men. The Stoics described a type of law that was linked to reason in the mind, and from which one could discern the best way to live, or a type of code of conduct (Horowitz, 1974). Thomas Aquinas, one of the most well-known early natural law theorists, theorised about an "eternal law" emanating from his god. He distinguished between natural law and customary law, or law arising from our conventions. In South Africa, we are familiar with the concept of African customary law arising from local customs and traditions. For Aquinas, the law should have both directive and coercive force (Finnis, 2021).

When we consider the rules of how we ought to live and whether law or ethics should take primacy, the social contract theory of Thomas Hobbes (1588-1679) is relevant to these questions. Social contract theory is the notion that we allow ourselves to be governed by certain laws and give up certain freedoms in exchange for order and predictability in society. This sacrifice of certain of our rights for the sake of consistent laws and social order is the social contract that we have entered into with the state. According to Hobbes, without the social contract, our lives would be lived in a "state of nature" and be "solitary, poor, nasty, brutish and short" (Hobbes & Plamenatz, 1991). This is because absolute freedom would include the freedom to commit wrongs against other members of society, e.g., murder and theft, and would result in an anarchic society without rules. In terms of this theory, government and its laws are not natural but result from arrangements such as elections and democracy, constructed by people. There are developments and early critiques of natural law and of social contract theory by philosophers such as Locke, Rousseau, and Rawls for the interested reader (Fosl & Baggini, 2020).

In contrast, utilitarian theories posit that what a society should strive for is the greatest good for the greatest number of people. We tend to find utilitarian ethical theories applied in public health arguments around the rationing of scarce health resources, as occurred in the *Soobramoney* case, discussed below, about access to dialysis in a public hospital. Some social contract theorists stipulate that we do not in fact yield complete control to governments and laws – there are certain implied conditionalities in the social contract. There is an assumption when we yield control to the state, that its laws are consensual, just, protect certain of our rights, and that there should be processes to meet these ends (Barnett, 1998). These conditions are important when we consider that the system of apartheid in South Africa was underpinned by a comprehensive system of laws and procedures for voting, health care, education, property ownership, expropriation of property, job reservation, access to schools and universities, ability to reside and travel in certain areas, etc. To put it simply, what is legal is not necessarily ethical.

1.2   WHAT ARE RIGHTS?

When we consider law and bioethics, we inevitably look to the nature of rights. This is especially so in a constitutional democracy such as South Africa's. Some theorists state that we do not possess absolute rights. Rather, to have a right means to have a *claim* to be *protected* from certain *harms*, while other rights are claims to be *provided* with certain *benefits* (Wenar, 2021). The former are *negative rights*, the latter are *positive rights*.

Rights impose moral and legal constraints on collective social goals, e.g., a patient's right to refuse treatment trumps a doctor's ethical duty to act in the patient's best interests. Rights can clash with ethical theories but also with other rights. An example of a clash of rights might be where a patient has a right of access to health care, but a doctor has a right to freedom of religion which interferes with the patient's access (Amnesty International, 2017). The SA Constitution requires that where there are opposing rights, we must carry out a "weighing up of rights" or proportionality review to assess whether a limitation of any right in favour of another is lawful (Rautenbach, 2014).

1.2.1   Types of rights

Rights can be classified according to their form, their function, who has them, or why someone might have them. Below, we have a basic system set out by Hope, Savulescu and Hendrick (2003):

- Claim rights: the subject of the right has a claim against another, e.g., claim in contract for sale of house;
- Liberty rights: the protective perimeter of duties on others not to infringe those rights, e.g., property rights;

- Powers rights: rights conferring powers to do things; and

- Immunities rights: rights conferring protection from others, e.g., the right to join a trade union against which the employer cannot object.

1.2.2 Human rights

In South Africa, given our political history, we often speak of human rights. Human rights are entitlements that people can claim relating to their basic needs because they are human. In the past, people were treated differently according to caste, religion, age, and gender. Bodily integrity was not respected – slavery persisted *de jure* until the late 1800s (Bales, 2004). Ideas about social equality and non-discrimination started to emerge in the 19th to 20th century. After World War II and Nazi atrocities, human rights were given international legal recognition. In 1948, the Universal Declaration of Human Rights was signed by all countries and enshrines human rights into international soft law.[2] Natural rights are negative rights, but human rights also include positive rights. Negative rights restrain conduct and positive rights place obligations on us to act in a certain way.

1.2.3 Opposition to rights theories

Not all philosophers find the concept of rights to be useful in ethical analysis. Jeremy Bentham (1843), in a famous attack on natural rights, stated:

> Right ... is the child of law: from real laws come real rights; but from imaginary laws, from laws of nature, fancied and invented by poets, rhetoricians, and dealers in moral and intellectual poisons, come imaginary rights, a bastard brood of monsters. Natural rights is simple nonsense: natural and imprescriptible rights, rhetorical nonsense – nonsense upon stilts.

According to Bentham, rights come from law and legal rights are to be respected when they lead to the greatest happiness of the greatest number, which is the foundation of morals and legislation. He preferred the term "securities against misrule" to rights that he was concerned would give power and acceptability to those acting out their personal desires (Schofield, 2003).

Real rights are established through a legal system that should aim for the greatest good for the greatest number. In society, laws are made in the general interest. The ends or objectives that the legislator should seek to attain are *security*,

---

2   Soft law means that an international declaration or treaty is only legally binding when it has been adopted into the law of a country, or "domesticated". Soft law has weak binding force.

subsistence, abundance, and *equality* (Bentham, 1843). Later critiques of human rights focus on their legitimacy in non-Western societies and on the imposition of Western power structures using the language of rights (Langford, 2018).

1.2.4   Interest-based theory of rights

Joseph Raz promotes perfectionist liberalism – an objective theory of the good life, or of human well-being and the belief that it is the business of the state to promote the good life of its citizens (Nussbaum, 2014). The theory is summarised below:

> My having a right to X means that I have an interest-based reason sufficient for imposing on others a duty to protect or promote my achieving X.
>
> To say that X is in a being's interest is to say that that being, on reflection, would thrive and flourish were it to have X.
>
> To say that X is in a being's interest is to say that that being, on reflection, would thrive and flourish were it to have X.

If the state is to promote the well-being of its citizens, it also has to intervene with citizens' actions that are not conducive to their well-being. Most perfectionist liberals try to avoid this by showing that paternalist state action is self-defeating, i.e., they try to show that the best way for the state to promote the well-being of its citizens is to restrain itself and let each individual strive for their good by themselves. Others hold that liberalism is compatible with some amount of paternalism.

1.3   SOURCES OF LAW

The law in South Africa emanates from several sources. These are the Constitution, Roman-Dutch law, English law, African customary law, academic writing by highly regarded legal authors, legislation (Acts and regulations), and the common law. The common law consists of legal precedents established by the courts in their judgements, as opposed to Acts that are created by Parliament. Roman-Dutch law consists of law principles created by 16th century Dutch jurists who wrote commentaries on Roman law. Roman-Dutch law was brought to the Cape Colony during the period of Dutch colonisation. Its influence remains in the law of persons, contract law, and the law of delict. Our common law system of precedent requires that judgments of higher courts, such as the Supreme Court of Appeal, must be followed by lower courts, such as High Courts in the provinces. In some instances, international law is also considered, as allowed by section 39(1)*(b)* of the Constitution.

It is important to note that all laws must be consistent with our Constitution and its values. Any law or policy that is inconsistent with the Constitution is invalid in terms of its section 2. The Constitution was drafted following widespread consultation and public constitutional forums throughout South Africa. In contradistinction to South Africa's pre-1994 dispensation, the Constitution promotes the values of dignity, equality, transparency, just administrative action, etc. The current constitutional democracy in South Africa replaced the system of parliamentary sovereignty inherited from the United Kingdom. South Africa became a self-governing dominion of Britain in 1910 (*SA History Online*, 2020). The influence of British law is most obvious in our laws of procedure and evidence. The distinguishing feature of the system of parliamentary sovereignty was that as long as the proper procedure was followed in making laws, their content or long-term effects could not be called into question. This of course resulted in many ethical quandaries for judges who were expected to apply laws that they disagreed with (Dugard, 1984). The South African constitution recognises customary law in section 39(2), but all laws "must promote the values that underlie an open and democratic society based on human dignity, equality and freedom". Thus, customary practices that are unfairly discriminatory, e.g., on the basis race or gender, would not be enforceable in South Africa.[3]

1.4   HOW LAWS ARE MADE

If a department, e.g., the Department of Health, decides that there is a need for legal regulation in a certain area of health, they will draft a bill and present it to Parliament. The bill will go through several consultative processes before it can be signed by the President of South Africa and become an Act. These processes include the publication of the bill for public comment, parliamentary portfolio committee hearings, and hearings by provincial legislatures. Statute law must be passed by both 'houses', the National Assembly, and the National Council of Provinces (NCOP). The state attorneys in the office of the President also assess whether new laws will pass constitutional muster, i.e., that they conform to the Constitution before the President signs them into law. Acts or statute law bills dealing with financial and revenue matters have a more complex process.[4] Even after the President has signed an Act, it must be promulgated in the *Government*

---

3   In the 2005 case of *Bhe v Magistrate, Khayelitsha*, the Constitutional Court held that the traditional system of excluding female heirs from intestate succession was incompatible with the equality and dignity sections of the Constitution.

4   This flow chart is a useful source describing law-making: https://www.parliament.gov. za/how-law-made

Gazette to become operational. Some Acts become operational in stages as government proceeds to set up systems for implementation.

In some instances, the South African Law Reform Commission may recommend new laws in light of a situation or a prevailing ethical problem. The Commission's report and proposals on euthanasia are good examples of such recommendations, although their suggestions were not implemented (SALC Project 86, 1998). Some Acts have their origin in Green Papers. In this process, an issue is identified by a government department and a discussion document, the Green Paper, is published for public comment and input by interested parties. This may lead to a White Paper on government policy, again published for public comment. In some cases, this process results in a bill which then follows the required parliamentary process for draft legislation.[5]

1.5   EXAMPLE OF AN UNPROCEDURAL LEGISLATIVE PROCESS

Since 1994, the legislative process in South Africa has been characterised by transparency and public consultation as required by the Constitution. In the 2006 case of *Doctors for Life v Speaker of the National Assembly*, Doctors for Life, the applicants, successfully challenged the validity of the Choice on Termination of Pregnancy Act (and certain other health-related legislation) because the NCOP had not invited written submissions and conducted public hearings as it was supposed to on four bills including the Choice Act (*DFL v Speaker*). The National Assembly had, however, followed the correct procedure. The Constitutional Court ruled that the invalidity of the Act was suspended for 18 months for Parliament to remedy the procedural defect by following the correct procedure and holding public hearings at provincial legislatures.

The issue of abortion is an interesting one, illustrating the intersection between ethics and law. The laws and policies of South Africa promote reproductive rights and access to abortion. Opponents of abortion initially attacked access by questioning the legal status of the foetus. When this was unsuccessful, they moved their focus to procedural matters such as NCOP consultation and they later attempted, also unsuccessfully, to insert other procedural requirements such as compulsory counselling and ultrasound. In the case of foetal legal status, the Court would not be drawn to pronounce on the ethics of abortion but instead analysed the arguments in relation to the provisions of the Constitution.

---

5   See https://pmg.org.za/page/legislative-process for a detailed description of this process.

1.6 CRIMINAL AND CIVIL LAW IN THE MEDICAL PROFESSION

There are several branches of the law. In this section, we consider two – criminal and civil law, in the context of the medical profession.

Criminal law is a branch of public law where the state takes action against an individual, following a police investigation. The state must prove that the accused person is guilty "beyond reasonable doubt" and the accused must attempt to raise doubt about their 'guilt' to escape conviction. The use of criminal proceedings in medicine has increased and become a controversial issue, with the Medical Protection Society (MPS) calling for the state to desist from launching criminal proceedings against doctors (Howarth, 2021; Ladher, 2018). Note that in medical negligence matters, a doctor can in theory be called upon to defend themselves at three levels simultaneously: civil proceedings, criminal proceedings, and disciplinary hearings at the Health Professions Council of South Africa (HPCSA), the regulatory body for health professionals. Howarth of the MPS recommends that criminal proceedings only be brought in cases where "there was clear recklessness" and "the clinician does what no other clinician would do under the circumstances" (Howarth, 2021).

Currently, criminal charges can be brought against a medical practitioner when they have been negligent even though not reckless, i.e., they should have fore-seen the harm that would result from their conduct or failure to act as they should, but they did not foresee the consequences, and harm ensued. There have been a number of recent cases of criminal charges being brought against doctors (*MedicalBrief*, 2021). These include charges against a paediatric surgeon and an anaesthetist following the death of a child after routine laparoscopy and against an obstetrician after the death during delivery of the pregnant woman (Lerm & Stellenberg, 2022). This is a conspicuous development in criminal law, as medical negligence matters have unfortunately been very common in the civil law environment, with burgeoning medical negligence claims against the state totalling R111.5bn in March 2020 (Bateman, 2021; Pienaar, 2016; Planting, 2021).

In medical ethics and law, civil actions usually occur around medical negligence actions. While criminal law involves action by the state against a person, civil actions involve one person, the plaintiff/applicant, bringing an action against another person, the defendant/respondent. The plaintiff must prove their case on a balance of probabilities. This is an easier standard to meet than in criminal matters, where the case must be proved "beyond a reasonable doubt". In civil matters, plaintiffs can claim damages, which may be for intangible harm such as pain, suffering, and the loss of amenities of life, e.g., the ability to enjoy certain hobbies. Compensation can also be for loss or damages which can be computed, known as patrimonial loss, such as for lost earnings due to the harm caused and medical expenses, past and future (Oosthuizen & Carstens, 2015).

In South Africa, obstetricians in private practice are struggling with unaffordable costs for professional indemnity insurance of around R1m per annum per practitioner (Erasmus, 2017). The reason for this exorbitant amount is that claims for high-severity injuries during the birth process, e.g., birth asphyxiation leading to brain damage lead to claims for lifelong medical care, specialised physiotherapy, occupational therapy, future pain and suffering, adaptive devices, and specialised education (Planting, 2021). This has of course led to an exit from the profession and situations where there are no practising obstetricians in private practice in small towns (Howarth & Carstens, 2014).

1.7 ETHICAL PRINCIPLES BECOME LAW AND POLICY

We have seen that ethical theories and legal systems have different origins but that laws are based upon certain ethical or value positions that we hold in society and that we want enforced, with sanctions for breaches of those legalised ethical boundaries. This applies squarely to the field of medical ethics. The ethical values of informed consent, confidentiality, and aspects of medical professionalism are examples of ethical principles which have become part of South African law.

1.7.1 The doctor-patient relationship

The age-old concept of the doctor-patient relationship is an instance of ethical requirements finding their place in law. There is an implied contract between the doctor or the provincial hospital authority and the patient. The doctor has a duty of care: to diagnose and treat according to generally accepted medical procedures in the patient's best interests. This ethical and legal duty will be limited in certain respects: by the availability of resources as well as the fact that patients can refuse care against their best interests. In private institutions, the contract is written, explicit, and signed. In terms of section 27(3) of the Constitution, no one may be refused emergency medical treatment. This means that even private health facilities must stabilise and provide emergency care, even to indigent patients. Once the patient's condition has been stabilised, they may move the patient to a public hospital.

1.7.2 Doctors' professional conduct

What is the difference between unprofessional conduct and negligence? Unprofessional conduct is not necessarily negligent, e.g., being rude to a patient may be unprofessional but it is not negligence. Negligence is conduct that the reasonable doctor would not have carried out. If there was a risk that the reasonable doctor would have foreseen and taken steps to avoid, but another doctor did not, that doctor was negligent. If that conduct caused damages of some kind to the patient, there are grounds for a medical negligence claim. Patients may choose to bring civil claims for medical negligence while they also lodge complaints of unethical or unprofessional conduct with the HPCSA. These complaints will first be assessed by the HPCSA's ombudsman, before being investigated by the HPCSA's relevant Professional Board for that area of medical practice.

1.7.3 Informed consent

This ethical concept is central to the health professional-patient relationship. Informed consent is based upon the ethical principle of respect for autonomy, in contradistinction to the 'doctor knows best' approach of earlier paternalistic times in medicine. Informed consent was first raised in medical case law in the United States in 1905 (*Mohr v Williams*). In South Africa, in 1926 already, the courts considered the importance of respect for patient autonomy (*Stoffberg v Elliot*). The common law principles relied upon were later set out in the Constitution and in the National Health Act. The patient can consent expressly or tacitly. Informed consent is now a central tenet of medical law. Section 6 of the National Health Act and section 12(2) of the Constitution both mandate informed consent which consists of providing information on

- the health status (unless this is not in the patient's best interests);
- the range of procedures and treatments available;
- the benefits, risks, and consequences of the procedures and treatments; and
- the right to refuse implications and risks.

In terms of section 7 of the National Health Act, there are exceptions to the requirement of informed consent. These are

- *failure to treat will result in a serious risk to public health;*
- if the user is unable to give consent but consent has been given by a proxy; and
- lack of treatment will result in death or irreversible damage and there has been no prior refusal.

In many areas of biomedical ethics, there are corresponding areas of law, policies, and guidelines.

TABLE 1.1 Corresponding areas of law, policies, and guidelines in biomedical ethics

Ethical issue	South African law
Circumcision of children	• Children's Act 38 of 2005: section 12
Confidentiality	• National Health Act 61 of 2003: section 14 • The Constitution: section 14
Euthanasia	• The crime of murder: Schedule 3 to the Criminal Procedure Act 51 of 1977
Informed consent	• National Health Act 61 of 2003: section 7 • The Constitution: section 12
Professionalism	• HPCSA Ethical Guidelines for Good Practice in the Health Care Professions
Research ethics	• National Health Act 61 of 2003: section 11 • Department of Health Guidelines: Ethics in Health Research
Stem cell use	• National Health Act 61 of 2003: sections 56, 57, and 68
Surrogacy	• Children's Act 38 of 2005: chapter 19
Termination of pregnancy	• Choice on Termination of Pregnancy Act 92 of 1996 • Department of Health National Guideline for the Implementation of the CTOP Act

1.8 FROM ETHICAL PRACTICE TO LAW: LEGAL CASES INVOLVING THE INTERSECTION BETWEEN ETHICAL PRINCIPLES AND THE LAW

In the summaries that follow, we illustrate the ethical values involved in various cases, where doctors, patients, and the state resorted to legal action to enforce moral principles embedded in the law.

■ *Traub v Administrator Transvaal, 1989: Duty to employer v duty to the patient*

This matter dealt with the right to be heard and the principle of legitimate expectation. The facts were that the provincial director of hospital services in the Transvaal (Gauteng) refused to appoint or re-appoint six qualified medical professionals as senior house officers. These doctors were refused employment by the director, despite recommendations by their Head of Department, because they had signed a letter exposing the conditions in medical wards at Baragwanath Hospital. There were insufficient beds, patients were sleeping on the floor, there was "horrendous overcrowding", and insufficient nurses were allocated to the wards. The doctors had refused to sign an apology as demanded by the provincial administrator. Most of the doctors had signed the apology to avoid personal victimisation. The six doctors had not been given a hearing before being refused employment. Given that this was a departure from the usual process where a HOD's recommendation was acted upon, the doctors had a legitimate expectation of a fair hearing before a decision on the appointments was taken. The decision of the administrator was overturned, and the administrator also lost their appeal.

This is a case of a dilemma known as dual loyalties: where there is a conflict of interest between the doctor's accountability to two or more different entities. In this case, the doctors were under ethical and professional duties to care for their patients and to report abuse but also needed to progress professionally. Another example is the threat of disciplinary action against Dr Tim de Maayer, who wrote an open letter to the Department of Health describing the dire and often fatal effects on children of the poor management at Rahima Moosa Hospital in Gauteng province (McQuoid-Mason, 2022).

▪ *Jansen v Kruger, 1993: Doctor's duty of confidentiality to patient*

In the case of *Jansen v Kruger*, we find the court deliberating on the doctor's duty of confidentiality to patients, especially patients with HIV. Medical confidentiality is an age-old concept, mentioned already around 3-5 BCE and later included in the Hippocratic Oath: "[W]hatsoever I shall see or hear in the course of my profession as well as outside my profession in my intercourse with men, if it be what should not be published abroad, I will never divulge, holding such things to be holy secrets" (Hippocratic Oath). The basis of this principle is that in order for a health practitioner to properly treat a patient, that patient must be able to freely disclose their symptoms without fear of disclosure. This is especially so in the case of diseases carrying social stigma such as sexually transmitted illnesses. In this case, in a small town, the doctor disclosed the patient's HIV status to a GP and to a dentist while playing golf. The patient had specifically asked the doctor not to tell anyone and the doctor had agreed to respect his privacy. Word spread quickly, and the patient soon discovered that his HIV status was being discussed in the social circles in the town. He launched a lawsuit that was unsuccessful in the High Court. He passed away, but his deceased estate continued with the matter and was successful upon appeal.

▪ *Soobramooney v Minister of Health, 1998: Allocation of scarce lifesaving resources*

Mr S was a 41-year-old man with diabetes, ischaemic heart disease, cerebravascular disease, and in the final stages of chronic renal failure. He sought renal dialysis to prolong his life, but hospitals can only dialyse limited patients and they have to ration the dialysis equipment for patients who are eligible for kidney transplants. Mr S did not qualify under their criteria but sued them on the basis of his right to emergency care, section 27(3) of the Constitution. Why did he not use section 27(1) of the Constitution, the "access to healthcare services" section? Section 27(1) is subject to the "progressive realisation" clause, i.e., there is a recognition that South Africa does not have sufficient health resources to meet the needs of patients but must work towards progressively building itself up in order to meet those needs. Section 27(3), which he tried to use, is an entitlement to immediate emergency care, but the Court found that chronic dialysis is not emergency care. His legal team used the emergency care section because it is not subject to progressive realisation. The Constitutional Court agreed with the utilitarian analysis used by the hospital for allocation of scarce resources. The Court found that the hospital had a rational plan to maximise the utility of its dialysis machines. The plan excluded access to people like Mr S, who would need dialysis indefinitely. They only dialysed those who had reasonable prospects of recovery, i.e., the principle of the greatest good for the greatest number was applied. In this matter, the principles of beneficence and non-maleficence clash with justice and utility.[6]

Christian Lawyers Association v Minister of Health, 1998: Constitutionality of abortion law

Despite abortion being widely recorded and practised in the ancient world, the morality of abortion is still one of the few intractable issues in ethical discourse (Peterson, 2012). In the 1800s in the US and parts of Europe, abortion went from being a woman's private matter to becoming a criminal offence. Until 1869, the Roman Catholic Church had allowed abortion before "quickening".[7] In South Africa, the Choice on Termination of Pregnancy Act was enacted in 1998 and, consequently, maternal deaths from sepsis were reduced by 91% (Jewkes & Rees, 2005). Since the Choice Act was implemented, it has faced several challenges from parties that are ethically opposed to it. Initially, these challenges were to the substance of its rights, and later, when the constitutional issues were clarified,

---

6   This illustrates a significant problem with the principlist approach to ethics where clashes between different principles often result in defaulting to a doctor-knows-best position. In this case, as in many resource-constraint ethical dilemmas, the court used a utilitarian analysis. For more on the lack of action-guidance in principlism, see Lewis and Schuklenk (2021) and Lee (2010).

7   In 1591, Pope Gregory XIV determined that "quickening or ensoulment" took place at 166 days of pregnancy. In 1869, Pope Pius IX stipulated excommunication for abortion at any stage (Noonan, 1965).

on procedural issues aimed at reducing access to abortion. An example, in 1998, was a case where the Christian Lawyers Association of South Africa brought an application against the Minister of Health to have the Choice Act struck down in its entirety. Their arguments were that the foetus has the right to life in terms of section 11 of the Constitution from the moment of conception and the Choice Act is therefore unconstitutional. The Court stated that it is not "the function of this Court to decide the matter on religious or philosophical grounds. The issue is a legal one to be decided on the proper legal interpretation of section 11". The Court agreed with the Canadian Supreme Court that "[m]etaphysical arguments may be relevant but they are not the primary focus of the enquiry".[8] Instead, the Court analysed the meaning of the words "child" and "everyone", the legislative history of the Constitution, and anomalies which might result, to decide whether the phrase "everyone has a right to life" applied to a foetus. It found that it did not. Thus, the Court did not debate the ethics of abortion, but analysed whether the right to life in the Constitution was applicable before birth.

▪ Naude & Von Mollendorff v MEC Health, Mpumalanga, 2008: Provision of antiretrovirals in the age of AIDS denialism

In the cases of Dr Malcom Naudé and Dr Thys von Mollendorff, there was a clash between their ethical duties to treat their patients with the best treatment available at the public hospital where they worked, and the instructions of the MEC for Health, Sibongile Manana (Bateman, 2008). The MEC had instructed that no doctors were to administer antiretrovirals as prophylaxis to rape survivors to prevent HIV infection. At the time, an NGO at the hospital was providing the medication free of charge, together with post-trauma counselling and care packages. Antiretroviral prophylaxis had already been scientifically proven to reduce HIV infection if administered within 72 hours of the rape. Manana even refused to make exceptions for child rape survivors (Naude v MEC Health). However, at the same hospital, staff who experienced needlestick injuries were allowed to follow a protocol of antiretroviral prophylaxis to reduce HIV infection. Von Mollendorff, who was the medical superintendent at the time, refused to prohibit the doctors at his hospital from providing effective prophylaxis to rape survivors. Both Naudé and Von Mollendorff were dismissed. Both doctors received substantial financial settlements after years of torturous legal battles in which one of the courts described their actions as that of "a deep-seated belief in the doctor-patient relationship" and "professional conscience and ethics" against the MEC's "irrational policy" and "dictatorial and tyrannical management style" (Naude v MEC Health).

---

8   Quoting the Canadian Supreme Court in Tremblay v Daigle (1989) 62 DLR (SC).

■ *Theron v Department Correctional Services, 2007: Professional duty to prisoner patients v duty to employer*

Doctors providing medical care to prisoners have for long been exposed to ethical dilemmas rising out of dual loyalties conflicts. Not all doctors or professional medical organisations put their duties to patients before the interests of their employers. In the Steve Biko case, it was clear that the doctors had placed their allegiance to their employer, the police services, above their professional ethical duties to their patient who died after being assaulted by the police.

In the case of Dr Paul Theron, the situation was reversed. He was severely penalised for reporting on the poor medical conditions at Pollsmoor Prison in 2007. The Inspecting Judge for Prisons is tasked with visiting and reporting on prison conditions, therefore, prisoner health care fell squarely within the remit of the Inspectorate. Dr Theron correctly believed that it was his ethical duty to inform the Inspectorate of sick or wounded prisoners being denied adequate health care. The Minister of Correctional Services launched a defamation suit against the doctor, and he was also suspended from work (ODAC [Open Democracy Advice Centre], 2015). Even when the Labour Court ordered his reinstatement, the prison guards barred his entry. Dr Theron was never reinstated at Pollsmoor Prison but transferred elsewhere. Despite the existence of the "whistleblower" law, the Protected Disclosures Act 26 of 2000, the doctor in this matter found himself being penalised by a large government department with deep pockets for acting according to his ethical conscience and his professional duty to his patients.

■ *Stransham-Ford v Minister of Justice, 2015: Physician-assisted suicide*

Euthanasia, like abortion, is one of the few ethical issues that are intractable to resolution through analysis and discussion. Euthanasia is illegal in South Africa despite progressive recommendations for legal change by the SA Law Reform Commission in 1998 (SALC Project 86, 1998). Proponents of euthanasia or physician-assisted suicide are concerned with alleviating human suffering caused by terminal illness and promoting dignity and autonomy in the dying process.[9] Opponents of euthanasia cite concerns around pressure on the poor and elderly, devaluation of human life, rifts in the doctor-patient relationship, and reduction in palliative care.

---

9   There are countries which allow assisted suicide in the absence of terminal illness. The procedural safeguards differ from country to country and usually involve requirements such as citizenship, mandatory waiting periods, diagnosis, repeated requests within certain time periods, assessment by independent doctors, physical or psychological suffering, etc.

In the Stransham-Ford case, we find a clash between the ethical position of the applicant, Advocate Stransham-Ford on euthanasia, and the criminal law in South Africa. Stransham-Ford had terminal stage-4 cancer and although he had tried palliative care, alternative remedies, and mainstream medicine, he continued to suffer in the final weeks of his life (McQuoid-Mason, 2017). He applied to the High Court which gave a ruling that his doctor would be allowed to assist him to commit suicide and the doctor's conduct would not be unlawful. Unbeknown to the judge and Stransham-Ford's lawyers, he had died a few hours before the ruling. When the judge gave reasons for his judgment four days later, he knew of Stransham-Ford's death but stood by his order. However, this judgment was overturned upon an appeal brought by the Ministers of Justice and Health, the HPCSA, and the National Director of Prosecutions. Two of the various reasons given were that (i) Stransham-Ford's death removed the cause of action and (ii) the issues of physician-assisted suicide and euthanasia were best left to the legislature, Parliament.

There has been a litany of cases in South Africa dealing with voluntary active euthanasia and assisted suicide with light sentences handed down for what is technically the crime of murder, as judges are forced to apply the criminal law as it stands, while at the same time having compassion for the suffering of the parties involved.[10]

▪ *EJ v Haupt, 2022: Surrogacy arrangements*

In a surrogacy pregnancy, the pregnant woman is usually not genetically related to the foetus conceived by artificial insemination. This method of conception can be used by infertile or homosexual couples to have children that are genetically related to one of them. In some instances, the ova of the surrogate mother are used. Technological advances in reproductive technology have led to ethical and legal debates around parental rights and the 'appeal to nature' fallacy. This fallacy states that the fact that something happens naturally has normative value. In the case of surrogacy or in vitro fertilisation, the argument would be that the conception process is unnatural and therefore unethical or bad. This fallacy is easy to debunk with examples of harmful things which occur in nature, e.g., viruses and natural disasters. Other ethical debates arise around commercialisation of pregnancy, payment of large sums of money, and potential exploitation of vulnerable women.

---

10   For example, in *S v De Bellocq* 1975 (3) SA 538 (T) 539D, the sentence was for her to be discharged on her own recognisance until recalled. In *S v Hartmann* 1975 (3) SA 532 (C), the sentence was a year's imprisonment of which all but the period until the rising of the court was suspended for one year. Both these were murder convictions.

It has occurred, albeit rarely, that the surrogate mother refuses to relinquish the baby to the commissioning parents. In *EJ v Haupt*, a same-sex female couple applied to Court for a declarator that section 40 of the Children's Act applied to same-sex couples. The Court granted the order that the sperm donor will have no rights or responsibilities towards the child and that both the mothers will have full parental rights from birth.

1.9 SUMMARY OF KEY POINTS

- Ethics forms the foundation of professional medical practice.
- Many ethical principles have become part of medical law in acts, guidelines; and the common law.
- Ethical principles may clash with each other and with the law.
- It is important to know and understand the ethical principles and laws relevant to one's area of medical practice.

Bibliography

Amnesty International. 2017. *Barriers to safe and legal abortion in SA*. 1 February. https://www.amnesty.org/en/documents/afr53/5423/2017/en/

Bales, K. 2004. *New slavery: a reference handbook*. Santa Barbara, CA: ABC-CLIO.

Barnett, R. 1998. *The structure of liberty: justice and the rule of law*. Oxford: Oxford University Press.

Bateman, C. 2008. Manana's costly machinations: Naude vindicated. *South African Medical Journal*, 98(12):916.

Bateman, C. 2021. Behind SA's medical malpractice billions. *Financial Mail*, 9 December.

Bentham, J. 1843. Anarchical fallacies: being an examination of the declarations of rights issued during the French revolution. In: *The Works of Jeremy Bentham*. Online Library of Liberty. https://bit.ly/3ADsRCw

Bracker, M. 1962. Warren favours ethics advisors. *New York Times*, 12 November.

Dugard, J. 1984. "Should judges resign?" A reply to Prof. Wacks. *South African Law Journal*, 286.

Erasmus, S. 2017. R1m bill: No-one left to deliver our babies? *Fin24*, 6 April. https://bit.ly/3i6fUL4

Finnis, J. 2021. Aquinas' moral, political and legal philosophy. In: Zalta, E. (ed.). *The Stanford encyclopedia of philosophy* (Spring). https://stanford.io/3OD0V7t

Fosl, P. & Baggini, J. 2020. *The philosopher's toolkit* (3rd edition). London: Wiley-Blackwell.

Hare, John. 2019. Religion and morality. In: Zalta, E (ed.). *The Stanford encyclopedia of philosophy* (Fall). https://stanford.io/3EUXGF5.

Hippocrates of Cos. 1923. The oath. *Loeb Classical Library*, 147:298-299. https://bit.ly/3Xv62un

Hobbes, T. & Plamenatz, J. 1991. *Leviathan*. Cambridge: Cambridge University Press.

Hope, T., Savulescu, J. & Hendrick, J. 2003. *Medical Ethics & Law*. London: Churchill Livingstone.

Horowitz, M.C. 1974. The Stoic synthesis of the idea of natural law in man: four themes. *Journal of the History of Ideas*, 35(1):3-16. https://doi.org/10.2307/2708739

Howarth, G. 2021. Coming into line with international practice on the criminalisation of doctors. *MedicalBrief*, 27 October.

Howarth, G. & Carstens, P. 2014. Can private obstetric care be saved in SA? *South African Journal of Bioethics & Law*, 7. https://doi.org/10.7196/sajbl.319

Jewkes, R. & Rees, H. 2005. Dramatic decline in abortion mortality due to the Choice on Termination of Pregnancy Act. *South African Medical Journal*, 95(4):250.

Ladher, N. 2018. Criminalising doctors. *BMJ*, 360. https://doi.org/10.1136/bmj.k479

Langford, M. 2018. Critiques of human rights. *Annual Review of Law and Social Science*, 69. https://doi.org/10.1146/annurev-lawsocsci-110316-113807

Lee, M.J.H. 2010. The problem of "thick in status, thin in content" in Beauchamp and Childress' principlism. *Journal of Medical Ethics*, 36. https://doi.org/10.1136/jme.2009.031054

Lerm, H. & Stellenberg, E. 2022. SA doctors call for law reform fearing a harsh penalty if patients die. *The Conversation*, 21 February. https://doi.org/10.5771/9783415071841-21

Lewis, J. & Schuklenk, U. 2021. Bioethics met its Covid-19 Waterloo: the doctor knows best again. *Bioethics*, 35(1):3-5. https://doi.org/10.1111/bioe.12840

McQuoid-Mason, D. 2017. Assisted suicide and assisted voluntary euthanasia: Stransham-Ford High Court case overruled by the Appeal Court – but the door is left open. *South African Medical Journal*, 107:381. https://doi.org/10.7196/SAMJ.2017.v107i5.12450

McQuoid-Mason, D. 2022. Is there a legal and ethical duty on public sector doctors whose complaints to hospital administrators have been ignored to inform the public about harm to child patients due to intentional maladministration, negligence or indifference at the local and provincial level? *South African Medical Journal*, 112:8.

MedicalBrief. 2021. Call for SA Law Reform Commission review on criminal charges against doctors. 10 March.

Noonan, J. 1965. *Contraception: a history of its treatment by the Catholic theologians and canonists* (2nd edition). Boston, MA: Harvard University Press.

Nussbaum, M.C. 2014. *Perfectionist liberalism & political liberalism*. Chicago, IL: Cambridge University Press. https://doi.org/10.1017/CBO9781139059138.004

ODAC (Open Democracy Advice Centre). 2015. Dr Paul Theron. In: *Heroes under Fire*. Cape Town.

Oosthuizen, W.T. & Carstens, P. 2015. Medical malpractice: the extent, consequences and cause of the problem. *Journal of Contemporary Roman–Dutch Law*, 78:269.

Parliamentary Monitoring Group. The legislative process. https://pmg.org.za/page/legislative-process [Accessed 15 March 2022].

Parliament of the Republic of South Africa. How a law is made. https://www.parliament.gov.za/how-law-made [Accessed 7 March 2022].

Peterson, A. 2012. From commonplace to controversial. *Origins: current events in historical perspective*. https://bit.ly/3V0ynar.

Pienaar, L. 2016. Investigating the reasons behind the increase in medical negligence claims. *Potchefstroom Electronic Law Journal*, 19. https://doi.org/10.17159/1727-3781/2016/v19i0a1101

Planting, S. 2021. The lesson from SA's medical malpractice disaster is that you can't manage what you don't measure. *Daily Maverick*, 6 July.

Rautenbach, I.M. 2014. Proportionality and the limitation clauses of the SA Bill of Rights. *Potchefstroom Electronic Law Journal*, 17(6):2229. https://doi.org/10.4314/pelj.v17i6.01

SA History Online. 2019, 23 July. Pass laws and the Sharpeville massacre. https://bit.ly/3V34kyL

SA History Online. 2020, 21 February. The Union of SA 1910. https://bit.ly/3i6ftAq

SALC Project 86 (SA Law Reform Commission Report). 1998. *Euthanasia and the artificial preservation of life*. https://bit.ly/3EX6vP1

Schofield, P. 2003. Jeremy Bentham's "Nonsense upon stilts". *Utilitas*, 15:1-26. https://doi.org/10.1017/0953820800003745

Warren, E. 1962. Speech at the Louis Marshall Award Dinner of the Jewish Theological Seminary, Americana Hotel, New York City (11 November).

Wenar, L. 2021. Rights. In: Zalta, E (ed.). *The Stanford encyclopedia of philosophy* (Spring edition). https://stanford.io/3OuxmVw

Case citations

Christian Lawyers Association of SA v Minster of Health 1998 (4) SA 1113 (T).

Doctors for Life International v Speaker of the National Assembly 2006 (6) SA 416 (CC).

Dr Malcolm Naude v Member of the Executive Council, Department of Health EJ v Haupt 2022 (1) SA 514 (GP).

Jansen van Vuuren NNO v Kruger 1993(4) SA 842 (AD).

Mohr v Williams 95 Minn 261 (1905).

Mpumalanga (2009) 30 ILJ 910 (LC).

S v Makwanyane 1995 (3) SA 391 (CC).

Soobramoney v Minister of Health 1998 (1) SA 765 CC.

Stoffberg v Elliott 1923 CPD 148.

Stransham-Ford v Minister of Justice and Correctional Services 2015 (4) SA 50 (GP). https://bit.ly/3gwI0P8

2

Universal Health Coverage, National Health Insurance, and Sustainable Workforce

Mariana Kruger

Keywords: equity; fairness; health care workforce; national health insurance (NHI) policy; right to health; sustainable; universal health coverage (UHC)

2.1 INTRODUCTION

Everybody has a right to health, which can be achieved by implementing access to universal health coverage (UHC), a key concept of the current century according to the World Health Organization (WHO) (Ottersen et al., 2014; WHO, 2014). Good health will ensure the pursuit of a wide range of life plans, which will affect all aspects of life such as education, income, and happiness (Daniels, 2008). Poor health is associated with limited well-being and often needs large payments for health services, impacting negatively on financial security. WHO encourages all countries to develop strategies to provide affordable, quality health care to their population (Ottersen et al., 2014; WHO, 2014).

The pursuit of health for all has been the important message since the 1978 Declaration of Alma-Ata (Declaration of Alma-Ata, 1978). Subsequently, several other documents stress the importance of health such as the Bangkok Statement on UHC in 2011 (*The Lancet*, 2012) and the recent global call to implement UHC (Barron & Koonin, 2021). UHC benefits society in general as improved population health impacts positively on country development. For example, healthy children learn better, while healthy adults contribute through their productive lives to economic growth. Investment in the health of a nation has therefore enormous benefits for the country.

UHC is defined as "all people receiving quality health services that meet their needs without being exposed to financial hardship in paying for these services" (Ottersen et al., 2014; WHO, 2014). UHC includes curative, preventive, rehabilitative, palliative, and promotive services (58th World Health Assembly, 2005; WHO, 2010). For effective UHC, the whole health system should be strengthened by improving service provision, ensuring adequate human-, physical- and financial resources, as well as good governance (WHO, 2000). The pursuit of UHC must be aligned with other strategies to improve social determinants such as housing, employment, education, and environment and should be aligned with the strategy of UHC implementation (Rio Political Declaration on Social Determinants of Health, 2011; WHO, 2008).

All countries must make judgements about what health care interventions they should implement to address their local health care needs. This does not mean all possible health services will be provided, as these services are subject to existing resource constraints. According to the WHO, countries should advance three dimensions in health care, namely expanding priority health services, including all people, and reducing out-of-pocket health care expenses (Ottersen et al., 2014; WHO, 2014). Numerous countries have embarked on the implementation of access to UHC, with the assistance of the WHO with implementation.

This chapter aims to address the following crucial questions: (1) Which services should be prioritised for expansion; (2) who should be included first; (3) how to move to prepayment; and (4) how to ensure fairness. Equity is especially of crucial importance. The actions taken by South Africa to move towards UHC will be discussed, as well as the planned South African NHI. Lastly, the need for a sustainable health care workforce will be discussed as this is crucial in the rollout of UHC and a major constraint in South Africa.

2.2   EXPANSION OF PRIORITY SERVICES

Health is an important good for society, but it is not the only good needed and there are always competing interests for the available resources. Choices must be made regarding priorities in health to ensure reasonable access to these resources. To justify these choices, decision-making should be based on good evidence and sound rationale (Daniels, Porteny & Urritia, 2016). Unfair distribution of resources must be limited with improvement in health equity. Safety, efficacy, and cost-effectiveness are usually assessed in the priority setting of health interventions but may not be enough according to Daniels et al. (2016), as they argue that there should also be "accountability for reasonableness" which include decisions that are transparent, relevant to resource allocation, can be revised with new evidence emerging, and enforceable (Daniels, 2008).

Health care service expansion necessitates the categorisation into high priority-, medium priority- and low-priority health care services (Ottersen et al., 2014; WHO, 2014). Criteria to be used in ranking such services include cost-effectiveness, protection against financial risk, and prioritising the worse-off. The key question for a country is which services should be expanded first and is best based on the burden of disease in the country. Significant morbidity and mortality causes of the population are important to consider. Interventions implemented should be population-based rather than based on individual services (WHO, 2010). In this context, both communicable and non-communicable diseases must be included with good reasons that are transparent to ensure public trust with accountability and corruption prevention (Glassman & Chalkidou, 2012). Successful prioritisation of health services has been implemented in the United Kingdom, Denmark, Sweden, Norway, and the Netherlands and common in their priorities are the objectives to improve population health with fair distribution of health services and proven cost-effectiveness (Sabik & Lie, 2008).

Cost-effectiveness is measured as either quality-adjusted life years (QALYs) saved, or disability-adjusted life years (DALYs) prevented (Gold, Stevenson & Fryback, 2002; Murray, 2012). Both QALYs and DALYs assist in developing a framework for priority setting and are utilitarian in nature with the aim to maximise benefit in society. Although useful in planning health services, critique of using QALYs and DALYs include the following: (1) priority cannot be given to the worse-off; (2) there may be discrimination against those with limited treatment options; and (3) cannot account for qualitative differences in outcome. To ensure fairness, countries need to find ways to overcome these issues and ring-fence budget allocation and services for certain predefined conditions affecting the worse-off or those with limited treatment options (Pinxten et al., 2012).

2.3   INCLUSION OF ALL/MORE PEOPLE

A key issue with implementation is to determine who should be included first as it is unlikely to be the whole population when embarking on UHC (Ottersen et al., 2014; WHO, 2014). The priority setting should probably address the needs of marginalised or low-income groups, rural populations, and other disadvantaged groups in terms of access to health care or coverage, especially in line with the burden of disease in a specific country. As mentioned above, the focus should be on groups rather than individuals, taking into consideration the conditions that affect the disadvantaged groups and should result in a reduction of inequalities of service coverage of the whole population (Jamison et al., 2013). It is important that all vulnerable groups of the population are included through a progressive implementation of UHC. In the process, health care workers must recognise human rights with a zero tolerance for discriminatory attitudes, while policymakers need to ensure the establishment of respectful services with effective dialogue between communities and health care providers (Tangcharoensathien et al., 2018).

2.4   REDUCTION OF OUT-OF-POCKET EXPENSES

Out-of-pocket payments for health services are common in many low- and middle-income countries, especially in Africa (Derkyi-Kwarteng et al., 2021). For impoverished communities, such payments cause a lack of access to health care, as often the out-of-pocket expenses place an enormous burden on the financial budget of the family with them refusing to seek such services, leading to a delay in diagnosis which in turn worsens the underlying condition. Only when these out-of-pocket expenses are less than 20% of health expenditure is the worsening of financial status prevented (WHO, 2010). Compulsory prepayment during the implementation of UHC is essential in the creation of a central fund to assist with prepayment of health care services. It is especially important to initially eliminate out-of-pocket expenses for high-priority services and to allow the worse-off to gain early access to these services (Ottersen et al., 2014; WHO, 2014). This compulsory prepayment must be in line with the increased income of households or individuals.

2.5   FAIRNESS AND EQUITY

Key ethical issues in UHC include fairness of distribution of health careservices with equity in access to health care (Frenz & Vega, 2010). Both fairness and equity address the benefit distribution and societal burdens (Ottersen et al., 2014; WHO, 2014). Fair access to health care services, however, should be based on need and not on the ability to pay. For fair distribution, the worse-off groups should be prioritised, and their health care needs must determine the services to be provided. However, in this context, utility should also be considered as only using worse-off as a single factor may lead to futile treatment without benefit, while others with less severe illnesses may potentially benefit more. It is therefore crucial to combine fair opportunity with utility to determine access to health care resources for society in general (WHO, 2014). But, fair contribution entails that prepayment is based on the ability of individuals to pay, and not on their health care needs. A fair equitable health care system will ensure that all have equitable access to these health care services, regardless of their prepayment contribution.

2.6   UHC SHOULD MAXIMISE BENEFITS

A cardinal aim of UHC is to maximise benefits for the whole population. These can be additional life years or improved quality of life. Cost-effectiveness is very important in this context as the benefits generated must justify the resources used. Benefit maximisation and fairness often go together as the sum of health benefits should also benefit those with the least access to health care or are worse-off (Jamison et al., 2013). The worse-off can be with regard to health, socio-economic status, well-being, or service coverage. However, the fairest of actions may not always maximise benefit. A good example is when the provision of health care services is prioritised for the rural population, but this may be too costly for a country, leading to prioritising the urban population first as it is more cost-effective (Chopra, Campbell & Rudan, 2012). Where the two objectives diverge, the WHO guideline suggests that countries should investigate alternative policies to achieve both objectives (Ottersen et al., 2014; WHO, 2014).

2.7   SUGGESTED WHO STRATEGY AND PATHWAYS

As mentioned above, the proposed steps to be undertaken should include (Ottersen et al., 2014; WHO, 2014):

1. Categorise health care services into priority categories. Aspects to take into consideration include the provision of priority to the worse-off persons, the cost-effectiveness of the interventions, and protection against financial risk.

2. Expand the high-priority health care services to all persons in the country, especially with the elimination of out-of-pocket expenses. Over a period of time, the compulsory prepayment should increase with a pooling in a central fund.

3. Ensure that the disadvantaged groups do gain access, especially low-income, marginalised, and rural people.

To ensure fairness, unacceptable trade-offs should be avoided, including the expansion of low- or medium-priority services prior to universal cover for high-priority services, the prioritisation of services resulting in small health benefits, the prioritisation of well-off groups with health cover before those impoverished groups without health cover, and to only include those that can contribute to the universal health fund (Ottersen et al., 2014; WHO, 2014).

Good governance, monitoring, and accountability in a UHC strategy are crucial to ensure success. Countries should carefully consider indicators to monitor the UHC process and invest in robust health information systems that can generate the necessary information needed to inform health policies that are linked to the priority-setting process, health outcomes, and protection of the central fund and coverage, while demonstrating equity and fairness.

2.8   SOUTH AFRICAN CONTEXT WITH REGARD TO UHC

Africa as a continent and South Africa specifically are faced with high burdens of infectious diseases such as multi-drug resistance tuberculosis and AIDS, as well as high mortality rates, malnutrition, and chronic non-communicable diseases (Modjadji, 2021). Furthermore, impoverished communities suffer more from diseases, including both communicable and non-communicable diseases (Ataguba, Akazili & McIntyre, 2011; Wong et al., 2021). This is further complicated by existing major inequalities within South Africa with regard to socio-economic status and access to health care services as part of the historical legacy of apartheid (Molepo, 2021). Health expenditure and resource allocation during the apartheid years have favoured the white population with most of the black population having far less allocated to them for health care (Harris et al., 2014). The health system has also favoured capitalist ideals, namely those who can pay have access to quality health care (Price, 1986).

The current South African health system is divided into a private and a public sector. This dual structure still has an unequal nature, whereby the more affluent members of society utilise private health care, whereas the majority rely on the under-resourced and overburdened public sector (Burger & Christian, 2018). About 16% of the population is served by the private sector versus 84% served by the public sector which has limited resources and is poorly managed. Also worsening the inequity is the fact that 30% of the health care workers serve the public sector versus 70% serving the private health care sector (Labonté et al., 2015). The health care worker shortage in the public sector is especially due to low remuneration, poor working conditions, and lack of career development versus the private sector with superior remuneration and working conditions (Rispel et al., 2018). Added to this, there is the 'brain drain' with health care workers emigrating (Labonté et al., 2015).

Since the change to a democracy in 1994, South African government spending is divided equally between the two sectors (Rispel, 2016). Current public health care is decentralised into the provinces with National Treasury providing the funding as conditional grants (Pauw, 2021). The allocation is based on the individual provincial risk characteristics, as well as health care facilities capacity (Roos, 2020). As medical costs are increasing in South Africa, private health care is becoming unaffordable, while quality health care access is compounded by an increasingly high unemployment rate and poor economic growth (Burger & Christian, 2018; Pauw, 2021; Tshoose, 2015).

2.9   SOUTH AFRICAN NATIONAL HEALTH POLICY

According to the World Bank, 9% of South Africa's gross domestic product (GDP) has been spent on health care in 2019, but by global standards return on investment is poor as demonstrated by the still existing health care inequalities mentioned above (World Bank, 2019a). Due to this inequity in health care and resource allocation, the South African health care system should be completely transformed with a focus on UHC (Giaimo, 2016).

The National Health Policy was introduced in May 1994 with a focus on both medical care and healthy lifestyles as the first steps in the improvement of health care for all with the introduction of the Primary Health Care (PHC) facilities to prevent disease, promote health, and provide primary health care (WHO, 2019). The National Health Act 61 of 2003 documents current national health policy and one of the major positive outcomes of this policy is the successful extensive antiretroviral treatment programmes implemented in South Africa (Hassim, Heyman & Honermann, 2008; Pauw, 2021).

As the roll-out of UHC is challenging with no single way to implement it, due to country differences in disease profiles, the South African government is embarking on an incremental process of UHC implementation through the improvement of public health infrastructure and services with subsequent improved public trust (Pauw, 2021; WHO, 2021).

2.10   NATIONAL HEALTH INSURANCE (NHI)

South Africa passed the National Health Insurance Bill in 2019 as a strategy to provide UHC to the South African population (National Health Insurance Bill, 2019) and is establishing National Health Insurance (NHI), which aims to provide affordable and high-quality health services for all South Africans (Navarro, 2007; Pauw, 2021; WHO, 2021). The NHI is a funding mechanism for the provision of health care for the whole population (Mash, 2020a; Pauw, 2021). The NHI will initiate a prepayment system with a public fund to cover health services to prevent personal expenditure on health care (NHI Bill, 2019). This funding mechanism will ensure that free health care services are provided if obtained from health care practitioners who meet predefined quality criteria and are registered for the NHI. The division of health funding between private and public sectors will be minimised, while the National fiscus will be responsible for obtaining funds from reallocation of medical scheme tax credits, the general tax revenue, a payroll tax (to replace current medical aid contributions), and a surcharge on personal income tax. The NHI funds will purchase medicines, health care services, and other related health products.

As the main aim of the NHI is to address the inequality in health care provision with improved quality health care to the whole population, it will cover health care services for South African citizens and permanent residents, refugees, and all children, regardless of origin (Mash, 2020a & 2020c). Other groups such as asylum seekers and illegal migrants will only be covered for emergency and notifiable diseases. All South African citizens will be required to register for the NHI, regardless of whether they have a medical aid or not. Patients will have freedom of choice regarding their primary health care provider and not be limited to either public or private sector (Mash, 2020b).

Both the current public and private health care sectors will serve as service providers, with a prescribed health care pathway. As PHC is the cornerstone of the NHI, the South African government plans to contract private health care providers in Contracting Units for Primary Health Care (CUPs). These CUPs will be combined with PHC to promote both prevention of disease as well as practice curative medicine (NHI Bill, 2019). The plan is to form District Health Management Offices to ensure good access to health care on a local level. The whole process of implementation needs good health service organisation and coor-dination, as well as restructuring of public health finances – both posing bureau-cratic challenges that must be addressed to ensure success (Michel et al., 2020).

The implementation of the NHI will be in three phases and the first phase has been the piloting of the NHI in ten PHCs with mixed successes (Genesis Analytics, 2019). These mixed successes are due to the existence of a strong political will with adequate human and financial resources in certain PHCs, while crucial challenges for the less successful implementation in PHCs are the lack of effective planning, limited resources, and poor communication with weak coordination and monitoring. Phase two is currently being introduced with the passing of the NHI Bill with amendments to existing legislation that may affect the implementation and the establishment of the NHI (NHI Bill, 2019). The third phase will implement resource allocation and the aim is to have all South Africans included into UHC by 2030 (BusinessTech, 2020b; NHI Bill, 2019).

The Minister of Health will be responsible for governance of the NHI while the National Department of Health will determine health policy and strategy. The NHI fund will be managed by a board of 11 members, who will be appointed by the Minister of Health, but nominated through public participation (Mash, 2020a; NHI Bill, 2019). Several advisory committees will provide guidance regarding the benefits to be covered, what payments should be for, and participation of stakeholders. Provincial health departments will oversee the services provided in their provinces, while existing private medical schemes will have to cover the health care services not covered by the NHI.

The South African Values and Ethics for Universal Health Coverage (SAVE-UHC) Working Group has developed a framework to use in South Africa for health priority-setting (Blaauw et al., 2022; Krubiner et al., 2022). There are 12 domains in the framework of which the first four are commonly used in health priority-setting, namely burden of disease, expected health benefits and harms, cost-effectiveness analysis, and budget impact. They describe a further eight ethical domains, namely respect and dignity, equity, ease of suffering, impact on safety and security, maintaining important personal relationships, impact on personal finances, solidarity, and social cohesion. A diverse group of stakeholders have accepted this framework.

There are currently major debates about whether NHI can be implemented effectively in South Africa as the policy is vague about what health services will be covered and what the tax individuals will have to contribute to the NHI (Pauw, 2019). Concerns about the roll-out of the NHI include issues such as corruption, poor leadership, poor management, and weak governance (Molepo, 2021; Rispel, 2016). The situation is further worsened by the infrastructure degradation, the lack of fully functional PHC facilities, limited resources, especially human resources in the public sector and a huge burden of disease (McIntyre, Doherty & Ataguba, 2014).

Learning from the experience of UHC implementation in Ghana, it is important to note that health care inequality is not reduced if participation is voluntary and not part of the tax system, as health care is still unaffordable for 60% (Kipo-Sunyehzi et al., 2020). South Africa therefore will introduce a tax-based NHI contribution, based on the ability of persons to contribute according to income (Pauw, 2020).

The Solidarity Research Institute conducted a survey in October 2019 to determine the health care workers' understanding and readiness to implement the NHI (Welthagen, 2019). The findings conclude that nearly 80% have an unfavourable opinion with apprehension whether government can ensure payment of health care services. The South African public is also not sure that government can deliver or successfully implement the NHI without corruption (Sekhejane, 2013). The Institute of Risk Management in South Africa reports that the government's inability to prevent corruption, public distrust in the health sector, inadequate service delivery, and inadequate number of health care workers pose major threats to the successful implementation of UHC through the NHI (Institute of Risk Management, 2020).

2.11   SUSTAINABLE HEALTH CARE WORKFORCE IN SOUTH AFRICA

The success of UHC access is crucially dependent on an adequate health care workforce (Rispel et al., 2018). This health care workforce includes all persons whose actions are intended to improve health, namely physicians, nurses, pharmacists, dentists, and other allied health care workers (dieticians, occupational therapists, physiotherapists) and support staff (Rispel, 2018; Soucat, Scheffler & Ghebreyesus, 2013). The health care workforce will include individuals working in either public or private sectors or on a voluntary basis. A sustainable health system needs balanced labour market dynamics with the right level of education. Core indicators of a sustainable health care workforce include the health worker density, the distribution by occupation or specialisation in regions including sex distribution, and the annual graduates of health care professions (number of graduates per 100 000 population per annum) (WHO, 2018).

2.11.1   Core indicator 1: Health care worker density in South Africa

The calculation of health care workers is easy to determine as these workers are registered with their professional boards and are used to compare the density of health care workers of different countries. The density is especially useful to monitor whether the workforce can provide the planned health care coverage. The most complete data exists for physicians, nurses, and midwives, but all other categories should be taken into account such as pharmacists, laboratory personnel, health managers, technicians, and others. The most recent health care worker density in South Africa is reported as 0.79 physicians per 1 000 people, while nurses and midwives are reported as 1.3 per 1 000 people by the World Bank (World Bank, 2019a, 2019b). This is in great contrast compared to the United Kingdom with a density of 5.82 physicians per 1 000 people, where existing UHC access through NHS is successfully implemented (World Bank, 2019c). However, even the South African reported density may be inaccurate as current data is obtained from the absolute numbers of health care professionals registered with their respective professional boards in South Africa, but it does not specify whether they are actively practising in South Africa, as many emigrating health care workers remain registered in South Africa (Rispel et al., 2018).

Although South Africa is currently in the top five countries in Africa with regard to the density of health care workers per 1 000 of the population, it is necessary to improve the density to achieve success with the rollout of UHC access. Rispel et al. (2018) recommend that a mapping should be done regarding the health care workforce capacity needs in all regions of South Africa (Rispel et al., 2018). Such a mapping exercise will assist in the planning of improving health care workforce density in regions currently underserved in South Africa and should take into consideration those health care workers actively working in South Africa and not rely on registration numbers from professional health care boards.

2.11.2 Core indicator 2: Health care worker distribution by occupation/specialisation/region/sex

Although South Africa is at the top when it comes to density, this is unfortunately not the case in the public health sector, especially in rural communities (BusinessTech, 2020a; South African Department of Health: Annual Report, 2017; WHO, 2018). For example, there are currently 16.5 medical specialists per 100 000 of whom 7 per 100 000 are employed in the public sector versus 69 per 100 000 in the private sector, while the Western Cape has 25.8 medical specialists per 100 000 versus the more rural Limpopo with 1.4 per 100 000 (BusinessTech, 2020a).

The National Department of Health aims to develop and implement staffing norms and standards for health facilities as part of the strategy towards UHC, based on the Workload Indicators of Staffing Need (WISN) method of the WHO (South African Department of Health: Annual Report, 2017; WHO, 1998). This method includes assessment of the health care worker's workload with time spent on each workload component in the different regions of a country. Unfortunately, the National Department of Health has only used the WISN method to address human resources in the health care sector and to date this method has not resulted in the planned improvement with existing inability to meet the targets for human resources improvement in primary health care (Rispel et al., 2018; Mabunda et al., 2021).

One of the major obstacles is the unaffordability to achieve the recommended health care workforce with appropriate distribution according to the WISN method. Other limitations include the major dependency on accurate annual service statistics with possible overreporting or underreporting and insufficient assessment of needs in rural regions. Improvements can perhaps be achieved through a combination of the WISN method with needs-based human resources planning methods for health care in the different regions (Birch, 2015). Such methods should include investigation into epidemiological changes regarding disease profile and regional needs, demography of health care workers, as well as their education and their productivity (ASSAf, 2018). According to Mumbauer et al. (2021), workplace conditions and remuneration packages are more important in employment decisions than location or employment sector in South Africa. Workplace condition improvements, together with the aforementioned health care worker density mapping exercise, may assist in the strategic planning and recruitment of staff to underserved areas in South Africa and a more equitable distribution of health care workers.

2.11.3   Core indicator 3: The annual number of health care graduates per annum

It is crucial to monitor the annual output of health care graduates in relation to the population per annum. Such data will assist in addressing the needs regarding all cadres, the underserved regions, and the number of foreign-trained graduates will indicate what needs exist to ensure self-sufficiency (WHO, 2018).

According to the Academy of Science of South Africa's (ASSAf) 2018 report, health care workers' education is excellent in South Africa, but is hampered by weak coordination, fragmented funding streams, inadequate infrastructure, inadequate clinical teaching platforms, lack of clinical teachers, and a decrease in health care workers pursuing careers in academic health sciences (ASSAf, 2018). Furthermore, health care student selection is hampered by a great variability in school education quality, poor career guidance, and inequity in financial and staff support at universities. The internship experience may negatively impact on the vision of future workplace choices. However, it seems that the compulsory community service programmes for health care workers have led to positive professional development.

The ASSAf report (2018) recommends that health care worker selection must use a broader set of criteria than currently used to attract a greater variety in culture and skills. Health care education should focus on addressing the existing inequity in health care access with a focus of support for the primary health care sector and increased supply of health care workers to rural areas. The existing academic institutions need strengthening to ensure an increase in the number of training health care professionals, utilising both the private and public sector. There is also a need for retaining training staff in academic institutions. A way forward is to implement a long-term national plan for the expansion of health care workforces through education with a pro-active strategy to retain the services of these graduates in South Africa through workplace improvements and remuneration packages, with opportunities for continual professional development and active mentoring in the workplace (Kovacs et al., 2017). This development of a sustainable workforce is, however, linked to improvement of other socio-economic circumstances such as job creation with reduced unemployment, improved housing and education, and other socio-economic factors that will improve the general well-being of the South African population and cannot be done in isolation, however, this is outside the scope of this chapter.

2.12 CONCLUSION

As health care is the right of every individual, governments should implement a UHC system to ensure equity in access to health care. The implementation of the NHI is, according to the South African government, the only potential way to achieve UHC for all persons with equity in the health sector. In countries where UHC has been successfully introduced, the population's health has improved, which has led to an improvement in the overall economy. However, the South African government needs to address the concerns of the South African population by ensuring transparency, clarity regarding public concerns, improve access to resources, especially sustainable human resources, and good governance with prevention of corruption. The roll-out of UHC should also be linked to other social determinants of health namely employment equity, housing, and education.

Bibliography

58th World Health Assembly. 2005. *Social health insurance: sustainable health financing, universal coverage and social health insurance.* Report by the Secretariat. Provisional agenda item 13.16.

ASSAf (Academy of Science of South Africa). 2018. *Reconceptualising health professions education in South Africa: Consensus study report.* Pretoria: ASSAf.

Ataguba, J.E., Akazili, J. & McIntyre, D. 2011. Socioeconomic-related health inequality in South Africa: evidence from General Household Surveys. *International Journal for Equity in Health*, 10(1):1-10. https://doi.org/10.1186/1475-9276-10-48

Barron, G.C. & Koonin, J. 2021. A call to action on UHC commitments. *The Lancet*, 397(10292):2335-2336. https://doi.org/10.1016/S0140-6736(21)01014-X

Birch, S. 2015. Improving the fiscal and political sustainability of health systems through integrated population needs-based planning. Seminar briefing #17. London: Office of Health Economics Research.

Blaauw, S.U., Chambers, C., Chirwa, T., Duba, N., Gwyther, L., Hofman, K. & Tugendhaft, A. 2022. Introducing an ethics framework for health priority-setting in South Africa on the path to universal health coverage. *South African Medical Journal*, 112(3):240-244. https://doi.org/10.7196/SAMJ.2022.v112i3.16278

Burger, R. & Christian, C. 2018. Access to health care in post-apartheid South Africa: availability, affordability, acceptability. *Health Economics Policy and Law* 15(1):1-13. https://doi.org/10.1017/S1744133118000300

BusinessTech. 2020a. South Africa faces massive healthcare worker shortage. 2 September. https://bit.ly/3EWnjph [Accessed 17 April 2022].

BusinessTech. 2020b. Government outlines NHI implementation schedule. 8 December. https://bit.ly/3EW7yhZ [Accessed 17 April 2022].

Chopra, M., Campbell, H. & Rudan, I. 2012. Understanding the determinants of the complex interplay between cost-effectiveness and equitable impact in maternal and child mortality reduction. *Journal of Global Health*, 2(1):010406. https://doi.org/10.7189/jogh.01.010406

Daniels, N. 2008. Just health: meeting health needs fairly, Chapter 1. Cambridge: Cambridge University Press. https://doi.org/10.1017/CBO9780511809514

Daniels, N., Porteny, T. & Urritia, J. 2016. Expanded HTA: enhancing fairness and legitimacy. *International Journal of Health Policy and Management*, 5(1):1-3. https://doi.org/10.15171/ijhpm.2015.187

Declaration of Alma-Ata. 1978. https://bit.ly/3GJjR2r [Accessed 9 April 2022].

Derkyi-Kwarteng, A.N.C., Agyepong, I.A., Enyimayew, N. & Gilson, L. 2021. A narrative synthesis review of out-of-pocket payments for health services under insurance regimes: a policy implementation gap hindering universal health coverage in sub-Saharan Africa. *International Journal of Health Policy and Management*, 10:443-461. https://doi.org/10.34172/ijhpm.2021.38

Frenz, P. & Vega, J. 2010. Universal health coverage with equity: what we know, don't know and need to know. Background paper for the Global Symposium on Health Systems Research.

Genesis Analytics. 2019. *Evaluation of the phase 1 implementation of the interventions in the National Health Insurance pilot districts in South Africa.* Pretoria: Republic of South Africa.

Giaimo, S. 2016. *Reforming health care in the United States, Germany, and South Africa: comparative perspectives on health.* London: Palgrave Macmillan. https://doi.org/10.1057/9781137107176

Glassman, A. & Chalkidou, K. 2012. *Priority-setting in health: building institutions for smarter public spending.* Washington, DC: Center for Global Development.

Gold, M.R., Stevenson, D. & Fryback, D.G. 2002. HALYs and QALYs and DALYs, oh my: similarities and differences in summary measures of population health. *Annual Review of Public Health*,

23:115-134. https://doi.org/10.1146/annurev.publhealth.23.100901.140513

Harris, B., Eyles, J., Penn-Kekana, L., Fried, J., Nyathela, H., Thomas, L. & Goudge, J. 2014. Bringing justice to unacceptable health care services? Street-level reflections from urban South Africa. *The International Journal of Transitional Justice*, 8:141-161. https://doi.org/10.1093/ijtj/ijt028

Hassim, A., Heywood, M. & Honermann, B. 2008. *The National Health Act 61 of 2003: a guide*. Cape Town: Siber Ink CC.

Institute of Risk Management. 2020. *IRMSA risk report: South Africa risks 2020*. https://bit.ly/3tRsel1

Jamison, D.T., Summers, L.H., Alleyne, G., Arrow, K.J., Berkley, S., Binagwaho, A. et al. 2013. Global health 2035: a world converging within a generation. *The Lancet*, 382:1898-955. https://doi.org/10.1016/S0140-6736(13)62105-4

Kipo-Sunyehzi, D.D., Ayanore, M.A., Dzidzonu, D.K. & Yakubu, Y.A. 2020. Ghana's journey towards universal health coverage: the role of the National Health Insurance scheme. *European Journal of Investigation in Health, Psychology and Education*, 10:94-109. https://doi.org/10.3390/ejihpe10010009

Kovacs, E., Girasek, E., Eke, E., Szocsk, M. & World Health Organization. 2017. Strengthening data for planning a sustainable health workforce: what data to collect for health workforce development and why. *Public Health Panorama*, 3(03): 497-504.

Krubiner, C.B., Barsdorf, N.W., Goldstein, SJ., Mosam, A., Potgieter, S., DiStefano, M.J. & Hofman, K.J. 2022. Developing and piloting a context-specified ethics framework for health technology assessment: the South African values and ethics for universal health coverage approach. *International Journal of Technology Assessment in Health Care*, 8(1). https://doi.org/10.1017/S0266462322000113

Labonté, R., Sanders, D., Thubelihle, M., Crush, J., Abel, C., Yoswa, D., Runnels, V., Packer, C., MacKenzie, A., Murphy, G.T. & Bourgeault, I.L. 2015. Health worker migration from South Africa: causes, consequences and policy responses. *Human Resources for Health*, 13(92):1-16. https://doi.org/10.1186/s12960-015-0093-4

Mabunda, S.A., Gupta, M., Chitha, W.W., Mtshali, N.G., Ugarte, C., Echegaray, C. & Joshi, R. 2021. Lessons learnt during the implementation of WISN for comprehensive primary health care in India, South Africa and Peru. *International Journal of Environmental Research and Public Health*, 18(23):12541. https://doi.org/10.3390/ijerph182312541

Mash, B. 2020a. National Health Insurance unpacked: Part 1. *South African Family Practice*, 62(1):a5094. https://doi.org/10.4102/safp.v62i1.5094

Mash, B. 2020b. National Health Insurance unpacked: Part 2: Accreditation of primary care facilities. *South African Family Practice*, 62(1):a5140. https://doi.org/10.4102/safp.v62i1.5140

Mash, B. 2020c. National Health Insurance unpacked: Part 3: Registration of patients at primary care facilities. *South African Family Practice*, 62(1):a5214. https://doi.org/10.4102/safp.v62i1.5214

McIntyre, D., Doherty, J. & Ataguba, J. 2014. *Universal health coverage assessment*. Global Network for Health Equity (GNHE). Cape Town, South Africa.

Michel, J., Tediosi, F., Egger, M., Barnighausen, T., McIntyre, D., Tanner, M. & Evans, D. 2020. Universal health coverage financing in South Africa: wishes vs reality. *Journal of Global Health Reports*, 4:1-12. https://doi.org/10.29392/001c.13509

Mkhize, Z. 2019. Opening address by Minister of Health. Presented at the Inaugural National Conference of the Health Professions Council of South Africa. South Africa.

Modjadji, P. 2021. Communicable and non-communicable diseases coexisting in South Africa. *The Lancet Global Health*, 9(7):e889-e890. https://doi.org/10.1016/S2214-109X(21)00271-0

Molepo, J.N. 2021. The South African health sector and the World Health Organization South Africa's health sector and its preparedness for the National Health Insurance (NHI): challenges and opportunities. *European Journal of Economics, Law and Social Sciences*. https://bit.ly/3OtlXWa

Mumbauer, A., Strauss, M., George, G., Ngwepe, P., Bezuidenhout, C., De Vos, L. et al. 2021. Employment preferences of health care workers in South Africa: Findings from a discrete choice experiment. *PLoS ONE*, 16(4): e0250652. https://doi.org/10.1371/journal.pone.0250652

Murray, C.J.L., Ezzati, M., Flaxman, A.D., Lim, S., Lozano, R., Michaud, C. et al. 2012. GBD 2010: design, definitions, and metrics. *The Lancet*, 380:2063-2066. https://doi.org/10.1016/S0140-6736(12)61899-6

National Health Insurance Bill. 2019. https://bit.ly/3gyXIZV [Accessed 29 March 2022].

Navarro, V. 2007. What is a national health policy? *International Journal of Health Services*, 37(1):1-14. https://doi.org/10.2190/H454-7326-6034-1T25

Ottersen, T. & Norheim, O.F. on behalf of the World Health Organization Consultative Group on Equity and Universal Health Coverage. 2014. Making fair choices on the path to universal health coverage. *Bulletin of the World Health Organization*, 92(6):389. https://doi.org/10.2471/BLT.14.139139

Pauw, T.L. 2021. Catching up with the constitution: An analysis of National Health Insurance in South Africa post-apartheid. *Development Southern Africa*, 1-14. https://doi.org/10.1080/0376835X.2021.1945911

Pinxten, W., Denier, Y., Dooms, M., Cassiman, J.J. & Dierickx, K. 2012. A fair share for the orphans: ethical guidelines for a fair distribution of resources within the bounds of the 10-year-old European Orphan Drug Regulation. *Journal of Medical Ethics*, 38(3):148-153. https://doi.org/10.1136/medethics-2011-100094

Price, M. 1986. Health care as an instrument of apartheid policy in South Africa. *Health Policy and Planning*, 1(2):158-170. https://doi.org/10.1093/heapol/1.2.158

Rio Political Declaration on Social Determinants of Health. 2011. https://bit.ly/3XujizF [Accessed 25 April 2014].

Rispel, L. 2016. Analysing the progress and fault lines of health sector transformation in South Africa. *South African Health Review*, 17-23.

Rispel, L.C., Blaauw, D., Ditlopo, P. & White, J. 2018. Human resources for health and universal health coverage: progress, complexities and contestations. *South African Health Review*, 2018(1):13-21.

Roos, E.L. 2020. Provincial Equitable Share Allocations in South Africa. Centre of Policy Studies/IMPACT Centre Working Papers g-298, Victoria University, Centre of Policy Studies/IMPACT Centre. https://bit.ly/3GE6Ln0

Sabik, L.M. & Lie, R.K. 2008. Priority setting in health care: lessons from the experiences of eight countries. *International Journal for Equity in Health*, 7:a4. https://doi.org/10.1186/1475-9276-7-4

Sekhejane, P.R. 2013. South African National Health Insurance (NHI) policy: prospects and challenges for its efficient implementation. *Africa Institute of South Africa*, 102:1-4. https://bit.ly/3gNLYTG

Soucat, A., Scheffler, R. & Ghebreyesus, T.A. (eds.). 2013. *The labor market for health workers in Africa: a new look at the crisis*. Washington, DC: The World Bank. https://doi.org/10.1596/978-0-8213-9555-4

South African National Department of Health. 2017. *Annual Report of the National Department of Health*. Pretoria: NDoH.

Tangcharoensathien, V., Mills, A., Das, M.B., Patcharanarumol, W., Buntan, M. & Johns, J. 2018. Addressing the health of vulnerable populations: social inclusion and universal health coverage. *Journal of Global Health*, 8(2):020304. https://doi.org/10.7189/jogh.08.020304

The Lancet. 2012. The Bangkok Statement on universal health coverage. *The Lancet,* 379(9815). https://doi.org/10.1016/S0140-6736(12)60212-8

Tshoose, C.I. 2015. Dynamics of public participation in local government: a South African perspective. *African Journal of Public Affairs,* 8(2):13-29.

Welthagen, N. 2019. *Healthcare workers' knowledge of, insight into and opinion of the proposed national health insurance.* Pretoria: Solidarity Research Institute. https://bit.ly/3u25nDe

WHO (World Health Organization). 1998. *Workload indicators of staffing need (WISN): a manual for implementation.* Geneva: World Health Organization. https://bit.ly/3ACCLnG [Accessed 17 April 2022].

WHO (World Health Organization). 2000. *Health systems: improving performance.* Geneva: World Health Organization. https://bit.ly/3grCnlo [Accessed 11 April 2022].

WHO (World Health Organization). 2008. *Commission on Social Determinants of Health. Closing the gap in a generation: health equity through action on the social determinants of health.* Geneva: World Health Organization. https://bit.ly/3GAgKdc [Accessed 11 April 2022].

WHO (World Health Organization). 2010. *The World Health Report 2010. Health systems financing: the path to universal coverage.* Geneva: World Health Organization. https://bit.ly/3Vig14o [Accessed 17 April 2022].

WHO (World Health Organization). 2014. *Making fair choices on the path to universal health coverage: final report of the WHO consultative group on equity and universal health coverage.* Geneva: World Health Organization. https://bit.ly/3U2Q6Nd [Accessed 30 March 2022].

WHO (World Health Organization). 2018. *World health statistics 2018: monitoring health for the SDGs, sustainable development goals.* Geneva: World Health Oranization. https://bit.ly/2USGTsT [Accessed 17 April 2022].

WHO (World Health Organization). 2019. *Primary health care.* https://bit.ly/2YNY2X6 [Accessed 17 April 2022].

WHO (World Health Organization). 2021. *Universal health coverage (UHC).* https://bit.ly/2QT9BLK [Accessed 30 March 2022].

Wong, E.B., Olivier, S., Gunda, R., Koole, O., Surujdeen, A., Gareta, C., Munatsi, D., Modise T.M., Dreyer, J., Nxumalo, S., Smit, T.K., Ording-Jespersen, G., Mpofana, I.B., Khan, K., Sikhosana, Z.E.L., Moodley, S., Shen, Y.J., Khoza, T. & Harilall, S. 2021. Convergence of infectious and non-communicable disease epidemics in rural South Africa: a cross-sectional, population-based multimorbidity study. *The Lancet Global Health,* 9(7):e967-e976.

World Bank. 2019a. *Physicians per 1,000 people - South Africa.* https://bit.ly/3OuIm5g [Accessed 19 April 2022].

World Bank. 2019b. *Nurses and midwives per 1,000 people - South Africa.* https://bit.ly/3tYTEoQ [Accessed 19 April 2022].

World Bank. 2019c. *Physicians per 1,000 people - United Kingdom.* https://bit.ly/3gwVjz4 [Accessed 19 April 2022].

3

Who Has the Right?

*Reproductive health and the termination of pregnancy
in contemporary South Africa*

Carike Noeth

Keywords: abortion; Choice on Termination of Pregnancy Act 92 of 1996; ethics; ethical challenges; ethical responsibility; reproductive health; reproductive rights; termination of pregnancy; women's rights

3.1   INTRODUCTION

Reproductive health in South Africa, like in any other country in the world, is by no means an easy topic to address, especially when it comes to the termination of pregnancy. While for some it is a complex ethical dilemma that leaves little or no room for the choice to terminate a pregnancy, for others it is about the right of a woman to choose what happens to her body. For many people, the question remains: who has the right to determine whether it is ethically justifiable to terminate a pregnancy? In contemporary South Africa, that question has a dual answer: on the one hand, the government made a decision, while on the other hand, the government's decision was that the final decision would rest upon the shoulders of a woman to choose whether or not to terminate a pregnancy. In this chapter, the aim is to provide information on reproductive health care in South Africa, more specifically, the termination of pregnancy in contemporary South Africa.

A brief overview of recent historical legislation regarding the termination of pregnancy in South Africa will be provided, focusing on the Abortion and Sterilization Act of 1975 and the Choice on Termination of Pregnancy Act 92 of 1996. This will be followed by a discussion of the reasons why the termination of pregnancy is regarded as an ethical dilemma in the 21st century. In this section, the argument will be made that some of the main reasons for the termination of pregnancy to be seen as an ethical dilemma include politics, technology, paternal rights, and religious conviction. The complexities and challenges of the termination of pregnancy will then be discussed to determine where the shortfalls are regarding the Choice on Termination of Pregnancy Act 92 of 1996. By determining the challenges with regard to the termination of pregnancy in contemporary South Africa, it will be argued that different role-players are key to accepting ethical responsibility when it comes to reproductive health in South Africa to ensure that policies, laws, and regulations are implemented practically. These include the acceptance of the ethical responsibility to ensure the implementation of the rights as set out by the laws of the country to secure the furtherance of gender equality, women's rights, and the right to reproductive health care.

The importance of the right to reproductive health care, the right to education, and the right to freedom can never be overestimated. It is crucial that these rights are not merely accepted as theories but lived experiences that allow women to live their lives according to their rights and not according to what society expects of them. To ensure that this happens, it is critical that ethical responsibility is accepted regarding reproductive health. In the absence of the practical implementation of these basic human rights, it will be argued that these human rights fail to be rights at all.

3.2   AN OVERVIEW OF THE TERMINATION OF PREGNANCY LAW IN SOUTH AFRICA

After the dawn of democracy in South Africa and the implementation of our new constitution, a new law on the termination of pregnancy was enacted in 1996. Not only was this a big step towards the rights of women in the country, but also meant that South Africa was committed to ensure that reproductive rights and reproductive health of women would align. In November of 1996, South Africa introduced the Choice on Termination of Pregnancy Act 92 of 1996 as a replacement for the outdated Abortion and Sterilization Act of 1975 which gave women an option for abortion, but not without the consent of at least two health care providers, among other rules that had to be adhered to.

The Abortion and Sterilization Act of 1975 made some advancements in terms of reproductive health, but still lacked the importance of the complete freedom of a woman's right to choose whether to terminate a pregnancy and it could easily be disallowed if consent was not obtained. This often led to self-induced abortion or illegal 'backstreet' abortion, leading to numerous cases of serious illness or even death among women. The Choice on Termination of Pregnancy Act 92 of 1996 that was implemented as part of the law of South Africa sets out specific conditions for the termination of a pregnancy as published in the *Government Gazette* of South Africa during November 1996. These conditions specify the three main categories for the termination of a pregnancy as follows:

> 2. (1) A pregnancy may be terminated–
>
> (a) upon request of a woman during the first 12 weeks of the gestation period of her pregnancy;
>
> (b) from the 13th up to and including the 20th week of the gestation period if a medical practitioner, after consultation with the pregnant woman, is of the opinion that–
>
>> (i) the continued pregnancy would pose a risk of injury to the woman's physical or mental health; or
>>
>> (ii) there exists a substantial risk that the fetus would suffer from a severe physical or mental abnormality; or
>>
>> (iii) the pregnancy resulted from rape or incest; or
>>
>> (iv) the continued pregnancy would significantly affect the social or economic circumstances of the woman; or
>
> (c) after the 20th week of the gestation period if a medical practitioner, after consultation with another medical practitioner or a registered midwife, is of the opinion that the continued pregnancy–
>
>> (i) would endanger the woman's life;
>>
>> (ii) would result in a severe malformation of the fetus; or
>>
>> (iii) would pose a risk of injury to the fetus. (RSA, 1996)

Between 1997 and 2002, after the implementation of the Choice on Termination of Pregnancy Act 92 of 1996, the mortality and morbidity cases found in post-abortion cases among women declined by 91% (Kaswa & Yogeswaran, 2020:1). According to Kaswa and Yogeswaran (2020:1) further amendments were made in 2004 and 2008 which led to an even greater decline in maternal mortality and morbidity during or after the process of the termination of pregnancy. The changes in law brought about by the government regarding the termination of pregnancy has had a big influence on the access to reproductive health care and rights of women in South Africa. As can be seen by the act, the Choice on Termination of Pregnancy Act 92 of 1996 allows a woman the right to choose whether to terminate a pregnancy up to the 12th week. During this time, the procedure can be done by either a trained nurse, a registered medical doctor, or a midwife, while only a registered medical doctor is allowed to perform a termination of pregnancy after the 12th week of a pregnancy (Kaswa & Yogeswaran, 2020:2). This period can be extended up to the 20th week of a pregnancy after the pregnant woman and a medical practitioner have had a consultation and have concluded that there may be mitigating factors to terminate the pregnancy (RSA, 2022). After the 20th week of pregnancy, a termination of pregnancy will only be conducted if the life of the mother or the life of the foetus is in danger or if there is a cause for serious concern regarding birth abnormalities (RSA, 2022).

Before and after the procedure, a woman has certain reproductive rights when it comes to the termination of a pregnancy, including the right to any information regarding the procedure, the right to choose as an individual whether to terminate the pregnancy, counselling, the various procedural options, and alternative options when women fall outside the window for a legal right to abortion (Kaswa & Yogeswaran, 2020:2). Mavuso and Macleod (2020:7-8) reiterate the importance of various forms of counselling that should be provided to ensure that women are exposed to the best possible information regarding reproductive health services and termination of pregnancy. They suggest that the following counselling options should be made available to assist women before and/or after a procedure: "decision-making counselling (for those who have not yet decided and would like assistance in talking through their options such as they may be), procedural counselling (where clients can elect to hear more details about the procedure), and pre- and post-procedural counselling (where clients may get emotional support prior to or after their procedure)" (Mavuso & Macleod, 2020:7-8).

Even though there have been great changes regarding the termination of pregnancy and women's rights in South Africa, there are still people who strongly oppose the right of a woman to choose to terminate a pregnancy.

3.3 WHY IS TERMINATION OF PREGNANCY STILL OFTEN CONSIDERED TO BE AN ETHICAL DILEMMA?

While this chapter is being written on termination of pregnancy in contemporary South Africa, the media is buzzing with the news from the United States of America (May 2022) on the very same topic. This is the result of a recent leak of official documentation from the Supreme Court of the United States wherein judges seem to have drafted a bill to overturn the notorious *Roe v Wade* decision of the Supreme Court that allows a woman to choose whether to terminate a pregnancy without legal interference from the government. This sparked anew an international debate on women's rights in general and a woman's right to specifically choose what happens to her body. Why is it then that in the 21st century, abortion is still considered to be such a controversial topic of discussion? Why is it still considered to be an ethical dilemma to so many people? Even more so in a country like the United States of America which is often regarded as the leader of the free world.

There are many reasons why people still object to the termination of pregnancy which make it such an ethical conundrum for people all over the world, including South Africa. From a moral and quite often a religious point of view, it is found that the exact moment of when life begins raises a lot of questions regarding the justification of the termination of a pregnancy. Some argue that life begins at the moment of conception, others argue that life begins the moment that there is a heartbeat, or that life only begins when a foetus is able to survive on its own outside a woman's protective uterus and is no longer dependent on the woman for its survival. There is still not consensus among individuals on when exactly life begins, and while this is the case, abortion will always be considered an ethical dilemma. Other influential ethical stances on the termination of pregnancy are often based on political and technological considerations, the rights of the father (Jones & Chaloner, 2007:46), or in some cases, religious reasons.

Politically, the most popular distinction in thinking regarding the termination of pregnancy is known as the pro-life and the pro-choice approaches. Scott Silk (1997:29) explains that these two perspectives are often viewed as the two main approaches to the termination of pregnancy. She calls pro-life an extreme approach that does not allow for any reason to terminate a pregnancy, even though there are very rare occasions that a termination of a pregnancy is allowed (Scott Silk, 1997:29). However, a basic or simplified understanding of the pro-choice approach allows a woman alone the right to choose whether to terminate a pregnancy or not as the law in South Africa currently stands (Scott Silk, 1997:29), even though the right of the woman to choose becomes a bit more complex after the 12th week of pregnancy since there has to be mitigating factors and medical practitioners involved to terminate a pregnancy after this period of time. People who relate more to the pro-life approach tend to believe that abortion is the equivalent of murder and therefore it should not be allowed, whereas people who relate more to the pro-choice approach tend to believe that only the person who is pregnant should have the right to decide whether to terminate the pregnancy or not, thereby allowing for the freedom and right of choice, up to at least 12 weeks of pregnancy without influence from unwanted external factors.

Technologically, there has also been some pushback on the termination of pregnancy due to "increased technological advances" (Jones & Chaloner, 2007:46) and what some label as unethical practices whereby tissue from aborted foetuses is used for "beneficent or therapeutic purposes" (Jones & Chaloner, 2007:46). Jones and Chaloner (2007:46) explain that this becomes an issue when considering the moral status of the foetus as a human life. This is further complicated by the conversation regarding embryonic stem cell research, gender selection, gene manipulation, and assisted reproductive technology. Ethical policies and laws are therefore crucial when it comes to technological advances and the challenges faced regarding the termination of pregnancy.

Another factor contributing to the ethical dilemma are the rights of the father of the foetus. There has been an increasing public outcry that the biological father of the unborn foetus should also have a say in the decision to terminate a pregnancy or not (Jones & Chaloner, 2007:46). It is especially the view of pro-life advocates that the biological father, as a contributor to the pregnancy, should have a right to have a say in the final decision. It is, however, mostly overruled in countries where a woman alone has the right to choose because she alone hosts the foetus.

As far as religion goes, termination of pregnancy has always been a contentious issue. Scott Silk (1997:36) notes that it is interesting that in ancient times a woman was given a set amount of time after conception to decide whether she wanted to continue with the pregnancy. She continues by claiming that most ancient cultures determined the timeframe for this decision to be made between conception and the first movement of the foetus (Scott Silk, 1997:36). The Stoics believed that life began at conception, but the soul of the foetus only came into existence at birth; Thomas Aquinas believed that a male foetus would receive its soul at 40 days and a female foetus at 80 days; and St Augustine believed that the soul was received at the first movement of the foetus (Scott Silk, 1997:36). According to Scott Silk (1997:37-40) religious beliefs regarding termination of pregnancy varies from very rigid points of view found among the Greek-Orthodox Church, the Roman Catholic Church, and Hinduism, to a slightly more refined view from Protestant and Muslim understandings. With most South Africans ascribing to some form of religious foundation, whether through upbringing or active religious affiliation, it would suffice to say that their stance on the termination of pregnancy may have been, or is still being, influenced by some form of religious conviction.

If politics, technology, the rights of the biological father, and religious conviction were all to be taken out of the equation and the only remaining factor determining the right of the woman to terminate a pregnancy was the law, then surely abortion should not face too many challenges in contemporary South Africa, one would think. This, however, is not the case.

3.4   UNDERSTANDING SOME OF THE CHALLENGES SURROUNDING TERMINATION OF PREGNANCY IN SOUTH AFRICA

Pickles (2017:496-497) acknowledges that South Africa has made great progress in valuing the rights of women in South Africa with the Termination of Pregnancy Act 92 of 1996, but also notes that the implementation of the act still faces some challenges in contemporary South Africa, especially regarding the lack of facilities with the necessary resources, the stigma that still clings to those who undergo the procedure, and abusive behaviour towards the person who opted for a termination of pregnancy. Overall, there is a generalised shame when it comes to sexual practices and reproductive health that may easily lead to ignorance or misinformation. This means that there are often situations where women are forced into a situation of self-inflicting a miscarriage or seeking illegal means to perform harmful and dangerous procedures that lead to increasing maternal morbidities and mortalities.

One of the ways to address these issues would be through education. This education should form part of primary school curriculums, at an age when children start to enter puberty. It is of the utmost importance that children be informed about the changes that occur in their bodies and how to be responsible and informed when it comes to issues of reproductive health. The stigma and shame surrounding sexual development, reproductive health, and sexual responsibility should never be a once-off conversation only but should rather become part of a responsibility-orientated approach whereby children are taught about the sexual changes and realities that they are facing throughout their developmental stages. This should not be seen as a means to encourage young girls to get abortions but should rather be seen as an opportunity to engage children in an open and honest conversation about reproductive health, sexual development, sexual responsibility, access to information, and an awareness of human rights. Of grave concern is the fact that information regarding reproductive health is either not being spread efficiently, or that the information made available is not received as it is aimed to. One example of this is that women reported that people are willing and open to discuss or even disclose their HIV status but are unwilling to do discuss termination of pregnancy (Orner, De Bruyn & Cooper, 2011:790).

Orner et al. (2011:781) stress the importance of investigation of the decisions and experiences of pregnant women who are HIV+ when it comes to sexual and reproductive health in South Africa. In a study conducted among women living with HIV in Cape Town, they found an extreme sense of judgement, social and economic difficulties, and a lack of information regarding reproductive health and more specifically South Africa's law on the termination of pregnancy up to 20 weeks of gestation (Orner et al., 2011:781-782). This means that women who are living with HIV who inadvertently become pregnant may seek illegal abortion options due to fear, shame, and being ill-informed about their reproductive rights. Where termination of pregnancy was sought, women often reported that they have experienced a feeling of being judged by their health care providers for being pregnant while living with HIV (Orner et al., 2011:782). Apart from feeling judged, these women also mention a lack of support within communities when a person living with HIV/AIDS fell pregnant and reached out to members of the community for assistance in deciding whether or not to terminate the pregnancy, they would not be supported (Orner et al., 2011:785).

Another complication with the termination of pregnancy concerns women seeking termination during the second trimester of their pregnancy. Harries, Orner, Gabriel and Mitchell (2007:2) state that an estimated 20% of the total number of termination procedures are conducted during the second trimester of a pregnancy. The chances of medical complications or maternal morbidity and mortality increase after the first trimester and is therefore considered to be of greater risk than first trimester terminations (Harries et al., 2007:2). While it may be a greater risk, it is still legal to undergo a termination procedure during the second trimester due to factors including socio-economic hardship, danger to the life of the mother (physical or mental), rape, or incest. However, during the second trimester any termination procedures must be conducted by a registered medical practitioner. Seeking reasons why women waited until their second trimester to opt for a termination of pregnancy, Harries et al. (2007:3) discovered that women often reported having a history of irregular menstrual periods and did not have any typical signs of being pregnant, and thereby realised only at a very late stage that they were pregnant. Most women are also not using any form of contraceptive medication to prevent them from falling pregnant, while those who did make use of a contraceptive pill, report that they did not use it consistently or as advised (Harries et al., 2007:3). Another reason that women sought a second trimester termination is because of the failure of an attempted, self-inflicted termination, after which they then approach legal facilities (Harries et al., 2015:2).

Adding to the challenges women face in seeking termination of a pregnancy, they reported receiving negative judgement or discouragement in certain cases by health care providers (Harries, Gerdts, Momberg & Foster, 2015:1). Women also reported the often very negative attitude of health care providers in their search for legal and safe options to terminate a pregnancy (Harries et al., 2015:1). Harries et al. (2015:2) add that legal and safe abortions are often lacking due to a shortage of trained staff and a shortage of legal facilities to accommodate these procedures. This not only hampers women's right to safe and legal abortion but can also lead to women seeking illegal options for the termination of a pregnancy or attempt to self-inflict termination which could have dire consequences for them. Unfortunately, this often seems to be the case in rural areas (Harries et al., 2015:2). This is worsened by the identification of an ever-growing network of termination of pregnancy providers who are not registered medical practitioners or legally trained to provide the service (Harries et al., 2015:2).

More recently, a study on the termination of pregnancy and refugees in South Africa concluded that refugees often face serious challenges in seeking legal and safe termination services. Munyaneza and Mhlongo (2019:1) say refugees are more likely to be on the receiving end of basic human rights violations than citizens in South Africa. Reports received from refugees suggest that they often experience "medical xenophobia and discrimination" (Munyaneza & Mhlongo, 2019:4) when they seek termination of pregnancy services. This was further complicated by the struggle to communicate properly due to language barriers between the refugees and the local service providers (Munyaneza & Mhlongo, 2019:4). Refugees often found legal termination services and service providers to be unprofessional because of a lack of health care information and sufficient care for the patient (Munyaneza & Mhlongo, 2019:4), while others mentioned that due to financial constraints as refugees, they were unable to afford private health care and struggled to access overcrowded public reproductive health care services where they felt like they were being judged for their decision to terminate a pregnancy (Munyaneza & Mhlongo, 2019:5). Taking the experience of refugees into account, it becomes crucial to address the issue of proper education and training in reproductive health care in South Africa. Refugees should not feel unsafe, unwelcome, or judged by health care providers in the same way that South Africans ought not feel unsafe, unwelcome, or judged for their reproductive health care decisions.

As a consequence of some of the challenges surrounding the termination of pregnancy, it becomes clear that more needs to be done to address these challenges. It has been 26 years since the Choice on Termination of Pregnancy Act 92 of 1996 has been enacted. It should not be regarded as a theoretical law but should rather be implemented responsibly and in the best interest of the patient in need of reproductive health care. This calls not only for an ethical awareness, but also for ethical responsibility and accountability when it comes to the furtherance of reproductive health care in South Africa.

3.5 ETHICAL RESPONSIBILITY AND REPRODUCTIVE HEALTH CARE IN SOUTH AFRICA

As seen by some of the challenges surrounding the termination of pregnancy in contemporary South Africa, the need for ethical responsibility and accountability regarding reproductive health care can no longer be evaded. As citizens, women, policymakers, academics, and politicians, we can no longer turn a blind eye to the desperate need for ethical responsibility in the reproductive health care sector. It is time for the Department of Health to look at the implication of the challenges faced surrounding the termination of pregnancy and to put policies and laws in place which seek to protect and advance the sexual reproductive health care rights of women – not only in theory or on paper, but by taking responsibility for the implementation of these policies and laws to create a safer and more just society wherein women are not shamed, judged, overlooked, frightened, or denied the right to reproductive health care. Macleod (2019:58) echoes the outcry for the practical implementation of reproductive health laws in stating that "there are a number of injustices that continue at both a micro- and macro-level, thereby hindering women's access to non-judgemental abortion services and, in some cases, jeopardising their health" (Macleod, 2019:58). Everyone, women and men alike, should have the right to feel safe, educated, and empowered by their right to reproductive health care. This should include the right to counselling and education to address "the dangers of clandestine abortions and the option of safe and legal abortion" (Orner et al., 2011:792).

Orner et al. (2011:781) reiterate the fact that the decision-making component when it comes to reproductive health in women who are living with HIV in South Africa are in a particularly troubled situation. The challenges regarding sexual reproductive health and women's rights are not only complex, but also severely neglected. South Africa has one of the highest HIV infection rates in the world and women are more often affected by this than men (Orner et al., 2011:781). Orner et al. (2011:781) ascribe this to the fact that contemporary South Africa is still very much an unequal society in terms of gender and socioeconomic rights. For women living with HIV, decision-making regarding pregnancy is extremely difficult, since they may likely not only be experiencing judgement about their HIV status, but also because they have fallen pregnant while living with HIV (Orner et al., 2011:781-782).

De Bruyn (2004:93) notes that there exists an unnoticed form of discrimination regarding living with HIV and access to information regarding reproductive health care in South Africa. Women's restricted access to responsible education and their inability to acquire the contraceptives of their choice further complicates the right to reproductive health care (De Bruyn, 2004:93). It is therefore critical to implement ethically sound policies that ensure women have access to proper education, reproductive health care resources, and safe services. The ethical importance of access to information regarding sexual reproductive health, the termination of pregnancy, and the laws surrounding it, cannot be stressed enough. This will not only lead to the furtherance of the practical implementation of women's rights, but also to safer and healthier reproductive health care services. If responsibility is not accepted for the implementation of basic human rights, there is no use for the existence of the human right concerned. Therefore, it can be said that a human right like access to reproductive health care is not a human right if the policies and laws do not ensure its practical implementation in the lives of citizens.

De Bruyn (2004:95) explains that, in the past, changes in terms of policies and laws that lead to the protection of women in society have come about through rigorous "lobbying by NGOs, researchers and members of the healthcare sector". It is the ethical duty of the same people who were lobbying for a change in policies, laws, and regulations to take responsibility along with the Department of Health in South Africa to make sure that these policies, laws, and regulations are thoroughly implemented. Where there is a lack of responsibility with regard to the practical implementation of the law, it can be stated that the "state should be held to account for its failure to respect, protect and promote women's rights in the context of abortion services" (Pickles, 2017:505). It is noteworthy that this effort to implement policies where needed never happens in isolation, but demands the involvement of different sectors of society. Bolarinwa and Boikhutso (2021:8) echo the "call for the attention of key stakeholders towards policy formation and development of behaviour and social intervention".

3.6   CONCLUSION

The termination of a pregnancy and the right to choose to terminate a pregnancy is without a doubt a difficult topic to discuss. It is however crucial to discuss this topic within the framework of reproductive health and reproductive health care services.

In this chapter on reproductive health, a brief overview is given on the most recent history of the laws regarding the termination of pregnancy in South Africa. This is done by briefly discussing the content of the Abortion and Sterilization Act of 1975 and the Choice on Termination of Pregnancy Act 92 of 1996. It is argued that the act of 1996 furthered the rights of women by allowing them the right to choose whether they want to terminate a pregnancy or not. This decision is left entirely in the hands of the women. It is then argued that although women have the legal right to choose whether to terminate a pregnancy or not, it never comes without challenges, whether it be political, technological, paternal rights, or religious conviction. The identification of some of the challenges leads to the demand that ethical responsibilities should be addressed. It is argued that women's rights, the right to reproductive health care, and the right to freedom cannot not be realised rights if they are not practically implemented. For this to happen, ethical responsibility for issues like education, access to information, and access to reproductive health care needs to be accepted.

Finally, although a woman has the legal right to decide whether or not to terminate a pregnancy, the practical implementation of the law falls somewhat short of securing women sole jurisdiction of their life choices.

Bibliography

Bolarinwa, O.A. & Boikhutso, T. 2021. Mapping evidence on predictors of adverse sexual and reproductive health outcomes among young women in South Africa: a scoping review. *African Journal of Primary Health Care & Family Medicine*, 13(1):1-10. https://doi.org/10.4102/phcfm.v13i1.3091

De Bruyn, M. 2004. Living with HIV: challenges in reproductive health care in South Africa. *African Journal of Reproductive Health*, 8(1):92-98. https://bit.ly/3OKTzij

Harries, J., Gerdts, C., Momberg, M. & Foster, D.G. 2015. An exploratory study of what happens to women who are denied abortions in Cape Town, South Africa. *Reproductive Health*, 12(21):1-6. https://doi.org/10.1186/s12978-015-0014-y

Harries, J., Orner, P., Gabriel, M. & Mitchell, E. 2007. Delays in seeking an abortion until the second trimester: a qualitative study in South Africa. *Reproductive Health*, 4(7):1-8. https://doi:10.1186/1742-4755-4-7

Jones, K. & Chaloner, C. 2007. Ethics of abortion: the arguments for and against. *Nursing Standard*, 21(47):45-48.

Kaswa, R. & Yogeswaran, P. 2020. Abortion reforms in South Africa: an overview of the Choice on Termination of Pregnancy Act. *South African Family Practice*, 62(1):1-5. https://doi.org/10.4102/safp.v62i1.5240

Mavuso, J.M.J.J. & Macleod, C.I. 2020. Contradictions in womxn's experiences of pre-abortion counselling in South Africa: implications for client-centred practice.

Nursing Inquiry, 27:1-9. https://doi.org/10.1111/nin.12330

Macleod, C.I. 2019. Expanding reproductive justice through a supportability reparative justice framework: the case of abortion in South Africa. *Culture, Health & Sexuality*, 21(1):46-62. https://doi.org/10.1080/13691058.2018.1447687

Munyaneza, Y. & Mhlongo, E.M. 2019. Challenges of women refugees in utilising reproductive health services in public health institutions in Durban, KwaZulu-Natal, South Africa. *Health SA Gesondheid*, 24:1-8. https://doi.org/10.4102/hsag.v24i0.1030

Orner, P., De Bruyn, M. & Cooper, D. 2011. 'It hurts, but I don't have a choice, I'm not working and I'm sick': decisions and experiences regarding abortion of women living with HIV in Cape Town, South Africa. *Culture, Health & Sexuality*, 13(7):781-795.

Pickles, C. 2017. Self-induced abortion in South Africa and Section 10 of the Choice on Termination of Pregnancy Act 92 of 1996. *South African Journal on Human Rights*, 40(3):496-506. https://doi.org/10.1080/02587203.2017.1394010

RSA (Republic of South Africa). 1996. *Choice on Termination of Pregnancy Act 92 of 1996*. https://bit.ly/3GNeQWx

RSA (Republic of South Africa). 2022. *Terminate pregnancy*. https://bit.ly/3grVMme [Accessed 31 May 2022].

Scott Silk, M.J. 1997. Aborsie. In: C. Jones, & L. Hulley (eds.). *Wonder jy ook oor...? Gedagtes oor omstrede kwessies van ons dag*. Kaapstad: Lux Verbi. 28-44.

4

Gender in Sport

Caster Semenya as a case in point

Juri van den Heever & Chris Jones

> Biologists may have been building a more nuanced view of sex, but society has yet to catch up. (Ainsworth, 2015:291)

Keywords: agriculture; discrimination; embryology; genetics; IAAF; international athletics; legal systems; neurobiology; Paralympics; physical reality; religion; sex and gender inequality; social reality; World Athletics

4.1 INTRODUCTION

In the social sphere, Western culture is still substantially influenced by the perception that, within the human sexual spectrum, there are only two possibilities. This paradigm dictates that one is either a heterosexual male or a heterosexual female, and Western legal traditions have, over time, reflected these assumptions, ostensibly drawing support from literalist readings of religious texts, superficial observations of the human body, and contingent decisions about physical and intellectual abilities. Despite clear advances in the legal perspective, overly simplified social perceptions about this matter still hold sway in the public mind.

It turns out that the binary interpretation of sexuality, long held as inviolate, is a social construct, whilst in reality, sex and gender differences manifest as a variable combination of factors, expressed as a spectrum of possibilities (see Figure 4.1).

Apart from popular belief generally favouring a binary approach, it appears also to be the position of choice of the International Association of Athletics Federations (IAAF), now World Athletics (WA), as to the legality of their decisions about the sex and gender of international athletes, as well as claiming sole jurisdiction in the prescription of chemical interventions.

South Africa has been in the spotlight because of the athletic prowess of Caster Semenya in international competitions. As the result of allegations about her sexuality, she refused chemical intervention to lower her testosterone levels and was subsequently banned from certain women's events at international competitions by WA.

However, it must be admitted that legal traditions throughout the ages have, through no fault of their own, attempted to adjudicate fairly with respect to social conventions and the perceived vagaries of human sexuality and gender, without the benefit of the solid, science-based biological approach currently recognised in, for example, the South African Constitution.

The phenomenon of intersexuality in its various forms has long been recognised in ancient cultures and religions as shown by often-portrayed subjects like the life-sized statue, *Sleeping Hermaphroditus*, of the Hellenistic and Roman periods, as well as the sexual proclivities of deities in the Greek pantheon.

That a spectrum of sex and gender differences have existed in nature since time immemorial is also shown by the behaviour of, among others, mammals in the wild, and within domestic herds. Logically, these observations should have led to the obvious conclusion that sex and gender preferences are variable, but instead, for a number of reasons, a simplistic and rigid binary system was settled upon, casting humans definitively as either male or female members of the two sexes.

More recently gender has, understandably, at times, been a controversial issue in the history of international sport. One memorable case that contributed to changes in administration at the international level concerned the amazing athletic prowess of two sisters. By the time the Soviet track and field athletes, Irina and Tamara Press, had accumulated 26 world records between them in international athletics, between 1959 and 1966, widespread doubts about their true sexuality started to circulate, causing them to be colloquially labelled in the Western media as the Press Brothers. Consequently, when the then IAAF instituted compulsory gender testing for women in international sport, commencing with the 1966 European Championships in Budapest, the sisters unexpectedly and permanently retired from international sport, shortly before the event.

The concept of a binary approach in human sexuality still exists in Western culture and, apparently, also within the executive echelons of WA as they continue to insist on the erroneous legality of their position. Meier, Koujer and Krieger

(2021:1) has noted that "[s]ince men's control of women's physical activity has been at the heart of masculine hegemony, sports have been a highly gendered social sphere".

Theberge (2000:322) points out that, historically, sport has been construed as a predominantly male endeavour and consequently males benefited markedly in terms of opportunities and rewards. "This arrangement is both the basis of, and a powerful support for an ideology of gender that ascribes different natures, abilities and interests to men and women" (Theberge, 2000:322). For her, the roots of contemporary sport were laid in the late 19th and early 20th centuries in Britain and North America. In Britain, the Victorian concept of masculinity was promoted through participation in physically tough, competitive games. "Games playing in the boys' public schools provided the dominant image of masculine identity in sports and a model for their future development in Britain and throughout the world" (Hargreaves, 1994:43).

The IAAF was established in 1912 for the sole purpose of advancing the participation of men in international sporting events. Women were excluded because "[t]he founder of the modern Olympic Movement, Pierre de Coubertin, thought women's sport was impractical, uninteresting, ungainly, and, I do not hesitate to add, improper" (Meier et al., 2021:2). Between World War I and II, increased participation of women in international events was permitted, but thereby hangs a tale, as noted by Meier et al. (2021:2): "Put simply, men wanted to maintain control over women's sport so it would not exceed the men's sport in popularity."

The aim of this contribution is to review the origins of gender discrimination, the agencies through which it has been perpetuated throughout history, and to offer a possible resolution to the quandary the WA finds itself in.

4.2   PHYSICAL REALITY AS OPPOSED TO SOCIAL REALITY

All life is inescapably subject to the physical realities of our solar system such as gravity, geology, geography, meteorology, and the rotational behaviour of our planet. As humans we are physically constrained and unable to jump over tall buildings in a single leap or run faster than a speeding bullet. In the same way, our sexuality and gender preferences are at the mercy of the physical realities of our embryonic development and intra-uterine influences. It is therefore a *fait accompli* that we are what our physical bodies deem us to be, and it is morally incumbent upon any society to recognise and respect the enduring embrace physical reality executes on the human condition in all its manifestations.

However, humans live in societies where we create our own social reality. We decide where the borders of countries lie, and which pieces of paper denote certain monetary values. Legal systems are socially constructed to serve specific moral conventions of the time and guide daily existence. Equally, religious groupings arise as social realities, each claiming single ownership of the ultimate truth, whilst allocating competitors to a future laced with fire and brimstone. Similarly, "[s]tudies show that wine tastes better if people believe it's expensive. Coffee labelled *ecofriendly* tastes better to people than identical, unlabelled coffee" (Barrett, 2020:111).

It is noteworthy also to realise that Western society is not alone in harbouring intransient views regarding transgenderism. Steven Spielberg's remake of the internationally acclaimed stage production of *West Side Story* has initiated negative reactions from the Arab world, because one of the actors portrays a transgender role and the film includes a kiss between two ostensibly male figures. As a result, the film has been banned in certain countries. According to *Netwerk24* (*Network24*) of 8 December 2021 (n.p.), censors in Kuwait and Saudi-Arabia apparently banned the film outright and refused to issue a certificate for distribution, whereas censors in Bahrain, Qatar, Oman and the United Arab Emirates requested the removal of certain scenes. When 20th Century Studios, the distributors of the film, refused to comply, these countries also banned the film. This attitude of a relentless refusal to accept the physical reality of the human condition for what it is and choosing rather to be guided by outdated and ambiguous social realities, generated by fundamentalist interpretations of religious texts, as well as misconceptions about human biology, is paradigmatic of either a perverse unwillingness to acknowledge the real world, or blissful ignorance of human physiology and sexuality. It seems paradoxical that whilst many Arabian countries are technologically advanced, they either prohibit or fastidiously ignore the essential biological basis of the human condition.

Human laws also represent a version of social reality and undergo radical changes at times. A good example in this case are the so-called laws of apartheid as well as the laws historically enacted in the United States of America restricting the civil rights of African Americans.

It is clear therefore that gender in sport is a biological issue and should be considered from a biological point of view in terms of a spectrum and not from the outdated view that humanity consists only of heterosexual men and women.

In discussing human sexuality and gender, there needs to be a distinct separation between physical and social reality, because for many social reality masquerades as a factual, fixed, and unchangeable guide to their life world. In reality, this is a misconception, because only physical reality allows us a factual approach, which can be tested. Thus, social reality reflects chosen protocols of time and place, all of which are subject to change. In this regard, human sexuality and gender lie within the parameters of physical reality and should be examined and judged as such.

4.3   THE ORIGINS OF DISCRIMINATION

The question remains as to when discrimination against women became histori-cally established, and by what means was it so successfully maintained. For this reason, it is necessary to briefly visit past human societies and their social practices.

It is illustrative to observe that in modern, mobile egalitarian hunter-gatherer societies there is a distinct lack of gender discrimination as decision-making and influence within such groups are most often equally divided between men and women. Dyble et al. (2015:1) has suggested that the egalitarian structure of modern, mobile hunter-gatherer groups reflects conditions pertaining to ancient human societies and can therefore offer constructive inputs, illuminating the phenomenon of sex equality. They link gender inequality to the rise of agriculture and pastoralism. Once heritable resources such as land and livestock became important determinants of reproductive success, sex-biased inheritance and lineal systems started to arise, leading to wealth and sex inequalities. "Understanding hunter-gatherer sex-egalitarianism and the shift from hierarchical male philo-patry typical of chimpanzees and bonobos to a multilocal residence pattern is key to theories of human social evolution" (Dyble et al., 2015:3).

Lewis and Maslin (2018:361) note that

> [w]hile modern-day hunter-gatherer societies are not the same as those living thousands of years ago, both historically and in modern times the evidence is they tend to be relatively egalitarian. The highly mobile groups that save no food or other resources are particularly equal. In these groups no person has authority over any other; this lack of authority also means a lack of dependency.

Alesina, Guiliano and Nunn (2013), investigating the origin of gender roles as related to agricultural practices in the pre-industrial era have shown that the transition from shifting cultivation, employing the hoe, and digging stick, tradi-tionally employed by women, to plough cultivation, represented a watershed with regard to gender roles.

> Unlike the hoe or digging stick, the plough requires significant upper body strength, grip strength, and bursts of power, which are needed

> to either pull the plough or control the animal that pulls it. Because of these requirements, when plough agriculture is practiced, men have an advantage in farming relative to women. (Alesina et al., 2013:470)

From this evolved the perception that men were more suitable to the physical tasks required by agriculture whilst women were best suited to the less arduous environment within the home. "These cultural beliefs tend to persist even if the economy moves out of agriculture, affecting the participation of women in activities performed outside the home, such as market employment, entrepreneurship, or participation in politics" (Alesina et al., 2013:471). More surprisingly, they note that:

> Our findings provide evidence that current differences in gender attitudes and female behaviour are indeed shaped by differences in traditional agricultural practices. Specifically, we have shown that individuals, ethnicities, and countries whose ancestors engaged in plough agriculture have beliefs that exhibit greater gender inequality today and have less female participation in non-domestic activities, such as market employment, firm ownership, and politics. In an effort to better identify a channel of cultural persistence, we examined the children of immigrants. We find that among these individuals who face the same labor markets, institutions, and policies, a heritage of traditional plough agriculture is still associated with more unequal gender attitudes and less female labor force participation. (Alesina et al., 2013:527-528)

Thus, the transition from mobile hunter-gatherer societies to pastoral and agricultural practices represented a watershed with reference to the position of women in society. Shifting perceptions within belief systems also increasingly contributed the establishment of gender inequalities during the transition from Polytheism to Monotheism.

Ancient Egypt evolved from a nomadic culture to a powerful state, dependent on slave labour. However, the highly complex State Religion remained polytheistic where natural objects like the sun and the moon were still, respectively, revered as Ra and Khonsu, together with a variety of animals that populated their pantheon of deities. This environment was not devoid of discrimination, but men and women were at least legally equal, which meant that for women like Hatshepsut and Sobekneferu it was possible to attain the executive position of Pharoah (Cornelius, 2022).

From Egyptian religious thought and other polytheistic world views, alternative religious world views, like Judaism, emerged, conflating and reinterpreting the then extant cosmic explanations and deities, clothing it with specific religious and political thoughts as necessary. Judaism, in turn, served as source material for the three Abrahamic religions, all of which included attitudes, beliefs, and myths condoning discrimination on the basis of sex and gender which are still functional in modern-day Christianity. Judaism itself evolved from polytheism, through monolatry (worshipping one deity but acknowledging the existence of many) to monotheism which acknowledged only one, true universal male god for all people, as does Christianity today.

In the polytheistic phase, the Hebrew God, Jehovah or Yhwh, had a consort or companion wife, Asherah, a deity primarily worshipped by women of the ancient near East. Dever (2005:188) attests to the fact that Asherah was "… long venerated in Canaan as patroness of mothers". According to Römer (2015:172):

> […] the goddess Asherah was associated with Yhwh as his *parhedros* [sitting beside or near] but she was also worshipped independently of him, especially by women in the form of the Queen of Heaven. It is only with the beginning of the reign of Josiah that we find Yhwh alone without his Ashera.

During the evolution of Jehovah from a warlike deity to a god of neighbourly love, as expressed by the third person of the Trinity, Ashera was systematically excised from the texts of the Old Testament, and thus also from religious observance, although the Christian Bible still contains 39 muted references to her existence. This literary manoeuvre further entrenched the subsidiary position of women in Hebrew and subsequent Christian societies. "To be the only true god means to have no partners. Thus, Yhwh is traditionally considered to be an 'unmarried' god, and the allusions to goddesses in the Bible, notably to Asherah, have been interpreted as referring to non-Yahwist cults. This is the way the editors of the Bible finally decided to present matters" (Römer, 2015:160).

Dever (2005:100) notes that the Hebrew word `ăšērāh occurs over 40 times in the Hebrew Bible. In addition, Römer (2015:161) points out that the word `ăšērāh is used 40 times in biblical texts "… mostly with the article" and that in places where the masculine plural is employed, it "… is an artificial creation of the editors of the Bible in order to avoid any possible allusion to the goddess Asherah". In sharp contrast to the biblical texts, "a close link between Yhwh and Asherah is attested in the inscriptions found at Kuntillet Ajrud and Khirbet el-Qom" (Römer, 2015:162).

The Catholic version of Christianity and its male-centred dogma is infamous for its transgressions against humanity, and particularly against women, whose position in society thereby further deteriorated. It created, from the religious perspective, a binary society with men dominating the existence of women, taking decisions about and for them, usually in their absence, on what is permissible in terms of behaviour in general, religious conduct, and more specifically, the ludicrous attempts by the allegedly celibate church hierarchy to dare to prescribe and pronounce on sexual conduct within marriage. It is interesting to note that the period of time when the Catholic Church virtually ruled the West is often sardonically referred to as the Dark Ages.

The unequal treatment of women by men continued through known history on multiple fronts, a case in point being women's suffrage, which is still not universally implemented. It appears evident then that gender inequality in sport constitutes only the tip of the iceberg that women still face, but it is of significant importance because international sport personalities are continually in the public eye and women athletes serve as role models on a variety of levels. Sex and gender inequality have developed over thousands of years and have been driven by social reality employing a variety of subversive tactics in establishing male dominance. Women have thus been wronged and subjugated by what is commonly referred to as the pillars of society, namely male representatives of mainstream religions, law, politics, the economic community, and, as this contribution attempts to show, long excluded from fair and free competition in international sporting events.

4.4   THE LEGALITY OF THE IAAF'S CLAIMS

Michele Krech, at the time a doctoral candidate at the New York University School of Law, served as consultant to the legal team of Caster Semenya in *Mokgadi Caster Semenya v International Association of Athletics Federations*, CAS 2018/O/5794. Krech (2019) succinctly outlines the misplaced burdens of gender equality in Caster Semenya's case against the IAAF and notes that "[t]he highly anticipated decision of the Court of Arbitration for Sport (CAS) in *Caster Semenya v International Association of Athletics Federations* (IAAF), has quickly become its most (in)famous" (Krech, 2019:66). The case revolves around regulatory issues which make it possible for the IAAF to block certain female athletes from competing on the grounds that they exhibit differences in sexual development. Krech (2019) has extensively analysed and concisely summarised the legal misinterpretations surrounding the case of Caster Semenya. Unfortunately, limitations of space prevent an extensive exposition of all her arguments. Consequently, we refer only to what we regard as a summary of her most salient points. For an in-depth exposition of her legal approach, interested readers are referred to Krech (2019:66-76).

Krech (2019:66) criticises the CAS findings as "tentative and incomplete" and lacking "conclusive authority". She accuses the CAS Panel of actually sidestepping the application of "… the widely recognised legal framework for the analysis of such claims" (2019:66) and in her view compromising the Panel's attempt at fair adjudication. "Instead, the decision in *Semenya v IAAF* makes clear that the CAS stamp of approval is no guarantee of human rights appliance" (2019:66).

According to Krech (2019:75), the IAAF maintains that it is exempt from international human rights laws, however "[t]he IAAF's position in this regard completely ignores the UN *Guiding Principles on Business and Human Rights* which delineate the responsibility of all business enterprises, including transnational ones such as the IAAF, to respect all internationally recognised human rights" (2019:76). The stated position of the IAAF, rather than complying with the UN *Guiding Principles on Business and Human Rights,* is to defend the CAS ruling, claiming that "CAS is competent to rule on all legal claims, including human rights claims, and it did so in its recent ruling, in favour of the IAAF" (2019:76).

Semenya confronted the CAS with the Eligibility Regulations for Female Classification, known as Differences of Sex Development Regulations (DSD), resulting in the CAS Panel conceding that the "… regulations at issue are prima facie discriminatory on the basis of protected characteristics, namely sex and gender …" The CAS Panel also acknowledged "… in principle, that the burden of proof shifts from the claimants (the athletes) – having established that the relevant regulations are prima facie discriminatory – to the defender of the regulations (the IAAF) to justify the discrimination" (Krech, 2019:67).

In her extensive legal analysis, Krech (2019:74) is pointedly at odds with the claimed legality of the assertions by WA, stating her arguments in convincing detail. However, in the interests of brevity we will restrict ourselves to a few brief and final comments. She points out that the Panel also failed to address discrepancies in the regulations which allow the same female athlete to compete as a male in some events and as a female in other events, and questions discrepancies in the regulations which the Panel failed to address properly, such as "… how it is reasonable and necessary that the DSD regulations apply to certain running events but not to the events in which the IAAF's own study shows the highest correlation between testosterone and performance benefit; hammer throw and pole vault" (Krech, 2019:73). Clearly at odds with the legal proceedings in the case, she unequivocally states that "[m]ore broadly speaking, the CAS decision in *Semenya* serves to underscore, rather than to address, the serious challenges of securing human rights – particularly gender equality – in the context of sport" (Krech, 2019:76), finally concluding that the CAS has

"… proven itself incompetent to conduct a full and proper human rights analysis" (Krech, 2019:76).

In summary, it would seem that the insistence of WA on the legality of their position represents a too narrow interpretation, relying overtly on the social reality of legal views, as opposed to the physical realities of human sexuality, a relevant point expressed by Krech (2019:70) as "[l]egal reasoning, especially when fundamental rights are at stake, must take account of the real world as it exists, as opposed to the hypothetical utopia we may hope to one day live in". In this respect, it is important to acknowledge that it is not incumbent upon the individual to conform to the social realities of the legal system, it is for the legal system to recognise, protect, and champion the physical reality of the biological basis of human sexuality and gender.

4.5   THE VIEW FROM BIOLOGY

4.5.1   Genetics

In the social environment, where sex is still perceived in binary terms, intersexuality remains problematic. "Few legal systems allow for any ambiguity in biological sex, and a person's legal rights and social status can be heavily influenced by whether their birth certificate says male or female" (Ainsworth, 2015:288). Medical researchers and doctors have long been aware of the complexities of sexuality:

> [...] doctors have long known that some people straddle the boundary – their sex chromosomes say one thing, but their gonads (ovaries or testes) or sexual anatomy say another. Parents of children with these kinds of conditions – known as intersex conditions or differences or disorders of sex development (DSDs) – often face difficult decisions about whether to bring up their child as a boy or as a girl. (Ainsworth, 2015:288)

Sex is therefore much more complicated than what it seems at first. The time is past when the presence or absence of a Y chromosome determined if an individual is a male or female. However, things are even more complicated than that. It is known now that the sex chromosomes do not have the last word, and in spite of what the sex chromosomes may suggest, the gonads (testes and ovaries) and the sexual anatomy can be indicators of a quite different scenario.

During the initial stages of development, the sex of the human embryo is indeterminate, so much so that at five weeks, the future external genitals are represented by a single external cellular *anlage*, the genital tubercle, which possesses the potential to develop into the external genitals of either of the two traditional sexes, boy or girl. At six weeks, the gonads differentiate into either ovaria or testes, each secreting the specific hormones that further drive internal and external development. At this time, testosterone facilitates a male developmental pattern, assisting in the regression of the female sexual attributes. When the ovaries release oestrogen in the absence of testosterone, it promotes the development of the female sexual system causing the regression of male sexual attributes.

> Changes to any of these processes can have dramatic effects on an individual's sex. Gene mutations affecting gonad development can result in a person with XY chromosomes developing typically female characteristics, whereas alterations in hormone signaling can cause XX individuals to develop along male lines. (Ainsworth, 2015:289)

It has also been shown that a DSD known as congenital adrenal hyperplasia (CAH) induces the production of abundant male sex hormones. Consequently, "... XX individuals with this condition are born with ambiguous genitalia (an enlarged clitoris and fused labia that resemble a scrotum)" (Ainsworth, 2015:290). It is therefore patently clear that the complexities of sex and gender are not binary and cannot be represented as a simple dichotomy.

4.5.2 Brain structure

Swaab and Garcia-Falgueras (2009) have contributed an extensive series of salient insights on the sexual differentiation of the brain, as it applies to gender identity and sexual orientation. Their argument clearly invalidates a binary approach, highlighting the role of the brain in the inherent complexity of human sexuality.

> Once the differentiation of the sexual organs into male or female is settled, the next thing that is differentiated is the brain, under the influence, mainly, of sex hormones on the developing brain cells. The changes (permanent) brought about in this stage have organizing effects later, during puberty, the brain circuits that developed in the womb are activated by the sex hormones. (Swaab & Garcia-Falgueras, 2009:17)

The observed structural differences in brain development results from reciprocal influences between hormones and developing brain cells. This phenomenon is regarded as

> [...] the basis of sex differences in a wide section of behaviours, such as gender role (behaving as a man or a woman in society), gender identity (the conviction of belonging to the male or female gender), sexual orientation (heterosexuality, homosexuality or bisexuality) and sex differences regarding cognition, aggressive behaviour and language organisation. (Swaab & Garcia-Falgueras, 2009:18)

To complicate matters further they reveal, in the same article that

> [t]he environment of a developing neuron is formed by the surrounding nerve cells and the child's circulating hormones, as well as the hormones, nutrients, medication and other chemical substances from the mother and the environment that enter the fetal circulation via the placenta. All these factors may have a lasting effect on the sexual differentiation of the brain. (Swaab & Garcia-Falgueras, 2009:17)

According to Swaab and Garcia-Falgueras (2009:18), the prenatal hormonal influences can, in effect, establish gender identity, although the uterine environment, in such a case, may be insufficiently equipped to allow complete genital differentiation. The sexual differentiation of the human brain adds further complications to sex and gender choices in that it is "… also expressed in behavioral differences, including sexual orientation (homo-, bi-, and heterosexuality) and gender identity, and in differences at the level of brain physiology …" (Swaab & Garcia-Falgueras, 2009:19). Thus, it is patently evident that gender is under the influence of numerous factors, which can lead to transsexuality.

Putting paid to an enduring myth, Swaab and Garcia-Falgueras (2009:21) make the important point that sexuality is not reversible, and that the sexuality of children raised by transsexual or homosexual parents will not be affected. In conjunction with a wide array of published research, they make a compelling case discussing an array of important prenatal factors that can influence sexual development during pregnancy. Phenobarbital and diphantoin prescribed for epileptic women during pregnancy add to the risk of delivering a transgender child (Swaab & Garcia-Falgueras, 2009:21). "Both these substances change the metabolism of the sex hormones and can act on the sexual differentiation of the child's brain" (Swaab & Garcia-Falgueras, 2009:21). Early development is also the time during which sexual proclivities are resolved, under the sway of our genetic make-up as well as factors affecting the interplay between the developing brain and the sex hormones (Swaab & Garcia-Falgueras, 2009:22). Prenatal causes of homosexuality, heterosexuality, or bisexuality can be the result of the intake of chemicals like nicotine, amphetamines, or thyroid medication. An extremely interesting phenomenon, known as the fraternal birth order effect, links the possibility of a boy being homosexual to the number of older brothers he has, and is "… putatively explained by an immunological response by the mother to a product of the Y chromosomes of her sons" (Swaab & Garcia-Falgueras, 2009:23). Excessive stress during pregnancy has also been identified as a contributing factor in producing a child with homosexual tendencies.

Swaab and Garcia-Falgueras (2009:22) make the telling statement that

> [s]exual orientation in humans is also determined during early develop-
> ment, under the influence of our genetic background and factors that
> influence the interactions between the sex hormones and the developing
> brain. The apparent impossibility of getting someone to change their
> sexual orientation is a major argument against the importance of the social
> environment in the emergence of homosexuality, as well as against the
> idea that homosexuality is a life-style choice.

Homosexuality has had an enduring presence throughout known history, right up to the present, and the questions most often asked are if its presence could possibly confer an evolutionary advantage in a population, and if so, by what means, as persons with homosexual orientation do not procreate. It is, of course, untrue as many homosexual males marry and have children, perhaps in an attempt to conform to the accepted behaviour dictated by society, only later to revert to an exclusively same-sex lifestyle. According to Swaab and Gardia-Falgueras (2009:23), an acceptable solution would be to show that the genetic features controlling homosexuality also have a positive effect on procreation. Camperio-Ciani, Corna and Capiluppi (2004:2217) have found just that and reported that "female maternal relatives of homosexuals have higher fecundity than female maternal relatives of heterosexuals".

4.5.3 Embryology[1]

Western culture has long favoured the binary concept of recognising only two sexes. It reflects the view of legal systems and clearly, the public at large, as this particular mindset is continually bolstered by linguistic expressions in common use, such as right or wrong, left or right, black or white, us or them, and him or her. In the real world, however, human sexuality is vastly more complex and interesting. Fausto-Sterling (1993:21) points out that

> [...] if the state and legal system have an interest in maintaining a two-party
> sexual system, they are in defiance of nature. For biologically speaking,
> there are many gradations running from female to male; and depending
> on how one calls the shots, one can argue that along that spectrum lie at
> least five sexes – and perhaps even more.

However, in the past and especially during medieval times, the options were clear in that sexuality was unambiguously binary, and hermaphrodites who strayed from their chosen sex and attempted to straddle the fence, did so at their own peril. Fausto-Sterling (1993:23) notes that

---

1   For an in-depth discussion, see Jones and Van den Heever (2021).

> [i]n Europe a pattern emerged by the end of the Middle Ages that, in a sense, has lasted to the present day: hermaphrodites were compelled to choose an established gender role and stick with it. The penalty for transgression was often death. Thus, in the 1600s a Scottish hermaphrodite living as a woman was buried alive after penetrating his/her master's daughter.

In view of the complexity of human sexuality, as currently understood, the binary approach is outdated and wrong, as is shown by the differential intra-uterine development of genetic, physiological, neurological, and anatomical features, culminating in a diverse spectrum of at least fifteen possible sexual options, sequentially interspaced between heterosexual males and heterosexual females.

4.6   A PRECEDENT AND AN ALTERNATIVE

It would be unfair of us to explicitly criticise the legality of the position of WA regarding the sexuality and gender preferences of international athletes, without suggesting what may be a plausible alternative. In this respect, the Classification Code of the International Paralympic Committee (IPC) comes to mind. This administrative body regulates a multitude of athletes, exhibiting bodily differences pertaining to intellectual, genetic, physiological, and anatomical aspects. Whilst no strict parallels can be drawn between these two international groupings, it is telling that the IPC appears to continually communicate in a respectfully supportive and non-judgemental manner with their members and charges. There appears also to be no coercive attempts at influencing athletes in any way with regard to the rules for competitive endeavour. In contrast, the WA is, rightly or wrongly, perceived as a vacillating and irresolute administrative body that hides behind suspect legal manoeuvres that they regard as inviolate, whilst attempting to coerce athletes in lowering their testosterone levels by chemical intervention.

Instead, the IPC has consulted widely over the years, and continues to do so, thereby delivering an extensive and detailed classification system that acknowledge the physical constraints of a wide variety of athletes, thusly providing a platform enabling paralympic athletes to experience the thrill and satisfaction of competing against peers at the international level. The IPC Classification Code outlines ten primary impairment types, eight referring to physical impairments, and one each to visual and intellectual impairment. The categories are further refined to include a large number of subdivisions, tailored to best showcase the athletic abilities of specific categories of athletes. We would like to think that the achievements of the IPC are not beyond the abilities of WA, and while the circumstances are not identical, relying on the perceived legality of their position, WA is in an untenable position and should consider alternative solutions that obviates the indignities and discrimination experienced by athletes during legal confrontations, because the burden of proof lies not with athletes, like Semenya, but with WA.

Spectrum of human sexual characteristics

Condition	typical sex chromosomes	gonads (○ female / ● male)	hormones — oestrogens (female) / androgens (male)	phallus — penis / clitoris	urination	menstruation	fertility	psychological sex
normal female	XX	○ ○	normal F / normal F	clitoris, normal size	normal	normal	+	F
simple constitutional masculinism	XX	○ ○	increased for female / increased for female	normal size	F	irregular or nil	+ or −	F
adrenogenital masculinism	XX	○ ○	increased for female / increased for female	enlarged	F	nil	−	F
female homosexual	XX	○ ○	normal F / normal F	normal or enlarged	normal or irregular	normal or irregular	−	M or F
female transvestism	XX	○ ○	normal F / normal F	normal or enlarged	F	normal or irregular	−	neutral or M
female intersex without adrenal disorder	XX	○ ○	normal F / normal F	enlarged clitoris	F	usually nil	−	F or M
true hermaphrodite	XX	● ○	normal F or low / normal F or low	normal penis or enlarged clitoris	F	usually nil	−	F or M
Turner's syndrome	XO	(small)	low	normal size	F	nil	−	F
pure gonadal dysgenesis	XY	nil		normal or enlarged	F	nil	−	F
male intersex testicular feminization syndrome	XY	●	normal M / normal M	normal size	F	nil	−	F
Klinefelter's syndrome	XXY	small ●	normal M ± M / subnorm-subnorm at for M	small to moderate	M	nil	−	neutral or M
male transvestism	XY	●	normal M ± M / subnorm-normal at for M	small	M	−	− or +	neutral or F
male homosexual	XY	●	normal M / normal M	normal size	M	−	+	M, F or both
adrenogenital feminism	XY	●	probably subnorm at for M / increased at for M	normal size	M	−	+	M
simple constitutional feminism	XY	●	subnorm-normal at for M	small	M	+	−	M or rarely F
male with hypospadias	XY	●	normal M / normal M	small (may resemble enlarged clitoris)	F	−	+	M
normal male	XY	●	normal M / normal M	normal size	M	+	−	M

FIGURE 4.1 Table summarising the spectrum of human sexual characteristics (Jost, 1971:104-105)

To us, the existence of the Paralympics creates both a precedent and a way out. We are convinced that it would be morally judicious not to chemically intervene with the naturally expressed spectrum of human sexuality. The essential differences between men and women dictate that they should not compete against one another. Therefore, there is no demand to masculinise women or feminise men to allow equal competition against one another.

A possible way out of the conundrum would be for WA to create further competitive categories to, at least, accommodate the five sexes, advocated by Fausto-Sterling (1993:21). An anticipated objection in this regard would be that the possible paucity of competitors in certain items would not justify a separate competition. For us, the answer would be to include these athletes in international events of WA, in separate categories. After all, in the binary system the two designated categories do not compete against one another, so why would a quinary system, albeit more complex, be any different? If such an arrangement seems propitious, it might even be acceptable in the future to consider inviting the Paralympic Movement to compete as a separate category, under the same umbrella.

We are satisfied that we have, to all intents and purposes, stated the case from biology as best we could, and have demonstrated, through the hard biological evidence of selected researchers, that a problem exists. It is natural to expect that this discrepancy should be investigated further and addressed in a humane and ethical way.

4.7   CONCLUSION

The acrimony that has ensued around the question of gender in sport has serious moral implications for how we view ourselves. Anton van Niekerk (2020:8), commenting on the nature of morality, has noted that "[i]t is the universal acknowledgement that all our actions can and ought to be submitted to the set of expectations known as the demand of obligation". From this, it follows that our deeds and behaviour have implications and will be evaluated and judged by society. "Yet if biologists continue to show that sex is a spectrum, then society and state will have to grapple with the consequences and work out where and how to draw the line. Many transgender and intersex activists dream of a world where a person's sex or gender is irrelevant" (Ainsworth, 2015:291).

Above all, to attempt legislation in the absence of necessary and relevant data on a subject as important as human sexuality, whilst the pertinent details have been available in the public domain for years, is tantamount to the worst kind of discrimination thinkable. Parallels in this regard would be the ludicrous defence of the legality of the apartheid laws, with the consent of both State and Church, all the while pointedly ignoring extensive and freely available biological data to the contrary. A more recent parallel is the unconscionable attitude of religious bodies, specifically, the Dutch Reformed Church in South Africa, pointedly denying the biological reality of human sexuality in favour of religious texts that were written and compiled by individuals who were totally ignorant of the psychological, physiological, anatomical, and genetic complexities of the human condition.

In this instance, the IAAF is guilty on at least two counts. Firstly, aiding and abetting an outdated and provably false conception of human sexuality and secondly, persisting to defend this interpretation whilst failing to implement necessary and humane changes, reflecting our biological heritage, abundantly supported by published data based on embryological, anatomical, physiological, and neurological research which unanimously attest to the physical reality of the human condition. With reference to the latest insights about sex and gender in general, Ainsworth (2015:288) notes that "[t]hese discoveries do not sit well in a world in which sex is still defined in binary terms. Few legal systems still allow for any ambiguity in biological sex, and a person's legal rights and social status can be heavily influenced by whether their birth certificate says male or female". We are not encouraging WA to comply with our suggestions, but merely stating that human inventiveness, sense of fairness, and originality has overcome many obstacles in the past. We are suggesting that the present attitude and declarations of WA are indeed suspect, and in our view, short-sighted and wrong. It is also true that competitions like the Paralympics exist to show that there are alternative decisions that can be made. The onus is on WA to, instead of continuing a controversial and decidedly wrong path, find alternative means to allow competition honestly and openly in the international world of sports.

Finally, we wish to underscore our initial statement that humans are in every respect biological entities, as is every other life form on the planet, and to plumb the depths of the human experience in all of its manifestations, all we have is the human body. We are our bodies and can only experience the world through our bodies. Our sexuality and gender are expressed within an extensive spectrum generated by the physical realities of our biology and should not be subservient to the inadequacies and ethereal misconceptions of social reality.

Bibliography

Ainsworth, C. 2015. Sex redefined. *Nature*, 518:288-291. https://doi.org/10.1038/518288a

Alesina, A., Guiliano, P. & Nunn, N. 2013. On the origins of gender roles: women and the plough. *The Quarterly Journal of Economics*, 128(2):469-530. https://doi.org/10.1093/qje/qjt005

Alexander, G.M. 2014. Postnatal testosterone concentrations and male social development. *Pediatric Endocrinology*, 5:1-6. https://doi.org/10.3389/fendo.2014.00015

Barrett, L.F. 2020. *Seven and a half lessons about the brain*. London: Picador.

Camperio-Ciani, A., Corna, F. & Capiluppi, C. 2004. Evidence for maternally inherited factors favouring male homosexuality and promoting female fecundity. *Proceedings of the Royal Society B*, 271(1554):2217-2221. https://doi.org/10.1098/rspb.2004.2872

Cornelius, I. 2022. Personal communication. 14 April, Stellenbosch. (Professor at the Department of Ancient Studies, Stellenbosch University).

Dever, W.G. 2005. *Did God have a wife: archaeology and folk religion in ancient Israel*. Grand Rapids, MI: William B. Eerdmans.

Dyble, M., Salali, G.D., Chaudhari, N., Page, A., Smith, D., Thompson, J., Vinicius, L., Mace, R. & Migliano, R.B. 2015. Sex equality can explain the unique social structure of hunter-gatherer bands. *Science*, 348(6236):796-798. https://doi.org/10.1126/science.aaa5139

Fausto-Sterling, A. 1993. The five sexes. *The Sciences*. New York Academy of Sciences, March/April. 20-25. https://doi.org/10.1002/j.2326-1951.1993.tb03081.x

Hargreaves, J.A. 1994. *Sporting females: critical issues in the history and sociology of women's sport*. London: Routledge.

Jones, C. & Van den Heever, J. 2021. Building blocks of sexuality. *HTS Teologiese Studies / Theological Studies*, 77(3):a6569. https://doi.org/10.4102/hts.v77i3.6569

Jost, A.D. 1971. Development of sexual characteristics. In: Human reproduction. *The Science Journal, Special Issue*. London: Paladin. 94-108.

Krech, M. 2019. The misplaced burdens of "gender equality" in *Caster Semenya v IAAF*: The Court of Arbitration for Sport attempts human rights adjudication. *International Sports Law Review*, 3:66-76.

Lewis, S.L. & Maslin, M.A. 2018. *The human planet: how we created the anthropocene*. London: Pelican Books. https://doi.org/10.2307/j.ctv2c3k261

Meier, H.E., Konjer, M.V. & Krieger, J. 2021. Women in international elite athletics: gender (in)equality and national participation. *Frontiers in Sports and Active Living*, 3:1-20. https://doi.org/10.3389/fspor.2021.709640

Netwerk24. 2021. 6 Lande in Midde-Ooste verbied Spielberg se 'West Side Story'. 8 December:n.p. https://bit.ly/3iPawfF

Römer, T. 2015. *The invention of God*. Cambridge, MA: Harvard University Press. https://doi.org/10.4159/9780674915732

Swaab, D.F. & Garcia-Falgueras, A. 2009. Sexual differentiation of the human brain in relation to gender identity and sexual orientation. *Functional Neurology*, 24(1):17-28.

Theberge, N. 2000, Gender and sport. In: J. Coakley & E. Dunning. *Handbook of Sport Studies*. London: Sage. 322-333. https://doi.org/10.4135/9781848608382.n20

Van Niekerk, A.A. 2020. Building the future in the 21st century: in conversation with Yuval Noah Harari. *HTS Teologiese Studies/ Theological Studies*, 76(1):a6058. https://doi.org/10.4102/hts.v76i1.6058

5

Ethics of Transplantation

Willie Koen

Keywords: artificial mechanical circulation; cadaver organ transplantation; Hippocratic oath; ethical challenges; lifesaving and non-lifesaving organ transplantation; living donor organ transplantation; stem cell transplantation; transplant waiting list; Xeno transplantation

5.1   INTRODUCTION AND GENERAL CONCEPTS IN TRANSPLANTATION

The first recorded attempt of human organ transplantation in 1934 opened a new chapter in the field of ethics. Transplantation is regarded as a medical procedure where the aim is, primarily, to improve the quality of human life and, secondarily, to improve the long-term outcome of the patient. The donor organ can be harvested either from a brain-dead human, also referred to as cadaver donor organs, or from a live human such as a family member, referred to as living related donor organs. In the case of cadaver organs, the donor organs can be harvested from a brain-dead, beating-heart donor or a non-beating-heart donor. Where a donor organ is harvested from a living donor, the donor can be either related or unrelated to the recipient.

Organs for transplantation can further be divided into solid organs such as heart, lungs, kidney, and liver, or non-solid organs such as bone marrow, corneas, or bone.

Lifesaving organ transplants include heart, lung, or liver transplants where a patient will not only have an improved quality of life but will also have the additional benefit of increased life expectancy. In non-lifesaving organ transplantation such as limb, face, uterus, and penis transplants, the patient can only expect an improvement in quality of life.

The main obstacle of successful human transplantation is donor organ rejection by the recipient. This is a phenomenon where the immune system of the recipient identifies the donor tissue as foreign and launches an immune response in an effort to remove this foreign tissue from the body. This is a similar response that the body will have to unwanted bacteria, viruses, or foreign bodies. This response eventually leads to the cessation of function of the transplanted organ. To counter this immune response, all transplantations require some form of suppression of the immune system. This is done by immunosuppressing medication, also referred to as anti-rejection medication. In the early days of transplantation, the main immunosuppressing medication was cortisone and the outcomes in, for instance, heart transplants, resulted in a one-year survival of hardly 30%. In 1984, a novel medication belonging to the group of calcineurin-inhibitors, namely cyclosporine, was discovered. This anti-rejection agent revolutionised the outcomes of organ transplantation and one-year survival rates of more than 90% have been seen since. Unfortunately, all anti-rejection medication has side effects, either due to direct toxicity or indirectly due to the long-term suppression of the immune system. This direct toxicity of these agents has a damaging effect on other organs, especially the kidneys. In contrast, the indirect complications of anti-rejection medication involve the suppression of the immune system, which prevents the immune system from functioning at its full capacity and leads to the inability to fight bacteria and viruses which eventually leads to infection. Furthermore, an important function of the immune system is to identify abnormal cells in the body such as rapid duplicating cells, more commonly referred to as cancer cells. As a result, anti-rejection medication can indirectly lead to cancer in the transplanted patient. For instance, in cardiac transplantation, malignancy and infections are the cause of 40% of the mortality by ten years after the transplant.

Therefore, finding a balance between under- and over-suppression of the immune system is a critical challenge in the management of the transplanted patient. As a result, these facts lead to a key question in transplantation: do the risks of the transplant with its subsequent complications, especially due to the immuno-suppressing agents, outweigh the risk of not performing the transplant?

5.2   CADAVER ORGAN TRANSPLANTATION

Before organs from a cadaver can be harvested from a deceased person, either in the case of a beating-heart or non-beating-heart situation, the necessary consent should be obtained from the donor (Groth, 1972). As the donor has ceased to exist as a person, the last wish of the donor should be considered. This wish of the donor could have been recorded at some stage in a legal document such as a will and, if not, the next of kin can give consent to proceed with the organ dona-tion process (Siminoff, Agyemang & Traino, 2013).

Due to factors such as the stability of the donor, the timeframe to harvest these organs is limited to hours. Therefore, waiting until the legal will of the patient is read and executed is not a practical option. For this reason, family consent is the norm in most transplanting countries, including South Africa. This is referred to as the "opt-in" system. Alternatively, with the "opt-out" system that is utilised in certain countries such as Spain, all citizens are regarded as organ donors unless there is an objection from the donor, for instance by a legal will of the donor. As many potential donors are lost due to failure to obtain consent, either due to difficulty in locating the family or due to a bereaved and traumatised family that cannot make a decision in this critical instance, the "opt-out" system leads to a higher donor organ yield. However, in countries such as South Africa, where there is a population with diversity in religion, cultures, and traditional beliefs, the "opt-out" system can, arguably, not be implemented, as it cannot be assumed that the general bias of the population is towards organ donation (Editorial, 2017).

In beating-heart organ donors, the donor is still in full physiological function but is brain dead. Brain death can be defined as irreversible brain damage with the loss of all brain stem activity and therefore voluntary or involuntary functions (Sarbey, 2016). This means that the patient is unable to breathe spontaneously (apnoea). For this reason, the donor is connected to a ventilator to maintain respiratory function, which is to supply oxygen to the blood. In the absence of oxygen in the circulation, also referred to as ischaemia, all organs will stop functioning over a period of minutes. For organs to be used in transplantation, these organs should be fully functional and undamaged, especially from ischaemia. In the case of non-beating-heart donors, the heart has already stopped, and organs are then harvested (Ridley et al., 2005). This situation occurs when the patient was unstable and cardiac function could not be maintained. This period where the heart has stopped has to be short as the absence of blood circulation will lead to organ ischaemia.

As the heart has the highest oxygen extraction rate of all organs in the donor, ischaemia will set in first in the heart and damage to the heart muscle starts seconds after the heart has stopped. Adding the time of the explanation proce-dure to this, which takes around an hour, the heart will sustain significant ischaemic damage. To overcome this delay, the patient can be connected to an extra-corporeal oxygenation mechanical circulation to minimise organ ischaemia.

Nevertheless, in cardiac transplantation, a non-beating-heart donor is a sub-optimal option and the outcomes of the transplant will be significantly compromised.

In contrast, in renal transplantation, the kidney can tolerate a short period of ischaemia better, although it is arguably still not an ideal situation. However, due to the shortage of organ donors, non-beating-heart donor organs are considered in many renal transplant centres around the world in special cases as an attempt to increase the donor organ pool. The dilemma faced by the renal transplant team is to weigh the risk of a non-beating-heart kidney against not performing the procedure at all. This is a debatable situation as the renal patient can still be maintained on a renal dialysis machine which serves as an artificial kidney and can maintain the patient. However, this dilemma can then be further complicated as there are only limited dialysis slots available due to the limited number of dialysis machines. It can therefore be argued that a patient who receives a kidney transplant will at least make a dialysis slot available for another patient in end-stage renal failure. Another consideration in non-beating-heart donation questions the absence of mechanical circulation oxygenation. In this situation, the absence of supporting the circulation of the non-beating-heart patient results in the ethics of the situation being challenged, because it is argued that the patient can still be neurologically not brain dead as brain dead testing requires a repeat evaluation 12 hours after the initial testing to confirm brain death (Mohamed, Verheijde & McGregor, 2007).

TABLE 5.1 Modified Maastricht classification of non-beating-heart donors (Kootstra et al., 1995)

Category I	Dead on arrival
Category II	Unsuccessful resuscitation
Category III	Awaiting cardiac arrest
Category IV	Cardiac arrest in a brainstem-dead donor
Category V	Unexpected cardiac arrest in a critically ill patient

5.3   LIVING DONOR ORGAN TRANSPLANTATION

In living donor organ transplantation, the organs are harvested from a live donor as opposed to cadaver organs as described earlier. For instance, as a patient has two kidneys and can function normally with one kidney, the other kidney can therefore be donated. However, in heart, liver, and lung transplantation, living donors cannot be used for obvious reasons. Nevertheless, part of an organ such as a lobe of the lung or liver can be donated (Broelsch, Testa, Alexandrou & Malagó, 2002).

As this is not the full organ, this portion or lobe will usually not be sufficient for an adult recipient and can be used, for instance, in a child or a very small adult.

The ethical dilemma lies in the relationship between the live donor and the recipient. In the case where there is a direct family relation or genetic relation, the motive for the donation of the organ by the donor can be assumed as benevolent. However, in the case where there is no family relation, benevolence cannot be assumed (De Groot, Van Hoek & Hoedemaekers, 2015).

This opens the discussion for donation of organs for compensation. Opponents of organs for compensation will argue that it can lead to exploitation of the poor and those in desperate need of money. Furthermore, organ trafficking is a reality where the donor is exploited to the advantage of the trafficker and the recipient. Even the donation of organs between wife and husband can later lead to a contentious situation after, for example, a divorce. However, proponents of organs for compensation will argue that it is not uncommon for employees to sacrifice their health for compensation, for example mine workers who are exposed to dust inhalation and subsequent pulmonary disease (Dalal, 2015).

5.4   ALLOCATION OF CADAVER ORGANS IN TRANSPLANTATION

When a potential donor is identified in a health facility, the donor organ procurement team is contacted. In South Africa, there is a network of organ donor coordinators in the five major cities of the country. The donor coordinator then liaises with the referring facility and gets the status of the donor. This includes the cause of brain death, confirmation that the necessary brain death testing has been carried out, as well as the donor's clinical status, weight, and blood group.

The coordinator usually obtains informed consent from the family. Once it has been confirmed that the patient fulfils the criteria to be a donor, the coordinator contacts the relevant organ transplant programmes. Each organ transplant fraternity has their own allocation system in South Africa. In the United States and Europe, there is a central organ registry that allocates organs. This means that the donor coordinator refers the donor organs to the central organ registry and on acceptance will allocate the organs to a recipient according to a protocol. The demographics, size of the country, and population distributions vary in different parts of the world and therefore different protocols are used. The type of organ referred is also allocated according to the protocol for that specific organ.

In South Africa, the vast differences and limited transplant programmes make the use of a single centralised organ allocation initiative unpractical. Each discipline, namely the cardiac, lung, and renal programmes, has their own collaborative allocation protocol which has been decided by each discipline. For instance, if a donor becomes available in a city, the heart will first be offered to the centre that procured the organ. The transplant surgeon can accept the heart unless there is an urgent priority listing at another centre. The priority listing is shared by all cardiac programmes and is updated weekly. Should the transplant surgeon not be able to use the heart for reasons such as a blood group mismatch or size mismatch, the organ will then be referred to the next programme in that city. Should this programme also not be able to use the organ, the organ will be referred to a programme in another province. As explanted organs have a limited safe timeframe before it has to be implanted, it makes sense that organs must be referred to local centres first. However, in the situation where there is a recipient on the urgent priority waiting list, the risk of the longer distance harvest will be considered and weighed against the urgency of the patient. Therefore, in organ allocation, the key consideration of risk of transplantation versus not doing the transplant comes to the fore again. This can lead to the dilemma of comparing the status of two urgently listed patients from different centres. In such a case, the surgeons of the respective programmes will contact each other and discuss the urgency of their listed patients to come to a mutual decision.

5.5   TRANSPLANT WAITING LIST

Age cut-off policies have been an ethical issue for decades in the transplant community. The argument is that in contrast to younger patients, older patients might have more risk factors for a transplant, have already enjoyed years of living, and are usually no longer the breadwinners. Furthermore, due to the shortage of donor organs, the bias is towards younger patients. For these reasons, the age cut-off for heart transplant recipients in North America and Europe is 60 years. However, in South Africa, due to the relatively smaller transplant programmes, a situation often arises that a donor heart cannot be used for various reasons among all the programmes. In this instance, the donor organ is sadly wasted. Also, as South Africa is the only country on the continent doing heart transplants, such a donor heart cannot be shipped to a neighbouring transplant country as is the case in Europe. To send the donor heart to, for instance, Europe is also not an option as the time frame of the donor heart outside the body is limited to four hours. For this reason, the age cut-off for heart recipients in South Africa is 65 years with the understanding by the recipient that younger patients could be considered first.

When a patient is confirmed to be a suitable recipient candidate, the next step is to add the patient to a waiting list. An important consideration is to establish the urgency of the need for the transplant and therefore a timing for the procedure can be envisaged. This is usually a 'wait-and-see' approach as patients can either deteriorate more rapidly than expected or even improve due to optimisation of the medication. For this reason, the patient on the waiting list must be assessed frequently to establish the clinical progression of the condition. In cardiac transplantation, this is a challenge as the progression of the underlying heart failure is temperamental.

With regard to considering when to put a patient on the waiting list, the fact that it can take up to one year for a suitable donor heart to become available must be considered. Centres often have an 'active' waiting list and a 'cold' list. Patients on the active waiting list are regarded to have a high mortality of 80% over the next year unless a transplant is performed. Should the joint view be that a patient has a stable condition with poor heart function but is still coping and should not have very high mortality in the next 12 months, then the patient will be placed on the cold list. When a donor heart becomes available, only patients on the active waiting list will be considered. However, should a patient's condition on the cold list deteriorate, then the patient can be moved onto the active waiting list.

To allocate a donor heart to a patient on the active waiting list requires some consideration. The blood group is the first consideration as this should be compatible. This is referred to as ABO-compatibility and represents the different classes of blood groups. The patients on the list that match the blood group will be considered. This sub-group will then be further assessed by using weight and size. It is important to use a donor heart of similar size to optimise the outcome. This will therefore eliminate more patients in the sub-group. From here, the remaining candidates will be considered according to the criticality of their conditions. The more critical patients will be considered. Should the patients be of the same clinical status, other factors such as the period on the waiting list, age, and social status of the patient and distance of harvesting will be considered. Therefore, contrary to common understanding, the patient who has been on the waiting list the longest is not necessarily the next candidate to receive the next donor heart. Unfortunately, this prioritisation of recipients can open an opportunity for manipulation and foul play (Connolly, 2013).

5.6   ARTIFICIAL MECHANICAL CIRCULATION

The search for a mechanical solution for end-stage cardiac failure started before the era of heart transplantation. However, since the first heart transplant, the majority of research continued in transplantation rather than finding a mechanical solution. Nevertheless, the rapid advances in technology have led to major progress in mechanical cardiac support. This research was also encouraged by the realisation that donor organ supply will always be a limiting factor and waiting periods for donor organs are a major disadvantage. This vision of having mechanical devices readily available on demand, as well as a gradual improvement in clinical outcomes, has developed to a point where mechanical heart implantation has the same two-year outcome as a human heart transplant.

The additional advantage of the mechanical device is that it can stabilise the recipient in desperate need of a heart and that the recipient can now safely wait for a donor heart. These devices are implanted into the heart but is still connected to an external battery-control system. This external hardware is a limitation to the patient as it needs daily charging. But, because these devices are made from biological inert material, rejection, which is encountered in organ transplantation, is not an obstacle and no anti-rejection medication is needed. These devices can support patients over several years and outcomes of over 10 years are often seen. Currently, the main indication for a mechanical heart device is a patient who is on the heart transplant waiting list and deteriorating, with the availability of an urgent donor heart not envisaged. Other indications would be other reasons for not qualifying for an organ transplant such as age cut-off or antibodies.

Once the patient has received a mechanical device, the patient can remain on the transplant waiting list. The dilemma then becomes whether the patient should have a lower priority for transplantation as the patient is now in a better clinical situation, or whether the priority should remain the same. As discussed earlier, the primary consideration to allocate a donor heart to the sickest patient can result in the patient who is now more stable on the mechanical device to face a much longer time waiting for a donor heart.

Arguably, a donor transplant is still the gold standard and mechanical devices do have complications of their own. Therefore, waiting to the point where complications set in as a result of the mechanical device can lead to the same initial dilemma of needing an urgent organ. It is therefore paramount that the patient on the mechanical device is frequently monitored to ascertain at which point the patient should be put back onto the active heart transplant waiting list, thereby having the same priority as other waiting recipients.

Another dilemma is that a mechanical heart could have been inserted into a patient where the patient was still within the age cut-off point. Should the patient have this device in for several years, it could take the patient over the cut-off age for transplantation, therefore the patient might not qualify according to the accepted age definition for a heart transplant. In these cases, the clinical status of the patient should be assessed, and should the patient still be eligible for an organ transplant, except for the age limit, most programmes will accept the patient onto the active waiting list regardless of age.

Another aspect of these devices is that a device can be implanted as a "bridge-to-transplant", meaning that it is a temporary strategy with transplantation as the end goal. The concept "destination therapy" refers to the strategy where a device is implanted but a later transplant is not planned.

A further dilemma is the cost of these devices. These devices are expensive, similar to that of a luxury motor vehicle. Being readily available and not governed like organ transplantation by the shortage of donor organs, many of these devices can be potentially implanted and can be a massive burden on a national health budget. For this reason, many countries, such as the United Kingdom, do not allow funding for mechanical devices as destination therapy unless it is privately funded. In such cases, it can be argued that destination therapy is only available to the wealthier society.

5.7   STEM CELL TRANSPLANTATION

The successful treatment of using human stem cells (hSC) is well recognised. Especially in bone marrow conditions and cancer treatment like leukaemia, this has proven a successful treatment modality (Chu et al., 2020). As stem cells have the potential to differentiate into other cell lines such as neural tissue, myocardial cells, or blood cells, the potential to use stem cell therapy in conditions such as heart failure, Parkinson's disease, and diabetes has been researched (Hwang, Varghese & Elisseeff, 2008).

Stem cells can be obtained from the person itself who requires the treatment and is referred to as autologous adult stem cell transplantation. In the case where stem cells are used from a different person, this is referred to as allogenic stem cell transplantation. Adult stem cells and stem cells from umbilical cord blood are multipotent cells, meaning they have the potential to differentiate, with the necessary manipulation, into other stem cell lines such as neural tissue or myocardial tissue. The practical principle of this treatment modality is to inject these cells into damaged areas such as the heart and allow the stem cells to differentiate into myocardial tissue and thereby repair the damaged areas (Gratwohl, Pasquini & Aljurf, 2015).

This strategy is still in an experimental stage and gives hope that eventually damaged organs can be repaired rather than transplanting the entire organ. However, there are also concerns with such treatment, for instance the risk that the stem cells might not differentiate into the desired tissue or can even lead to excessive differentiation which can lead to tumours (Kanagasundram & Amini, 2018). However, obtaining these adult cells is a relatively easier process than other forms of obtaining stem cells.

Stem cells can also be obtained from embryos, referred to as human embryo stem cell transplantation (hESC). However, this strategy is fraught with ethical issues. In contrast to adult stem cells, these cells have a better potential to differentiate into the desired tissue line. With hESC, the stem cells are obtained from the early stage of an embryo. After the fertilisation of the oocyte, the cells duplicate to form an early embryo also known at this stage as a blastocyst which usually contains five to six cells. It is from this stage onwards that the main lines of human tissue develop. This process can be done as an in vitro process in a laboratory (Vazin & Freed, 2010). Nevertheless, it still requires a human oocyte which has to be donated by the female human. It is at this point where the ethical dilemmas in hESC transplantation come to the fore.

The first argument is that an embryo is an early human being and therefore human life is sacrificed. The debate continues – at which stage does an embryo become a person? This debate has been going on for decades as there is strong public support that once an oocyte is fertilised, human life has begun. This view has been challenged by the fact that these cells often do not continue to grow, can form into multiple cells (in the case of twins), and cannot be defined as a person at that early point. The debate goes on (Assen, Jongsma, Isasi, Tryfonidou & Bredenoord, 2021).

The irony in many of these debates is the fact that it overlooks the situation where a large percentage of females in the world are using oral contraceptives for birth control. These contraceptives have different mechanisms of action, whereby one such action prevents the fertilised oocyte from attaching to the inside of the uterus (endometrium) and therefore preventing a pregnancy. The human oocyte is therefore also sacrificed (Rivera, Yacobson & Grimes, 1999). Therefore, the view of "sacrifice life to save life" is still a contentious debate in the world of hESC research.

A further ethical problem involves informed consent for the donation of tissue for stem cell research. As there is a wide difference in opinion of members of the public on stem cell research, it cannot be assumed that all members of the public agree on all the modes of stem cell research. For instance, a person might agree on research for cancer treatment but might not necessarily agree on aspects such as financial gain from this research. These aspects should be included in the informed consent given by the donor (Caulfield, Ogbogu & Isasi, 2007). A further dilemma is confidentiality in stem cell donation. Donors have the right to confidentiality of personal information which could be used in later discrimination towards donors by anti-stem cell activists (Snyder & Loring, 2006).

Another strategy in stem cell research is the reprogramming of the oocyte (egg cell) by transplanting the genetic DNA from the nucleus of a donor cell into the recipient oocyte. As a result, an embryo with a different genetic code can develop. This process is referred to as somatic cell nuclear transfer (SCNT). This has been successful and had wide media coverage when Dolly the sheep was cloned in 1996 (Campbell, McWhir, Richie & Wilmut, 1996). In 2013, the first human embryonic stem cells derived by somatic cell nuclear transfer were described (Tachibana et al., 2013). This reprogrammed oocyte can then be transferred back into a surrogate and allowed to develop to maturity. An application of this strategy could be used to produce animals such as pigs with a gene code of which organs can be used to be transplanted into humans.

It is evident that there are many ethical dilemmas to be considered in SCNT. One such dilemma could be to ask to what extent can the oocyte be reprogrammed and what would be the purpose of the end creature that is developed. This could for instance lead to the development of an embryo and subsequently a mature animal with two sets of DNA also known as a chimera. This process of chimerism is well established and already in clinical use in human stem cell treatment in bone marrow transplantation. This is a process where the diseased bone marrow of a patient is replaced by donor bone marrow to produce blood cells. After the transplant, the patient with their DNA will have circulating blood cells with a different DNA (Bader, Niethammer & Willasch, 2005). The ethical dilemma comes when the chimerism is between two different species and the possibility to create a 'half man, half beast'. This is referred to as interspecies chimerism. Although the motive behind this form of chimerism is intended for medical treatment, such as producing organs or body parts for humans to be grown from animals, the fear of abuse of this science cannot be overlooked.

5.8   XENO TRANSPLANTATION

Cross-species organ transplantation is referred to as Xeno transplantation. The idea of using animal organs to improve the lives of humans has already been described in 1667 when French physician, Jean-Baptiste Denis, transfused 12 ounces of blood from a lamb into a feverish young man (*Encyclopaedia Britannica*, n.d.). In the 1960s, Keith Reemtsma implanted 13 human patients with chimpanzee kidneys (Reentsma et al., 1964). During the same period, James

Hardy implanted the first chimpanzee heart into a human. The organ failed after a few hours (Hardy et al., 1964).

In 1977, Christiaan Barnard implanted two animal hearts into two patients. The first was a baboon heart which failed some hours after the implant and the second was a chimpanzee heart which was implanted as a heterotopic transplant. The patient died after four days as the patient's own heart did not recover (Barnard, Wolpowitz & Losman, 1977; Brink & Hassoulas, 2009).

The reason why xenografts fail and have not yet become a recognised source for human transplantation is that the animal organ excites a strong immune response in the human against this foreign tissue and leads to acute rejection. The current anti-rejection strategies and medication used in human-to-human transplantation are not effective to ensure a viable transplanted xenograft.

In 2022, the first pig-to-human heart transplant using a heart from a genetically modified pig was performed. At the time of writing, the patient was still doing well after the surgery (Reardon, 2022).

As the main limitation in the field of transplantation is the shortage of donor organs, this latest breakthrough in Xeno transplantation has given this field new hope as a future option in organ supply. However, this latest strategy to use genetically modified animal organs will have to prove itself against existing modalities such as human organ transplant and readily available mechanical heart options. The current outcome of a human/mechanical heart has a one-year survival of more than 90% and a two-year survival of 85%. The question is whether genetically modified animal organs will ensure similar results. It would be ethically difficult to implant a patient if these other two methods are available in the absence of long-term results of xenografts. Until it has proved itself, genetically modified xenografts can only be used when the other two options are not available or contra-indicated.

As far as animal rights and ethics in the use of animals as organ donors are concerned, the two main groups of animals considered for Xeno transplantation are the non-human primates such as chimpanzees, gorillas and baboons and large non-primates such as pigs. In the first group, the concern is that these animals have a closeness to humans and more developed feelings. They breed slowly and err on the brink of extinction and are not sacrificed for human consumption but rather conserved. In the latter group, these animals are too distant to evoke the same feelings and can breed rapidly. Currently, pigs are the most consumed large animal in the world. It can be expected that fewer ethical dilemmas will arise in using the latter group as a source of donor organs. As the field of Xeno transplantation was to date purely a field of research, recent breakthroughs will elicit the need for interfraternal discussions and the publication of guidelines to address these challenges.

5.9   NON-LIFESAVING ORGAN TRANSPLANTATION

When organs are transplanted to improve the quality of life rather than saving the life of the patient, it is generally referred to as non-lifesaving transplantation. This form of transplantation includes limb, face, penis, and uterus transplantation. As mentioned earlier in this chapter, all forms of transplants are subjected to the process of immunorejection and will require anti-rejection medication to ensure a viable implant. However, these drugs come with their own complications such as renal toxicity, hepatic toxicity, and neuro toxicity. It also has secondary complications due to the suppressed immune response and predisposes the patient to infections and malignancies. The primary consideration in all forms of transplants holds here too, namely: the risk of the procedure vs the benefit.

5.9.1   Penile transplantation

The first penis transplant was reported in 2006 but the procedure was reversed only fourteen days after the transplant (Hu et al., 2006). In 2015, Andre van der Merwe performed the world's first successful penis transplant in Tygerberg Hospital, Cape Town, South Africa. The patient had a speedy recovery and could have sexual intercourse after three months. No major complications were reported in the first 24 months other than reversible anti-rejection agent induced renal impairment (Van der Merwe et al., 2017).

As the indication for penile transplantation is not necessarily lifesaving, many debates have followed since the first procedure. The risks of a long-protracted operation which can include septicaemia and even death have been raised in addition to the side effects of anti-rejection medication which include renal failure, sepsis, and malignancies. However, the protagonists point out that the absence of a penis not only increases the risk of urinary tract infections but may also have psychological impacts on a person. This could lead to lifelong psychological trauma and even suicide. In certain cultures, such as traditional Chinese thinking, the penis is seen as the 'life-spring' essential to carrying on the ancestral line. The following guiding principles have been suggested by Zhang, Zhai and Hu (2010):

1.   Penile transplantation should be performed only in patients with severe damage to the penis.

2. Penile transplantation should be done in appropriate institutions under the protocols approved by institutional review boards.

3. Institutions should have surgical and transplantation expertise, and transplantation teams should include multidisciplinary experts such as plastic surgeons, immunology/transplant specialists, infectious disease and oncology specialists, medicolegal experts, physical therapists, pharmacology specialists, patient advocates, and media relations representatives.

4. Appropriate selection criteria should be established, and the risk/benefit ratio must be considered for each individual patient.

5. Patients and their families should be presented with special informed consent documents explaining the risks, benefits, alternatives, and innovative nature of the procedure.

6. Candidates for penile transplantation should undergo a thorough psychiatric and psychological evaluation, including evaluation of their psychosocial support system.

7. Patients with known psychological and psychiatric diagnoses, poor coping skills, poor support systems, or a history of noncompliance are poor candidates for penile transplantation.

8. Due to the novelty of the procedure, proceeding in incremental steps and gathering more evidence from research done in the field are necessary to ensure its appropriate application.

9. Peer review of the penile transplantation procedure is mandatory to ensure compliance with medical standards of care and objective assessments of the outcomes.

10. The ethics of performing a new procedure with unknown outcomes must be carefully assessed and weighed against potential benefits to the selected group of patients with severe penile damage following the evaluation of such candidates for penile transplantation by medical ethics specialists.

Therefore, the ethical consideration in penile transplantation will be again the basic question: is the benefit worth the risk? From the considerations mentioned above, it is clear that the importance of a penis can be viewed by the individual differently. This difference in views will depend on the age of the patient, culture, and also the joint view of not only the patient but also the partner. It will be important to view each case individually rather than having a dogmatic approach. A multidisciplinary panel approach is key in the consideration of this treatment.

5.9.2 Facial transplantation

In 2005, the first partial face transplant was reported in France on a 39-year-old woman whose face was mauled by a dog. Her nose, lips and chin were transplanted from a cadaver donor, and she required anti-rejection medication (Rifkin et al., 2018). Her face was reported to have been rejected ten years later. She died a year later from cancer which was reported as a complication from anti-rejection therapy (Jouan, 2016). Since this initial ground-breaking procedure, many more facial transplants which also included full-facial transplants were performed. The ethical dilemma in this case boils down to the question if the face transplant was worth the nine years of survival just to die at the age of 49. This was nine years of intense immune therapy, a high-cost burden with a relative improvement in facial appearance. During this period, she could not bear children as it is contra-indicated in patients on anti-rejection therapy, required to frequently attend the transplant clinic which entails numerous blood tests and investigations. One can also ask if other options such as reconstructive surgery was not an alternative?

Nevertheless, a patient still possesses autonomy in decision-making but with the proviso that the patient was fully informed of the outcomes before giving consent to such therapy. Also, how much weight can be placed on a patient's ability to make decisions in a traumatised psychological state and the role of the health care worker with the professional foreknowledge which can assist her decision at the time.

5.9.3 Uterus transplantation

Another form of non-lifesaving transplantation is the transplantation of a uterus for the purpose to bear a child. The main indications include an absent uterus, or malformed or diseased uteri. The first successful transplant of a uterus to bear a healthy child was reported in 2014 (Akouri, Maalouf & Abboud, 2020).

In 2021, it was reported that since the first successful implant, 45 uterus transplants have been performed worldwide with nine live births (Jones, Saso & Bracewell-Milnes, 2019). Other options for acquiring motherhood include surrogacy and adoption. Ethical questions that have been raised include, for instance in the UK, the number of children put up for adoption is increasing in contrast to the decreasing number of adoptions (Department for Education England, 2019). Surrogacy is well established, and thousands of children have been brought into life with this strategy (Perkins, Boulet, Jamieson & Kissin, 2016). Uterus transplantation can also be extended to transgender individuals or even men which will allow them to bear children. In the case of uterus transplantation into men or transgender women, new concepts of being a 'mother' or 'father' will need to be defined (O'Donovan, Williams & Wilkinson, 2019).

As the uterus transplant is a temporary undertaking, anti-rejection agents with known long-term complications such as renal failure and malignancies become less contentious as the anti-rejection medication is a temporary requirement.

5.10 CONCLUSION

The field of transplantation is fraught with ethical challenges. However, these challenges can be addressed and overcome by using the fundamental question of "risk versus benefit". Furthermore, the first part of the Hippocratic oath of the medical profession still forms the basis of any medical intervention namely, "do no harm". Doctors are brought up to always consider the four main principles of medical ethics: *respect for autonomy*, *beneficence*, *non-maleficence*, and *justice*.

Bibliography

Akouri, R., Maalouf, G. & Abboud, J. 2020. First live birth after uterus transplantation in the Middle East. *Middle East Fertility Society Journal*, 25:a30. https://doi.org/10.1186/s43043-020-00041-4

Assen, L.S., Jongsma, K.R., Isasi, R., Tryfonidou, M.A. & Bredenoord, A.L. 2021. Recognizing the ethical implications of stem cell research: a call for broadening the scope. *Stem Cell Reports*, 16(7): 1656-1661. https://doi.org/10.1016/j.stemcr.2021.05.021

Bader, P., Niethammer, D. & Willasch, A. 2005. How and when should we monitor chimerism after allogeneic stem cell transplantation? *Bone Marrow Transplant*, 35:107-119. https://doi.org/10.1038/sj.bmt.1704715

Barnard, C.N., Wolpowitz, A. & Losman, J.G. 1977. Heterotopic cardiac transplantation with a xenograft for assistance of the left heart in cardiogenic shock after cardiopulmonary bypass. *South African Medical Journal*, 52:1035-1039.

Brink, J.G. & Hassoulas, J. 2009. The first human heart transplant and further advances in cardiac transplantation at Groote Schuur Hospital and the University of Cape Town – with reference to: the operation. A human cardiac transplant: an interim report of a successful operation performed at Groote Schuur Hospital, Cape Town. *Cardiovascular Journal of Africa*, 20(1):31-35.

Broelsch, C.E., Testa, G., Alexandrou, A. & Malagó, M. 2002. Living related liver transplantation: medical and social aspects of a controversial therapy. *Gut*, 50(2):143-145. https://doi.org/10.1136/gut.50.2.143

Campbell, K.H.S., McWhir, J., Richie, W.A. & Wilmut, I. 1996. Sheep cloned by nuclear transfer from a cultured cell line. *Nature*, 380:64-66. https://doi.org/10.1038/380064a0

Caulfield, T., Ogbogu, U. & Isasi, R.M. 2007. Informed consent in embryonic stem cell research: are we following basic principles? *Canadian Medical Association Journal*, 176(12):1722-1725. https://doi.org/10.1503/cmaj.061675

Chu, D.T., Nguyen, T.T., Tien, N., Tran, D.K., Jeong, J.H., Anh, P.G., Thanh, V.V., Truong, D.T. & Dinh, T.C. 2020. Recent progress of stem cell therapy in cancer treatment: molecular mechanisms and potential applications. *Cells*, 9(3):563. https://doi.org/10.3390/cells9030563

Connolly, K. 2013. Mass donor organ fraud shakes Germany. *The Guardian*. [Online]. 9 January.

Dalal, A.R. 2015. Philosophy of organ donation: review of ethical facets. *World Journal of Transplantation*, (2):44-51. https://doi.org/10.5500/wjt.v5.i2.44

De Groot, J., Van Hoek, M. & Hoedemaekers, C. 2015. Decision making on organ donation: the dilemmas of relatives of potential brain dead donors. *BMC Medical Ethics*, 16:a64. https://doi.org/10.1186/s12910-015-0057-1

Department for Education England. 2019. *Children looked after in England (including adoption), year ending 31 March 2019.* London: Department for Education.

Editorial. 2017. Organ donation: opting in or out. *British Journal of General Practice*, 68(667):62-63. https://doi.org/10.3399/bjgp18X694445

Encyclopaedia Britannica. n.d. The strange, grisly history of the first blood transfusion. https://bit.ly/3AELEx6

Gratwohl, A., Pasquini, M.C. & Aljurf, M. 2015. One million haemopoietic stem-cell transplants: a retrospective observational study. *The Lancet Haematology*, 2:e91-e100. https://doi.org/10.1016/S2352-3026(15)00028-9

Groth, C.G. 1972. Landmarks in clinical renal transplantation. *Surgery, Gynecology & Obstetrics*, 134(2):323-328.

Hardy, J.D., Kurrus, F.D., Chavez, C.M., Neely, W.A., Eraslan, S., Turner, M.D., Fabian, L.W. & Labecki, T.D. 1964. Heart transplantation in man: developmental studies and report of a case. *JAMA*, 188:1132-1140. https://doi.org/10.1001/jama.1964.03060390034008

Hu, W., Lu, J., Zhang, L., Wu, W., Nie, H., Zhu, Y., Deng, Z., Zhao, Y., Sheng, W., Chao, Q., Qiu, X., Yang, J. & Bai, Y. 2006. A preliminary report of penile transplantation. *European Urology*, 50(4):851-853. https://doi.org/10.1016/j.eururo.2006.07.026

Hwang, N.S., Varghese, S. & Elisseeff, J. 2008. Controlled differentiation of stem cells. *Advanced Drug Delivery Reviews*, 60(2):199-214. https://doi.org/10.1016/j.addr.2007.08.036

Jones, B.P., Saso, S. & Bracewell-Milnes, T. 2019. Human uterine transplantation: a review of outcomes from the first 45 cases. *BJOG*, 126(11):1310-1319. https://doi.org/10.1111/1471-0528.15863

Jouan, A. 2016. "Décès d'Isabelle Dinoire, première greffée du visage" [Death of Isabelle Dinoire, first facial grafted]. *Le Figaro (in French)*. [Accessed 6 September 2016].

Kanagasundram, S. & Amini, F. 2018. Late complications of allogenic stem cells transplantation in leukaemia. *Tissue Engineering and Regenerative Medicine*, 16(1):1-9. https://doi.org/10.1007/s13770-018-0157-3

Kootstra, G., Daeman, J.H. & Oomen, A.P. 1995. Categories of non-heart-beating donors. *Transplantation Proceedings*, 27(5):2893-2894. https://pubmed.ncbi.nlm.nih.gov/7482956/

Mohamed, R.Y., Verheijde, J.L. & McGregor, J. 2007. "Non-heart-beating" or "cardiac death" organ donation: why we should. *Journal of Hospital Medicine*, 2(5):324-334. https://doi.org/10.1002/jhm.204

O'Donovan, L., Williams, N.J. & Wilkinson, S. 2019. Ethical and policy issues raised by uterus transplants. *British Medical Bulletin*, 131(1):19-28. https://doi.org/10.1093/bmb/ldz022

Perkins, K.M., Boulet, S.L., Jamieson, D.J. & Kissin, D.M. 2016. Trends and outcomes of gestational surrogacy in the United States. *Fertility & Sterility*, 106:435-42.e432. https://doi.org/10.1016/j.fertnstert.2016.03.050

Reardon, S. 2022. First pig-to-human heart transplant: what can scientists learn? *Nature*, 601:305-306. https://doi.org/10.1038/d41586-022-00111-9

Reemtsma, K., Mccracken, B.H., Schlegel, J.U., Pearl, M.A., Pearce, C.W., Dewitt, C.W., Smith, P.E., Hewitt, R.L., Flinner, R.L. & Creech, O. 1964. Renal heterotransplantation In Man. *Annals of surgery*, 160(3):384-410.

Ridley, S., Bonner, S., Bray, K., Falvey, S., Mackay, J. & Manara, A. 2005. The Intensive Care Society's working group on organ and tissue donation. UK guidance for non-heart-beating donation. *British Journal of Anaesthesia*, 95(5):592-595. https://doi.org/10.1093/bja/aei235

Rifkin, W.J., David, J.A., Plana, N.M., Kantar, R.S., Diaz-Siso, J.R., Gelb, B.E., Ceradini, D.J. & Rodriguez, E.D. 2018. Achievements and challenges in facial transplantation. *Annals of Surgery*, 268(2):260-270. https://doi.org/10.1097/SLA.0000000000002723

Rivera, R., Yacobson, I. & Grimes, D.1999. The mechanism of action of hormonal contraceptives and intrauterine contraceptive devices. *American Journal of Obstetrics & Gynecology*, 81:1263. https://doi.org/10.1016/S0002-9378(99)70120-1

Sarbey, B. 2016. Definitions of death: brain death and what matters in a person. *Journal of Law and the Biosciences*, 3(3):743-752. https://doi.org/10.1093/jlb/lsw054

Siminoff, L.A., Agyemang, A.A. & Traino, H.M. 2013. Consent to organ donation: a review. *Progress in Transplantation*, 23(1):99-104. https://doi.org/10.7182/pit2013801

Snyder, E.A. & Loring, J.F. 2006. Beyond fraud: stem-cell research continues. *The New England Journal of Medicine*, 354:321-324. https://doi.org/10.1056/NEJMp058323

South African National Health Act. 2008. Regulations regarding the general control of human bodies, tissue and organs for transplantation. *Government Gazette*, 7 March:16.

Tachibana, M., Amato, P., Sparman, M., Gutierrez, N.M., Tippner-Hedges, R., Ma, H., Kang, E., Fulati, A., Lee, H.S., Sritanaudomchai, H., Masterson, K., Larson, J., Eaton, D., Sadler-Fredd, K., Battaglia, D., Lee, D., Wu, D., Jensen, J., Patton, P., Gokhale, S. & Mitalipov, S. 2013. Human embryonic stem cells derived by somatic cell nuclear transfer. *Cell*, 153(6):1228-1238. https://doi.org/10.1016/j.cell.2013.05.006

Van der Merwe, A., Graewe, F., Zuhlke, A., Barsdorf, N., Zarrabi, A., Viljoen, J.T., Ackermann, N.W., Spies, P.V., Opondo, D., Al-Qaoud, T., Bezuidenhout, K., Nel, J.D., Bailey, B. & Moosa, M.R. 2017. Penile allotransplantation for penis amputation following ritual. *The Lancet*, 390(10099): 1038-1047. https://doi.org/10.1016/S0140-6736(17)31807-X

Vazin, T. & Freed, W.J. 2010. Human embryonic stem cells: derivation, culture, and differentiation: a review. *Restorative Neurology and Neuroscience*, 28(4):589-603. https://doi.org/10.3233/RNN-2010-0543

Zhang, L.C., Zhao, Y.B. & Hu, W.L. 2010. Ethical issues in penile transplantation. *Asian Journal of Andrology*, 12(6):795-800. https://doi.org/10.1038/aja.2010.88

6

Ethical Issues in the HIV-positive to Positive Transplant Setting

Elmi Muller

Keywords: clinical decision-making; deceased donation; end-stage renal disease; evidence-based medicine; HIV; renal failure; transplantation

6.1   INTRODUCTION

This chapter is written from a personal perspective, highlighting some of my experience as a transplant surgeon while starting a programme to transplant HIV-positive patients with end-stage renal failure (ESRF) with kidneys that came from HIV-positive deceased donors. I would like to try and show the ethical issues which had to be considered before and immediately after the first transplants were done at the end of 2008.

When I started working in transplantation, my youngest son had just been born. Four years later, I met a patient to whom I will refer as Sarah.[1] I was particularly moved by her situation. She was a 29-year-old mother with a four-year-old boy – also the age of my son – who accompanied her to the renal unit. The child was a typical four-year-old who ran around and demanded his mother's attention while she was talking to me. The mother was a beautiful, kind, graceful woman. She didn't speak good English, so we used short sentences and made do with minimal vocabulary. After a while, I called a translator, our social worker who had first introduced me to the patient. He told me that Sarah had been diagnosed with HIV and renal failure at the same time, about three months before. She was not aware of her HIV status until she presented symptoms of ESRF and was

---

1   Fictional name.

tested for HIV. After testing positive, the presumption was that she had HIV-associated nephropathy (HIVAN) as a cause of her kidney disease – something we used to see quite commonly in South Africa when antiretroviral therapy was not available to all patients with HIV. Sarah was turned down for dialysis. She was in the prime of her life, socially responsible in her duties of motherhood, in a good state medically except for HIV and renal failure. How could this happen, and what did it mean?

The second story is about a patient I will refer to as Peter.[2] He was 36, living with his older brother in Cape Town, selling sweets to make a living. They fled Uganda just before the 2006 elections when President Museveni was re-elected. Peter supported the opposition candidate in Uganda who had spent much of his campaign period in jail. After Museveni's re-election, Peter and his brother feared for their lives. Civil war, although it waxed and waned in intensity, had been an enduring aspect of life in Uganda for 20 years. When Peter came to South Africa, he applied for refugee status. Two years later, he was granted a permanent visa to remain in South Africa. Although he was struggling financially, compared to life in Uganda he was much better off. He and his brother managed to rent a small flat in Cape Town. Prior to 1994, immigrants from elsewhere in Africa faced discrimination and even violence in South Africa, though much of that risk stemmed from the institutionalised racism of the time due to apartheid. After democratisation in 1994, contrary to expectations, the incidence of xenophobia in South Africa increased. Peter still feared for his life every day in South Africa. Struggling to make ends meet, he and his brother worked tirelessly to continue to afford their accommodation in Cape Town. They were too scared to move to a cheaper area or township, as they could speak none of the native South African languages.

In July 2008, Peter started to feel unwell. He was tired, short of breath, and felt very stressed. He was wondering whether the psychological burden of living in dismal circumstances was affecting him. His brother accompanied him to the emergency room at Groote Schuur Hospital (GSH), where he was turned away as he did not live in the catchment area for GSH. After being told to go to the GF Jooste Hospital's outpatient clinic, he was seen a week later and diagnosed with HIV and ESRF. He was referred back to the GSH renal unit (the only state dialysis unit in a 30km radius for Cape Town) – and was presented at the Renal Unit Assessment meeting early in August 2008. At this stage, his creatinine was climbing – he was not feeling well, and his legs were permanently swollen. Having survived civil war and political persecution in Uganda and xenophobic violence

---

2   Fictional name.

and structural racism in South Africa, Peter was turned down for dialysis. He was just one of many patients in category 3 – deemed unsuitable for transplantation – who would be turned down that week.

Again, I ask the question: How could this happen, and what does it mean? I will try to make sense of the predicaments these two individuals found themselves in, and the ethical choices provoked by their respective plights.

6.2   THE ECONOMY VERSUS THE "ETHICS OF POSSIBILITY"

In his essay, "Ethics: An Essay on the Understanding of Evil", the French philosopher Alain Badiou (Badiou, 2001) writes:

> There is no ethics in general. There are only – eventually – ethics of processes by which we treat possibilities of a situation. There is not, in fact, one single Subject, but as many subjects as there are truths, and as many subjective types as there are procedures of truths. The modern name for necessity is, as everyone knows, 'economics'. The logic of Capital. It consists of turning the spectacle of the economy into the object of an apathetic public consensus.

I want to use Badiou's radical perspective on ethics, his "ethics of processes" and the "possibilities of the situation" as opposed to the inertia of ethics as ideology to outline some of the choices I had to make in Cape Town, South Africa, when I started the world's first HIV-positive to positive transplant programme in 2008.

Constituted as subjects by the truths of their personal histories, fears, and ambitions, neither Sarah nor Peter was looked upon as viable economic projects – Badiou's "logic of capital" – in the truth of hospital or Department of Health budgets. Although the circumstances of both individuals strongly affirmed their subjectivity through their choices – the caring mother, the resilience to live – both came up against the logic of a system in which money decided what can and cannot be done to save their lives.

Like physicians the world over, we were forced to think of our vocation as Badiou states, "a bureaucratic medicine that complies with ethical ideology that depends on 'the sick' conceived as vague victims or statistics". Of course, other than point out that this is what happens when patients like Sarah and Peter test the possibilities of inadequate health care provision in developing countries, I cannot suggest easy solutions to the intractable problems of 'managing' health care from considerations that are radically external to genuinely medical situations. What I will do with the help of Badiou is suggest how being faithful to the genuinely medical situation – as opposed to the bureaucratic and managerial situation – enables doctors to treat the clinical situation as one that is faithful to the notion of an affirmative humanity as opposed to one based on humanity as statistics. Importantly, I argue here through these case studies and my subsequent programme of transplanting patients with HIV, that it is when doctors allow themselves to be overwhelmed by urgent, singular situations of need, that ethical decision-making happens.

6.3   THE ISSUE OF SCARCE RESOURCES

As a transplant surgeon in a relatively small unit at GSH (we did about 60-70 kidney transplants per year), I was called for every potential deceased donor and recipient in 2008. Generally, the transplant coordinator would phone me when consent had been obtained from a deceased donor's family and I would then be asked to get the preservation fluids, ice box, and instruments ready that we need to go and do the procurement operation. Sometimes the donor was in my own hospital, sometimes I had to drive to one of the peripheral hospitals, and sometimes I had to fly to, for instance, the Eastern Cape or Northern Cape, to do the procurement.

During preparation, the blood results we needed for the transplant would become available and I would be continually updated on these results. In 2008, HIV was a contra-indication to being a donor or to receive a transplant in South Africa, and should it happen that the donor's results would show that he/she was HIV-positive, we would decline that donor for transplantation. We would inform the family that some tests indicated that we could not use the organs. We would not necessarily disclose the HIV status of the donor to the family – only if he/she had a wife/husband or partner: where we felt from an ethical point of view the person needed to know the status of their loved one. Between 2005 and 2007, I declined many potential donors who were HIV-positive.

Of course, transplant surgeons work very closely with general nephrologists, who are the professionals who make the medical decisions related to transplantation. Like all medical professionals, general nephrologists in state hospitals in South Africa have to take into account policy that enables collective responsibility and allow them to make life and death decisions every week. In weekly meetings, all sorts of decisions will be taken about patients with renal failure. Nephrologists have to accept, every week, that patients cannot be treated at our hospital because they do not meet the medical/procedural requirements for dialysis. The reasons we have medical criteria are less medical, and more economic. Patients are classified according to three categories (Moosa, Meyers, Gottlich & Naicker, 2016):

Category 1 represents the perfect transplant candidate: no end organ disease, no social concerns, no cardiac or chronic problems – basically an otherwise perfectly healthy and socially adjusted patient with end-stage renal failure. These patients will be acceptable dialysis patients. They will also possess the necessary legal residency papers and contribute to the South African Revenue Service. For every one patient in this group, there will be five patients (or sometimes more) who are classified as either category 2 or category 3.

Category 2 patients are those with a well-controlled additional disease besides renal failure. This could potentially be a patient with hypertension, asthma, well-controlled psychiatric problems, etc. However, this patient would only receive dialysis if there were a vacant place on our programme. With 300 dialysis slots serving a population of ±2 million people, the odds were stacked against even category 2 patients receiving dialysis. But in 2008, when I met Sarah and Peter, HIV was classified as a category 3 disease. In our context, this meant 'untransplantable'. I say 'in our context', because patients seen as 'not fit for transplantation in the South African context' would qualify for transplants in other places. These patients included type 1 diabetics, HIV-positive people, and people who did not attend follow-up and was stamped non-compliant. It would also include the teenager who experimented with drugs or alcohol when they were 16. In South Africa, if you were in this group and presented with renal failure, you would be sent home to die. In short, nephrologists' tasks in state hospitals in South Africa included decisions on which ill people in the South African medical system were to be treated, and which – because the budget and public opinion demanded it – were to be sent away to die.

Coming face-to-face with Sarah and Peter in 2008, I made a decision to respond to the needs of these individuals instead of the exigencies of the health care situation and how it had been set up to make Sarah and Peter into statistics. As a mother of a four-year old myself, I could not regard the beautiful Sarah as a category 3, or a category anything. To me, she was a mother with a child who deserved to live. Similarly, Peter, with his determination to live and to make a living, was an extraordinary individual rather than an anonymous category.

Meeting these individuals, I took the decision that I would investigate using HIV-positive deceased donor kidneys to transplant HIV-positive recipients turned down for dialysis in Cape Town. It was a decision that would change their lives, and mine. Before I return to a consideration of the ethics of my decision, and to make any consideration of this decision as an ethical one possible, it is necessary that I make a rather lengthy detour and explain the background to the HIV crisis in South Africa, the implications of this crisis for patients requiring transplantation, the medical risks of transplanting HIV-positive patients, the way in which we addressed these risks by our selection of donors and recipients, and the status quo of the programme.

6.4   THE BACKGROUND IN SOUTH AFRICA AND WHY THIS PROBLEM NEEDED TO BE ADDRESSED

South Africa has a large group of patients who are HIV-positive. The incidence of HIV in South Africa is two to ten times higher than in the rest of the world (Shisana, Rice, Zungu & Zuma, 2010). For a long time, the political climate in South Africa was one of denial and most politicians denied the impact that this virus had on the country. In Thabo Mbeki's opening address to the 13th AIDS conference in Durban, he pleaded with scientists to respect "the politician's point of view" (Horton, 2000). He acknowledged that South Africa has a health crisis of enormous proportions and concluded: "we cannot blame everything on a single virus". He emphasised that the world's biggest killer and the greatest cause of ill-health and suffering across the globe (including South Africa) is extreme poverty.

When the HIV-positive to positive programme was started, South Africa had 50.5 million people of which 5.38 million people were HIV-positive. In people between the ages of 15 and 25, the incidence was even higher: 21% of our population (Connolly, Shisana, Colvin & Stoker, 2004). These statistics were based on antenatal clinic statistics in the country as we do not have a register for HIV in South Africa. Important to note is that a large part of our population (84%) have no medical insurance and depend on the state for their health care (Mayosi & Benatar, 2014). It is this group of patients that was severely affected by the policies around HIV and renal care in the country.

In 2008, the situation was as follows:

1. Antiretroviral therapy (ART) was now available since four years ago;

2. The number of people on treatment grew rapidly, but not rapidly enough with only about 12 000 people on treatment by the end of 2006; and

3. In all state hospitals across the country, HIV-positive patients were declined for dialysis programmes.

A major problem is that a large percentage of HIV-positive people will develop HIVAN – HIV-associated kidney disease – the classic kidney disease associated with HIV infection. Working with the statistic of a 20% incidence of HIV in the country, we can reason that 1:5 people in the country has HIV. HIVAN will develop in approximately 20-27% of the untreated population and 8-22% of the treated ones (Banu, Banu & Saleh, 2013; Wearne et al., 2012). This means a conservative estimate would be that 1 in every 5 HIV-positive patients will develop HIVAN.

Histologically, HIVAN is a collapsing form of focal sclerosing glomerulosclerosis (FSGS), which can be distinguished from idiopathic FSGS by the presence of microcystic tubular dilatation and interstitial inflammation (Okpechi et al., 2011). HIVAN classically presents with proteinuria, but it seldom develops in HIV-positive people who are treated correctly and where the virus is controlled from a very early stage. Therefore, one can reason that HIVAN is the direct result of our health care system failing HIV-positive patients.

6.4.1   Options for HIV patients with renal failure in the South African context

The question in 2008 was what to offer these South African patients who were dying of renal failure. For medical practitioners, there were a few options available:

1.   Continue to let the HIV-positive people with ESRF die;

2.   Increase the available dialysis slots to treat more HIV-positive patients with renal failure;

3.   Use HIV-negative deceased or living donors to transplant HIV-positive patients (as had been done in the USA); or

4.   Utilise a new unique source of donors that has never been used before, the HIV-positive donor.

All four of these options had a unique set of ethical and logistical problems.

6.4.1.1   Continue to let the HIV-positive people with ESRF die

In a context with limited resources and a huge demand to provide primary health care, this was by default the position physicians, surgeons, and society found themselves in. By not accepting HIV-positive patients into renal replacement programmes, we managed to maintain a degree of stability in a crisis situation. Because dialysis had limited availability, HIV was one of the clearcut ways to lower the burden on this treatment option. Interestingly, because of the stigma the disease carried, the fact that very few patients in South Africa were prepared to make their HIV status known and the reality that HIV-positive patients were generally poor and had limited access to resources like the media, this 'status quo' situation was never questioned and never debated.

6.4.1.2   Increase dialysis slots to treat HIV-positive patients with renal failure

Before 2008, but also in the subsequent years in Cape Town, dialysis slots remained stable or increased only marginally (Moosa, Meyers, Gottlich & Naicker, 2016). In terms of the population with ESRF, dialysis remained a totally under-resourced utility. In the state sector, which serves 75% of this population, we only have about 300 dialysis slots in the larger Cape Town area. Increasing these slots would in all likelihood have had a small impact on the treatment of the HIV population as such, as there was a huge need for both HIV-positive as well as HIV-negative patients for dialysis.

Furthermore, data confirmed that HIV-positive patients did not do as well on dialysis as with a transplant (Morales Otero, Molina & González, 1991). In a study done to compare dialysis and transplantation in HIV-positive people, transplanted patients had a much better outcome in terms of life expectancy as well as quality of life, compared to dialysis.

6.4.1.3   Using HIV-negative donors

The USA had been using HIV-negative deceased donors for transplantation into HIV-positive recipients with excellent graft and patient survival rates for about five years before 2008 (Roland et al., 2008). Rejection and infection rates were higher than for HIV-negative counterparts, but in general results compared with high immunological risk HIV-negative recipients. Transplanting HIV-positive patients with HIV-negative kidneys was a very safe option. The results from the USA were encouraging and although this would have been an easy solution, in South Africa it was also a very impractical one. Because of a severe shortage of deceased donors, the impact of this procedure on the HIV-negative waiting list would have been dramatic. Not only would the small number of deceased donors in the country have had to be shared with a new and quite large group of HIV-positive patients, but the unutilised source of donors, namely the HIV-positive donors, would also remain a lost resource.

Using HIV-negative living donors for recipients who would seem to be higher risk patients for infective and rejection risk than the average HIV-negative patient did not seem ethical or responsible at that stage. Living donation should only take place in circumstances where outcomes of recipients had already been researched and proven to be optimal.

This made the use of living or deceased HIV-negative donors for HIV-positive recipients morally and ethically questionable in a country where there was no experience yet with transplantation for HIV-positive patients.

6.4.1.4 Using HIV-positive deceased donors

In a country where many referred braindead patients were found to be HIV-positive, it made sense to try and think about a way to incorporate this pool of potential deceased donors into the pool of confirmed or utilised deceased donors. But certain questions needed to be asked first and the most important was: What will happen when you introduce a second viral strain into an HIV-positive patient by transplanting a kidney from an HIV-infected donor? There was no transplant model for this, so when I started the programme, I reviewed the literature that reported on sex workers who obtained a second viral strain through intercourse. The outcomes and reports of these HIV-positive patients with super infections were difficult to interpret as there were many methodological difficulties that often yielded conflicting results (Pernas et al., 2006; Smith et al., 2004).

The different types of dual infections might depend on the timing of the introduction of the second viral strain. When a patient with low viral load is exposed to a second viral strain, a superinfecting strain may be detectable for only a short period of time. Viral fitness and the ability of a viral strain to replicate effectively in a given environment may play a role to determine whether the two different strains will eventually become undetectable in standard resistance tests or whether outgrowth of a different virus from the baseline or a novel recombinant virus will become detectable. Judging the situation after a transplant would rely on this data.

In 2008 in South Africa, we had a unique situation because we had low ART resistance rates. Most patients who failed second-line ART in South Africa had wild-type virus and resistance rates remained less than 5%.

Observational studies suggested that after four and eight years' access to ART in the Mankweng and the Bela Bela communities respectively, drug resistance mutations in the native population remained low (Nwobegahay et al., 2012; Waters & Smit, 2012). With this information available, the suggestion was that the risk for transplanting a resistant second viral strain was low in the South African context.

Utilising HIV-positive deceased donors made sense in our context (Muller, Barday, Mendelson & Kahn, 2012). Using deceased donors did not expose an HIV-negative living donor to a risky operation in a population group where we did not have significant experience in transplantation in South Africa yet. And using this group of donors opened up a new stream of potential organs that could never be utilised before. Besides this, the risk with this in the South African context seemed low because of our low viral resistance rates and fairly homogenous subtype C virus throughout the country. In 2008, looking at the literature and at outcomes after a second viral strain had been introduced to an already HIV-positive patient (for instance through unprotected intercourse), we knew that these patients could potentially get a flare up of viral load, or possibly a new recombinant virus. But one could argue that we didn't know how patients would behave in the kind of controlled circumstances of a transplant, a situation where we could time the introduction of the second viral strain and where viral load could be monitored closely following the procedure. We anticipated the virus to be completely suppressed by ART immediately after transplant and did not anticipate a flare up or a new recombinant virus. One could therefore argue that there was no evidence that this situation would be harmful to the patient. But there was also no evidence that the situation would not be harmful to the patient.

6.5. THE ISSUE OF RISK WHEN TRANSPLANTING HIV-POSITIVE PATIENTS

6.5.1 The risk of rejection

Rejection rates in the HIV-positive population are about three times higher than the HIV-negative population. Acute allograft rejection is associated with impaired long-term survival because of the increased risk of developing chronic rejection and it is estimated that the impact on long-term graft survival is to decrease the allograft half-life by 34% (Stock et al., 2010). Two major issues are probably associated with high rejection rates in this population. One is the dysregulated immune system that HIV-positive patients have, and the second is the challenge of managing the drug interactions between the antiretrovirals and the immunosuppressants. Many of the antiretrovirals either induce or inhibit the cytochrome P450 liver enzymes resulting in the need for either very high doses or very low doses of immunosuppression. Managing these drug interactions require regular trough levels and even slight dose modifications might change the exposure of the patient to immunosuppressive drugs. This results in higher rejection rates than in patients with less complicated drug regimens as highlighted in the next section.

6.5.2 The risk of drug interactions

Drugs can influence the cytochrome P450 enzyme in two different ways. First, the inhibitors of this enzyme will decrease the metabolism of substrates and generally lead to increased drug effects. This is the result of the inhibitor competing with the other drug for the enzyme-binding site.

Second, the inducers will increase the metabolism of substrates and therefore lead to decreased drug effects. Thus: inducers will either stimulate more enzyme protein or enhance the enzyme's binding capacity.

There are some antiretroviral drugs in both these two groups (inhibitors and inducers) (Frassetto et al., 2003). Ritonavir is a strong inhibitor resulting in a fivefold increase in the drug exposure and an 80% or more decrease in clearance of the drug. Evafirenz and Nevirapine are both inducers of the cytochrome P450 enzyme, needing higher doses than normal of calcineurin inhibitor to obtain the same drug concentrations than in HIV-negative people.

When we started the HIV transplant programme, we switched a lot of patients to a Ritonavir-based drug regimen. The reasons for this were that

(a) it would reduce the amount of immunosuppressants needed dramatically and result in a much cheaper regimen of drugs; and

(b) Ritonavir-based drug regimens were second line treatment in South Africa and therefore it meant that the new incoming viral strain would be very likely to be suppressed if it was exposed to first line treatment in the past.

However, the side effects of the calcineurin inhibitors become more pronounced and some patients on this regimen developed features of calcineurin toxicity on their biopsies. This resulted in a poorer graft survival in some patients.

6.5.3 The risk of induction therapy

Because of the very high overall rejection risk HIV-positive patients have, all patients in our group receive induction therapy with Thymoglobulin (Sawinski et al., 2017). Thymoglobulin is a T-cell depleting agent that is efficient in both blood and peripheral lymphoid tissue because of complement-dependant cell lysis. The effect of the Thymoglobulin induction therapy on the CD4 count is very dramatic and lasts a long time. The median CD4 counts in our study group has dropped from 340 (with an interquartile range of 324 to 511) as measured on the day of admission to 180 (with an interquartile range between 172 and 516) as measured at one year (Muller et al., 2020).

In the next few years after the transplant, CD4 counts do recover and all patients have an upward trend after their transplant.

Weighing up the risk of acute and severe rejection at the time of the transplant versus the long-term well-being and risk for infection over the next few years was a very difficult clinical decision. Informed consent meant that patients should be made aware of the use of lymphocyte depleting medication and the long-term side effects of the drug. As most patients knew they would die if they did not get renal replacement therapy, the choice was fairly easy for them. However, as the treating physician, the decision to prevent rejection in a way that was not possible to revert was difficult. Guided by the experience in HIV-positive patients who received HIV-negative kidneys in the USA, and their very high rejection rates, a decision was made to use induction therapy and to follow-up patients very carefully after the transplant. The result was that patients were required to come to a weekly post-operative clinic for the first three months and that several prophylactic agents were used to prevent infection with tuberculosis, pneumocystis, and viral and bacterial infections as I will highlight in the next section.

6.5.4   The risk of infection

Opportunistic infection is a general risk when you receive a transplant, even with minimal immunosuppression (Muller, Barday & Kahn, 2015). If you are HIV-positive, receive Thymoglobulin, and are maintained on fairly potent immuno-suppression, the risk for infection increases. Therefore, all HIV-positive patients need prophylactic therapy to prevent opportunistic infections.

This includes lifelong antibiotic treatment for pneumocystis pneumonia, lifelong isoniazid to prevent tuberculosis as well as Valganciclovir for three to six months to prevent cytomegalovirus infection. Patients therefore not only sign up for immuno-suppressive drugs with potential side effects, but also for several antibiotics and antiviral drugs, resulting in a large medication burden. After a transplant there has to be careful patient education so that people don't get overwhelmed with the pill burden.

As a result of this post-operative infection risk, this patient population needs constant monitoring for urinary tract infections, respiratory infections as well as serious opportunistic infections like tuberculosis and meningitis. During the Covid-19 pandemic, there were four patients in this transplant cohort who died before the vaccines were made available. Even after the vaccine was on the market, Covid-19 remained a serious risk to immunosuppressed patients as their response to a vaccine was limited because of a reduced capacity to make antibodies because of their immunosuppression. Patients needed third doses of Pfizer and second doses of the Johnson and Johnson vaccine before any immune response was noted.

The decision to receive a transplant does have long-term effects on your health and carries the risk of infection. This is the reason why a careful conversation, weighing up these sometimes even unknown future risks with the risk of not receiving a transplant takes place. (We did not even think of a pandemic like the recent Covid-19 pandemic when we consented patients in the past.) In the case of kidney failure and no access to dialysis, this decision is fairly logical. However, if there are options for treatment outside of this scenario where a patient is doomed to die, the ethical argument becomes less clear.

6.5.5   The risk of the second viral strain

When the transplant programme started in 2008, there was no way to be sure that the introduction of a second viral strain would not cause a flare up of viral load or a recombinant new virus that might be resistant to ART. For the first year, all patients received regular monthly viral loads post transplantation. If a viral load would flare up, the plan was to switch the ART, although some of the new classes of drugs were not yet available at that time. We saw no patients with detectable viral loads after the transplant and we also saw no patients who had a flare up of clinical problems with the new HIV strain post-operatively. This was very reassuring.

During 2014, we started doing a detailed sequencing of all donors and recipients to look at the viral strain for each patient (Selhorst et al., 2019). It was technically very difficult to do as the recipients had undetectable viral loads because of the ART they received. However, we found no patients where the virus changed and reported these results in 2019. As time went on, it became easier to reassure patients about the safety of using HIV-positive donors. It is also because of the scientific work we reported, that policy to use HIV-positive donors changed in other countries, like the USA.

In 2017, the Hope Act was signed by President Obama in the USA and, since then, HIV-positive donors could be used in this country as well. Before this time, it was prohibited by law. Similarly, policies changed in England and Europe, resulting in many places now offering HIV-positive donors to HIV-positive recipients (Durand, Segev & Sugarman, 2016).

6.5.6   The risk of death

Not only do patients need to be informed about infections and rejection when receiving a transplant, they also need to know that if severe opportunistic infections occur, there is a risk of death (Muller, 2015). Most patients in this study faced death in any case, because of the general lack of dialysis slots. Even after dialysis policies changed and HIV patients were allowed to dialyse, there was still a limited number of patients who could be helped because of the resource constraints in South Africa.

Several incidences of death occurred in the study group (Muller, Barday, Mendelson & Kahn, 2015). One patient died one month after transplant when he became septic with chronic pancreatitis as well as a duodenal perforation. A second patient had recurrent gram-negative septicaemia due to recurrent urinary tract infections and grew a carbapenem-resistant klebsiella pneumoniae on blood culture. Another example of a patient who died four months after his transplant was a 45-year-old male who developed rapidly progressive invasive aspergillosis of his lung. These are examples of patients who died early after transplant and where the immunosuppression resulted in a very high risk for invasive infection.

There are also examples of patients who died later after a transplant. Some of the causes of death was unrelated to the immunosuppression, for instance a myocardial infarction and a metastatic squamous lung carcinoma.

When using potent immunosuppression, the risk of death should be considered and therefore any patient who consents to this treatment should be fully informed about this risk. This complicated discussion should also take place with family members, if possible, as many patients are not able to fully comprehend this risk when faced with a decision like this.

6.6 SELECTION PROCESS FOR DECEASED DONOR ORGANS

How did we select donors? We tried to select them according to the lowest possible clinical risk for a donor-derived disease or illness in the recipient (Muller & Barday, 2018). In other words, donors were chosen to minimise serious harm to the recipient, keeping in mind that the *potential* risk of harm to the recipient should be kept as low as possible. What is unique in this argument was that we accepted that there would be some risk to recipients, who were informed about this risk. In a world where patients as consumers are used to demanding a risk-free environment, this was perhaps unique.

One could argue, however, that this was not that different from using a marginal donor for a recipient and discussing this in the informed consent. Or when one buys a generic medicine, and you know that this preparation is not the one tested in the laboratory as part of the original research. A generic drug product is comparable to an innovator drug product in dosage form, strength, route of administration, quality, performance characteristics and intended use, but it is not exactly the same. To bring a generic drug into the market, bioequivalence needs to be shown, but nothing more. Thus, consumers buying this product do so in the full knowledge that they are buying a cheaper alternative, willingly accepting the complications of this choice should there be any. In the case of using a marginal organ, the patients as consumers can make this same decision if they are fully informed about the risk.

In the South African study, we selected our donors to be either naïve to ART or on first-line treatment with no sign of resistance. Later on in the study, we could do more tests to prove if a donor was on ART by using mass spectrometry. However, when we started, we relied on the clinical records of the patient to make this decision. We also wanted the donors to have a normal serum creatinine. Sometimes braindead patients had a temporary spike in their creatinine level because of the trauma or short-term issues with acute tubular necrosis of the kidney at the time of death. However, there was usually a record of a fairly normal creatine before the time of death which could guide us about the long-term well-being of the donor's kidney. We avoided donors with significant proteinuria as this was a possible sign of damage to the donor kidney by the HIV he or she had as well. As we did protocol biopsies on reperfusion of all the transplanted kidneys, we learned a lot about the assessment of the donor through the years and we also noted that HIVAN sometimes improved when on the correct treatment. There were some biopsies that showed mild signs of change as a result of the donor's own HIV and with time these changes disappeared and gave no clinical problems.

To avoid any donor-derived infection in the recipients, we did not use anyone who had an active viral, fungal, or parasitic infection as a donor. We also avoided using a donor with any malignancy.

6.7   A REFLECTION ON THE HISTORIC EVENTS IN VIEW OF CURRENT RESULTS

Until today, we have done almost 60 HIV-positive transplants from HIV-positive recipients and have published our results at several time points over the years.

The cumulative patient survival at one year is almost 90% and this is compatible with higher risk HIV-negative recipients. There are some patients who lose their grafts because of chronic rejection resulting in a one-year graft survival of around 90% as well. Overall, the outcomes are such that we have continued to use HIV-positive organs for HIV-positive recipients without any problems.

Looking back at September and October 2008, when I transplanted the first four HIV-positive patients with HIV-positive kidneys, I also want to keep my first two patients, Sarah and Peter, in mind. The reaction from the hospital and the provincial administration was to impose a moratorium on HIV-positive to positive transplant procedures. I was asked to submit a formal study protocol to the University of Cape Town's ethics committee and to get separate funding and support for this study to continue. I was asked to do a detailed cost analysis, look at the impact of these patients on dialysis slots and report back to the provincial Department of Health. I also received a disciplinary warning for flouting the policies and procedures of the Western Cape Provincial Administration.

Over the next 12 months, my professional and personal life were dominated by the fall out of my decision to transplant Sarah, Peter, and two more patients with HIV-positive kidneys. The institutional response to these transplants was, in many respects, quite brutal. And yet, two years later, as a result of these transplants, the dialysis policies in the Western Cape were changed. Doing the transplants had changed the basis of argument, the conditions of possibility for these procedures.

Badiou would say: Being faithful to the fidelity of a truth process, by linking the known (that these patients would die without the procedures) to the unknown (what would happen if they were transplanted) and by persevering in addressing this unknown. HIV patients were accepted into the state dialysis programmes. They became not only eligible to receive HIV-positive organs, but also HIV-negative organs. In August 2009, the HIV-positive to positive programme could be restarted.

During the period of the moratorium, four HIV-positive patients with ESRF died because I was forced to decline the use of four kidneys. While I was being disciplined and investigated for transplanting four patients who would have died and were now leading healthy lives, no one was held accountable for these deaths, even though they were preventable.

6.7.1 Who decides what is the right thing to do?

Alain Badiou writes about the constitution of a subject, a becoming-subject through truth processes that depose constituted knowledges and thus opposes opinions (Badiou, 2001). These opinions, he writes, are representations without truth, the anarchic debris of circulating knowledge. In practice, I understand this to mean that certain situations, if they are approached as consistent encounters with other subjects, hold the power to expose patterns of thinking or behaviour as limited. Badiou would probably say 'evil', but I would hesitate to go so far. Thus, the truth of life for Sarah or Peter exposes the anarchic debris of constituted knowledges circulating as policies born of fear and neoliberal economic common sense. And yet, it is important for me to reflect what the opening up to such encounters could mean practically, and not only philosophically.

The situation in which I performed my transplants in 2008 involved many parties: a conservative medical community, a larger university community consisting of ethicists and philosophers, policymakers, administrators, the community of HIV-positive patients, and the community of patients with renal failure. This was a situation where the system uncertainties were high and where epistemological and ethical issues were multiple. In these circumstances, the traditional domination of hard facts over soft values often gets inverted. In this situation of a high level of uncertainty, approaching sheer ignorance, I realised that I would never be able to solve the situation unless I simply jump in. Not on the basis of hard facts, but on the basis of personal need of each and every individual patient.

My first enquiries to the university ethics committee about my idea of using HIV-positive donors for HIV-positive recipients, elicited the following two responses:

> ... I see this as therapeutic care in this population and not research ...
> ... off label use of medicines and procedures fall under the responsibility of the clinician ...

This seemed to put me in the clear to proceed. I did not plan these transplants as research when I started – I was simply trying to increase the organ donor pool. Therefore, it seemed to me that my plans were similar to the clinical decisions we had to make when using donation-after-cardiac-death donors, older donors, and donors with other infections that could potentially flare up in the recipients.

But after I had performed the transplants, the hospital authorities and some of my colleagues no longer accepted these arguments. So, the programme had to be submitted as a study and all the consent forms and protocols reviewed by the University of Cape Town Research Ethics Committee. I was initially informed that the transplant programme would only be acceptable if the patients could also get access to dialysis. Providing transplantation without a dialysis programme, the argument went, would be unacceptable from an ethical point of view. The reasoning here was that patients who receive a transplant that for instance did not work, should be able to fall back onto dialysis. There was also the assumption that only patients who have access to dialysis could safely consider the risk that a transplant with an HIV-positive donor would hold. I was therefore asked to facilitate discussions in the state sector to make dialysis accessible for HIV-positive patients and also to ensure that HIV-positive patients were listed on waiting lists for HIV-negative donors. It was made clear to me that it would only be acceptable to enrol patients into the study if they were willing to take an HIV-positive kidney as an alternative form of treatment to either an HIV-negative kidney or dialysis. This basically left me in a position where I could, in the next few months, only accept patients who were able to access dialysis in the private sector but chose to accept an HIV-positive kidney on my programme. As dialysis policies took another six to twelve months to change in the state sector, I was unable to transplant any state dependent patients during this time. HIV-positive people were only accepted for state dialysis programmes at the end of 2009.

To my way of thinking as a surgeon who saw people die because of the time it took for these decisions to be taken, the timing and pace of change became a very real part of the process of ethical decision-making. What would be for Badiou the *event* that effects a break from a particular order of doing things, has a temporal dimension. It is not, in other words, all the same to the individuals concerned whether changes happen fast or slow. It is this temporal dimension of decision taking, the event that forces the break in the situation, that needs to be closely scrutinised not only for its ethical implications, but for the structural understanding it allows of the complexity of ethics.

In *The New Yorker* of 29 July 2013, Atul Gawande writes about slow ideas (Gawande, 2013). Why is it that some ideas spread swiftly, and others spread slowly? He uses the example of Bigelow and Morton's discovery of ether and chloroform reported in the Boston Medical and Surgical Journal in 1846 versus Lister's innovative idea of carbolic acid for cleansing which resulted in lower rates of sepsis and death published in *The Lancet* a few years later in 1867.

The idea of a painless anaesthetic spread like a fire and within a year the whole of Europe and large cities in the rest of the world adopted these new anaesthetic practices. However, it took a whole generation to implement aseptic technique as suggested by Lister. The author then proposes that the visible and immediate problem of pain forms a stark contrast with the invisible problem of germs. He also proposed that both these practices made life easier for patients, but that only one made life easier for doctors. Listerism was tedious; the dilution he suggested burnt surgeons' hands and asked a sacrifice from the surgeon. So, he proposes that it is for this reason that behaviour took so long to change.

In my case, changing the criteria for dialysis and transplantation to benefit HIV-positive people would make things difficult for the nephrologists who need to constantly worry about the budget of state hospitals and furthermore it would make it impossible for the health care system as they would suddenly have to cope with a new set of patients accessing the health care facilities. In one meeting with a state official, I was told "transplantation is of no benefit to us – every patient you transplant opened up a new slot on dialysis and now we have to pay for two patients – one on immunosuppression and a second new one on dialysis".

In this complex system where it was unclear where control was located (the university, the clinical peer group, the ethics committee, the provincial administration, the courts) and unpredictability and contradictions therefore multiplied, I had to ask myself: Can I solve this problem with the traditional problem-solving strategies like going back to core science and applying it, or by simply relying on professional consultancy? Badiou (2001) answers the question as follows:

> To be faithful to an event is to move within the situation that this event has supplemented, by *thinking* (although all thought is a practice, a putting to the test) the situation 'according to' the event. And this, of course – since the event was excluded by all the regular laws of the situation – compels the subject to *invent* a new way of being and acting in the situation.

Key here is the notion of inventing new ways of being and acting in situations that require immanent breaks in processes through the sheer intractability of the paradoxes and unpredictability resulting from the complexity conditions. Where applied science is mission orientated, professional consultancy is client serving. Where core science is curiosity motivated, the situation created by the dire medical prospects of Sarah and Peter was issue driven. A policy for HIV-positive patients could therefore not proceed on factual predications, as there were none. But the impact of these transplants would be universal, long term, novel but also complex and variable. Facts were uncertain, values were in dispute, stakes were high, and decisions were urgent as patients were dying.

In his essay on ethics, Badiou actually writes about medical ethics:

> [...] there is only one medical situation, the clinical situation, and there is no need for an 'ethics' (but only for a clear vision of this situation) to understand that in these circumstances a doctor is a doctor only if he deals with the situation according to the rules of maximum possibility – to treat this person who demands treatment of him as thoroughly as he can, using everything he knows and with all the means to his disposal, without taking anything else into consideration. And if he is to be prevented from giving treatment because of the State budget, because of death rates or laws governing immigration, then let them send for the police! (Badiou, 2001)

While most of us can agree, in principle if not in pragmatic terms, to the notion that the benefit of patients should take precedence of bureaucratic considerations like budgets, immigration laws, or statistics that Badiou so contemptuously refers to, Sarah and Peter also ethically challenged me in a way that made Badiou's phrase "everything he knows" ring somewhat hollow. The fact was, I did not know, and nor could I. Sometimes decisions are made on intuition or individual knowledge rather than on the basis of evidence-based medicine. The situation in South Africa asked for a change – something needed to be done to give hundreds of people with HIV and renal failure hope. And transplanting them with HIV-positive organs turned out to be a successful and positive step forward. In the USA, new legislation was adopted in 2013 to make it possible to use HIV-positive donors there as well. This was a major step forward for the HIV-positive population in the USA.

6.8   CONCLUSION

For me, the use of HIV-positive donors was something I needed to do to give people hope, but also to address some of the barriers in the medical community in South Africa regarding the disease of HIV. And for these patients, who often had no other options, it was a lifesaving procedure. Starting a research project in a field where there were no clear guidelines, often relying on intuition rather than scientific evidence, was difficult. But the use of high-risk donors in South Africa was a new form of treatment that overcame many medical and social barriers: a risk I feel comfortable with in retrospect today. The complexity of the situation I was presented with included ethical considerations, the historical and social weight of Western medicine in South Africa, badly articulated administrative and managerial structures, scientific consensus favouring evidence-based medicine and the varied kinds of risk associated with tackling this complexity with a combination of clinical experience and expertise, scientific rigor, common sense and empathy for patients that had to bridge the gap between what was knowable and what was not. Progress, I want to suggest, depended in this situation on risks not incompatible with an understanding of clinical decision-making as also complexity-driven, and not only evidence-based. It is this principle that confirms medicine as a domain of research that is not post-human, but humane.

Bibliography

Badiou, A. 2001. *Ethics: an essay on the understanding of evil.* London: Verso.

Banu, S.G., Banu, S.S. & Saleh, F.M. 2013. HIV-associated nephropathy (HIVAN): a short review of different authors. *Mymensingh Medical Journal,* 22(3):613-617.

Connolly, C., Shisana, O., Colvin, M. & Stoker, D. 2004. Epidemiology of HIV in South Africa: results of a national, community-based survey. *South African Medical Journal,* 94(9):776-781.

Durand, C.M., Segev, D. & Sugarman, J. 2016. Realizing HOPE: the ethics of organ transplantation from HIV-positive donors. *Annals of Internal Medicine,* 165(2):138-142. https://doi.org/10.7326/M16-0560

Frassetto, L., Thai, T., Aggarwal, A.M., Bucher, P., Jacobsen, W., Christians, U., Benet, L.Z. & Floren, L.C. 2003. Pharmacokinetic interactions between cyclosporine and protease inhibitors in HIV+ subjects. *Drug Metabolism Pharmacokinetics,* 18(2):114-120. https://doi.org/10.2133/dmpk.18.114

Gawande, A. 2013. Slow ideas. *The New Yorker,* 29 July. https://bit.ly/3ijguoY

Horton, R. 2000. Mbeki defiant about South African HIV/AIDS strategy. *The Lancet,* 356(9225):225. https://doi.org/10.1016/S0140-6736(00)02489-2

Mayosi, B.M. & Benatar, S.R. 2014. Health and health care in South Africa: 20 years after Mandela. *The New England Journal of Medicine,* 371(14):1344-1353. https://doi.org/10.1056/NEJMsr1405012

Moosa, M.R., Meyers, A.M., Gottlich, E. & Naicker, S. 2016. An effective approach to chronic kidney disease in South Africa. *South African Medical Journal,* 106(2):156-159. https://doi.org/10.7196/SAMJ.2016.v106i2.9928

Morales Otero, L.A., Molina, M. & González, Z.A. 1991. Incidence and fate of HIV-positive dialysis and transplant patients. *Transplant Proceedings,* 23(2): 1841-1842.

Muller, E. 2015. Transplantation in resource-limited setting: using HIV-positive donors for HIV-positive patients. *Clinical Nephrology,* 83:S39-S41. https://doi.org/10.5414/CNP83S0039

Muller, E. & Barday, Z. 2018. HIV-positive kidney donor selection for HIV-positive transplant recipients. *Journal of the American Society of Nephrology,* 29(4):1090-1095. https://doi.org/10.1681/ASN.2017080853

Muller, E., Barday, Z. & Kahn, D. 2015. HIV-positive-to-HIV-positive kidney transplantation. *The New England Journal of Medicine,* 372(21):2070-2071. https://doi.org/10.1056/NEJMc1503288

Muller, E., Barday, Z., Mendelson, M. & Kahn, D. 2012. Renal transplantation between HIV-positive donors and recipients justified. *South African Medical Journal,* 102(6):497-498. https://doi.org/10.7196/SAMJ.5754

Muller, E., Barday, Z., Mendelson, M. & Kahn, D. 2015. HIV-positive-to-HIV-positive kidney transplantation: results at 3 to 5 years. *The New England Journal of Medicine,* 372(7):613-620. https://doi.org/10.1056/NEJMoa1408896

Muller, E., Botha, F.C.J., Barday, Z.A., Manning, K., Chin-Hong, P. & Stock, P. 2020. Kidney transplantation in HIV-positive patients: current practice and management strategies. *Transplantation,* 105(7):1492-1501. https://doi.org/10.1097/TP.0000000000003485

Nwobegahay, J., Selabe, G., Ndjeka, N.O., Manhaeve, C. & Bessong, P.O. 2012. Low prevalence of transmitted genetic drug resistance in a cohort of HIV infected naïve patients entering antiretroviral treatment programs at two sites in northern South Africa. *Journal of Medical Virology,* 84(12):1839-1843. https://doi.org/10.1002/jmv.23348

Okpechi, I., Swanepoel, C., Duffield, M., Mahala, B., Wearne, N., Alagbe, S., Barday, Z., Arendse, C. & Rayner, B. 2011. Patterns of renal disease in Cape Town South Africa: a 10-year review of a single-centre renal biopsy database. *Nephrology Dialysis Transplantation,* 26(6):1853-1861. https://doi.org/10.1093/ndt/gfq655

Pernas, M., Casado, C., Fuentes, R., Perez-Elias, M.J. & Lopez-Galindez, C. 2006. A dual superinfection and recombination within HIV1 subtype B 12 years after primoinfection. *Journal of Acquired Immune Deficiciency Syndrome*, 42(1):12-18. https://doi.org/10.1097/01.qai.0000214810.65292.73

Roland, M.E., Barin, B., Carlson, L., Frassetto, A.L., Terrault, N.A., Hirose, R., Freise, C.E., Benet, L.Z., Ascher, N.L., Roberts, J.P., Murphy, B., Keller, M.J., Olthoff, K.M., Blumberg, E.A., Brayman, K.L., Bartlett, S.T., Davis, C.E., McCune, J.M., Bredt, B.M., Stablein, D.M. & Stock, P.G. 2008. HIV-infected liver and kidney transplant recipients: 1- and 3-year outcomes. *American Journal of Transplantation*, 8(2):355-365. https://doi.org/10.1111/j.1600-6143.2007.02061.x

Sawinski, D., Shelton, B.A., Mehta, S., Reed, R.D., MacLennan, P.A., Gustafson, S., Segev, D.L. & Locke, J.E. 2017. Impact of protease inhibitor-based anti-retroviral therapy on outcomes for HIV+ kidney transplant recipients. *American Journal of Transplantation*, 17(12):3114-3122. https://doi.org/10.1111/ajt.14419

Selhorst, P., Combrinck, C.E., Manning, K., Botha, F.C.J., Labuschagne, J.P.L., Anthony, C., Matten, D.L., Breaud, A., Clarke, W., Quinn, T.C., Redd, A.D., Williamson, C. & Muller, E. 2019. Longer-term outcomes of HIV-positive-to-HIV-positive renal transplantation. *The New England Journal of Medicine*, 381(14):1387-1389. https://doi.org/10.1056/NEJMc1903013

Shisana, O., Rice, K., Zungu, N. & Zuma, K. 2010. Gender and poverty in South Africa in the era of HIV/AIDS: a quantitative study. *Journal of Women's Health*, 19(1):39-46. https://doi.org/10.1089/jwh.2008.1200

Smith, D.M., Wong, J.K., Hightower, G.K., Ignacio, C.C., Koelsch, K.K., Daar, E.S., Richman, D.D. & Little, S.J. 2004. Incidence of HIV superinfection following primary infection. *JAMA*, 292(10): 1177-1178. https://doi.org/10.1001/jama.292.10.1177

Stock, P.G., Barin, B., Murphy, B., Hanto, D., Diego, J.M., Light, J., Davis, C., Blumberg, E., Simon, D., Subramanian, A., Millis, J.M., Lyon, G.M., Brayman, K., Slakey, D., Shapiro, R., Melancon, J., Jacobson, J.M., Stosor, V., Olson, J.L., Stablein, D.M. & Roland, M.E. 2010. Outcomes of kidney transplantation in HIV-infected recipients. *The New England Journal of Medicine*, 363(21):2004-2014. https://doi.org/10.1056/NEJMoa1001197

Waters, L. & Smit, E. 2012. HIV-1 super-infection. *Current Opinion in Infectious Diseases*, 25(1):42-50. https://doi.org/10.1097/QCO.0b013e32834ef5af

Wearne, N., Swanepoel, C.R., Boulle, A., Duffield, M.S. & Rayner, B.L. 2012. The spectrum of renal histologies seen in HIV with outcomes, prognostic indicators and clinical correlations. *Nephrology Dialysis Transplantation*, 27(11):4109-4118. https://doi.org/10.1093/ndt/gfr702

7

The South African Legal Response to Organ Trafficking and Transplant Tourism in International Perspective

Rosaan Krüger

Keywords: altruism in organ donations; human trafficking; non-commercialism; organ trade

7.1 INTRODUCTION: A LEGAL FRAMEWORK TESTED

Between 2001 and 2003, a record number of kidney transplantations took place in private hospitals in South Africa (Moosa, 2019:236-238). The dramatic increase over the previous years was the result of an illegal international organ and human trafficking scheme that operated at the time. It resulted in 224 kidney transplantations taking place between June 2001 and November 2003, when the scheme dramatically unravelled (Allain, 2011:117; Ambagtsheer, 2021; *Daily News* report, 2010; Scheper-Hughes, 2011:55; Slabbert & Oosthuizen, 2011:740).

In November 2003, organ broker Meir Sushan called the South African Police Service to report that a thief was about to leave South Africa for Israel with $18 000 that the thief had stolen from him. During the report, Sushan also mentioned a missing kidney. This call set in motion an investigation which uncovered an international network that facilitated illegal kidney transplants in hospitals of the Netcare private hospital group.

Sushan's phone call led to the immediate arrest and questioning of the would-be Israeli donor/seller, who fled from Netcare's St Augustine hospital in Durban shortly before his kidney was about to be removed, his wife, and the would-be recipient/buyer of the kidney.[1] The statements of these individuals confirmed their involvement in a scheme to buy and sell a kidney. On the strength of their evidence, the police obtained a search warrant and collected evidence from the hospital, including statements from staff, logs of operations, and details of donors and recipients. The evidence showed that an organ transplantation programme for Israeli recipients was being run in parallel with a national programme and that it involved multiple compatibility tests for Israeli recipients.

An Israeli organ broker, Ilan Perry, was the kingpin and initiator of the international scheme. Sushan, who made the phone call to the police in November 2003, joined the scheme later as a second broker. Through a liaison – nephrologist Jeffrey Kallmeyer, based at St Augustine's Hospital, Durban – Perry arranged for his clients, who were paying Israeli citizens in need of kidney transplantations, and their willing donor/sellers of kidneys, to travel from abroad to undergo nephrectomies and transplantations respectively at hospitals in the Netcare group in return for up-front payment for the operations to the hospital. Netcare was estimated to have profited by more than R22 million from the operations.

Wealthy Israeli citizens who needed kidney transplantations paid up to $120 000 to the organ brokers to procure the kidneys from willing sellers and to arrange for the kidneys to be transplanted to the recipients in Netcare hospitals in South Africa. The brokers employed recruiters who would look for willing kidney sellers, initially in Israel, and later in Romania and Brazil.[2] On finding blood type matches, the brokers would arrange for the intended recipients and the would-be donors to be chaperoned during their travel to South Africa. On arrival, further tests for compatibility were conducted prior to the ultimate nephrectomy and transplantation of every kidney. The network included translators, recruiters of donors/sellers, chaperones, and local brokers, including Netcare employees, who were to ensure smooth functioning of the scheme. The Netcare employees were also responsible for falsifying evidence of family relationships between the recipients and donors of the kidneys.

---

1   In March 2003, the police received information from a whistle-blower doctor regarding suspected illegal kidney transplants being performed at Netcare's St Augustine's Hospital in Durban. The police set up a surveillance operation which was slow to yield results.

2   At the beginning of the scheme, donors/sellers were recruited from Israel. These participants in the scheme were paid $20 000 for a kidney. In 2002, Perry secured prospective donors/sellers from Brazil and Romania who were willing to accept $8 000 or less for a kidney, thus increasing his profit margin.

In 2010, after an investigation that took more than seven years to complete, the prosecuting authorities in South African brought charges against Netcare Kwa-Zulu (Pty) Ltd, two of the organ brokers involved, the two transplant coordinators in the employ of the hospital, the nephrologist, four transplant surgeons, three interpreters, and a patient. An attempt to have Perry extradited to South Africa from Germany was unsuccessful. He later agreed to testify against Netcare on the condition that the charges against him were dropped.

The charges against the accused included contravening the Prevention of Organised Crime Act 121 of 1998[3] by acquiring or benefiting from the proceeds of crime, assault with intent to do grievous bodily harm, and fraud. They also faced charges relating to the contravention of the Human Tissue Act 65 of 1983 related to removing the organs of minors, in this case 19-year-old donors/sellers.[4] A further offence related to a contravention of a Ministerial Policy which required the approval of an organ donation between genetically unrelated living persons (Slabbert & Oosthuizen, 2007:307)[5] and the approval for the transplantation of an organ into a non-South African citizen or permanent resident.

In spite of having denied complicity in the scheme for years, Netcare Kwa-Zulu admitted that it played a role in facilitating the illegal transplants. It entered into a plea and sentence agreement[6] with the prosecuting authority and pleaded guilty to 109 charges, which included those listed above, namely the removal of the organs of minors, receipt of payment for the transplantation of those organs in contravention of the Human Tissue Act, the transgression of the policy requiring authorisation from the Minister of Health for the transplantation of an organ of an unrelated living person into another person, and for the contravention of the policy requiring authorisation for the transplantation of an organ into a non-South African citizen. There were another 91 charges relating to receiving the proceeds of unlawful activities as prohibited by the Prevention of Organised Crime Act. As a sanction for the criminal conviction, Netcare agreed to pay a

---

3   Section 6.

4   Section 19(c)(ii) read with section 34.

5   The policy applied at the time meant that South African hospitals accepted donations from living donors who were related "by blood to the patient seeking a donation, or if the patient's spouse donates an organ. If the source of the donation is a friend or an altruistic acquaintance, an application has to be made to the Department of Health, which will investigate the matter and determine that it is not for financial gain and only then will permission be granted for the operation to be carried out". Magda Slabbert and Hennie Oosthuizen "Establishing a market for human organs in South Africa part 2: shortcomings in legislation and the current system of human procurement" (2007) *Obiter* 304 at 307.

6   In terms of section 105A of the Criminal Procedure Act 51 of 1977.

fine of R4 million and to forfeit assets worth R3.8 million to the state, being the proceeds of crime.

The charges against some of the individuals who had been arrested in 2004 and 2005 for their involvement in the scheme were resuscitated in November 2010. Kallmeyer and an interpreter concluded plea and sentence agreements with the prosecution in December and November 2010 respectively.[7] The two Netcare transplant coordinators and four transplant surgeons were similarly summoned to appear in court in November 2010. After three postponements, the surgeons and former Netcare employees approached the High Court for a permanent stay of prosecution, which the Durban High Court granted in December 2012.[8]

The criminal conviction of Netcare Kwa-Zulu (Pty) Ltd by the Durban Commercial Crimes Court is the only criminal conviction of its kind against a hospital in the world. Despite this unique feat, the investigation of the operation of the scheme and formulation of appropriate charges against all role-players were hampered by an inadequate legal framework (Allain, 2011:117; Ambagtsheer, 2021). For example, while the Human Tissue Act prohibited the sale of organs,[9] it did not prohibit the purchase of organs, nor did it regulate living donations in any way. At the time, South Africa also did not have any legislation outlawing human trafficking. Investigators and prosecutors were thus constrained in their investigation and prosecution of the case.

Since the prosecution of this matter, the National Health Act 61 of 2003 has replaced the Human Tissue Act. South Africa has also ratified the United Nations Convention Against Transnational Organized Crime and its accompanying protocols, including the protocol which prohibits human trafficking of persons for purposes of organ removal.[10] To give effect to its international law commitments under the protocol prohibiting human trafficking, Parliament enacted the Prevention and Combating of Trafficking in Persons Act 7 of 2013.[11]

---

7 Kallmeyer had by then fled to Canada but pleaded guilty to 90 charges and was fined R150 000 for his involvement in the scheme. The interpreter, Samuel Ziegler, was sentenced to pay a fine of R50 000 or three months' imprisonment. In addition, a five-year prison sentence was suspended.

8 *Robbs and five others v Deputy Director for Public Prosecutions, KZN* (case number 13510) KwaZulu-Natal High Court, Durban (14 December 2012) unreported judgment on file with author.

9 Section 28 read with section 34.

10 South Africa signed the Convention and the Protocol to Prevent, Suppress and Punish Trafficking in Persons, especially Women and Children; and Protocol against the Smuggling of Migrants by Land, Sea and Air on 14 December 2000 and ratified these on 20 February 2004.

11 Act 7 of 2013. It came into operation on 18 July 2004.

In this chapter, I outline the international standard relating to organ trafficking and transplant tourism before setting out the current South African legal framework. While the proverbial book on the Netcare organ trafficking and transplant tourism scandal was closed more than a decade ago, I conclude this chapter by returning to the scandal. With the benefit of the new legal framework, I view the charges and outcomes that those who were involved in the scheme at that time could have faced under the new legal framework. At the same time, I assess the compatibility of the new South African legal framework with the international standard.

7.2   THE INTERNATIONAL LAW FRAMEWORK

7.2.1   Altruism and non-commercialisation as the point of departure: World Health Organization Guiding Principles

Despite the absence of evidence regarding trade in organs at the time, the 1980s saw the adoption of the general principle that the buying and selling of organs is morally and ethically improper (De Jong, 2017:30).[12] This principle was first adopted in the United States of America. After a congressional hearing in 1983 to address the shortage of organs for transplantation, and in firm rejection of a proposal to permit the sale of organs, Congress passed the National Organ Transplant Act of 1984 which criminalises the sale of human organs and sets liability on conviction of a fine of up to $50 000 and/or a sentence of imprisonment of up to five years.[13] This legislation remains in place and affirms the principle that organ donation, whether from deceased or living donors, ought to be motivated by altruism alone.

Following the US example, the World Health Organization (WHO) condemned trade in organs in 1987 (De Jong, 2017:31; WHO, 1987)[14] and adopted Guiding Principles in 1991 which have served as a basis for national legal and ethical frameworks regulating organ transplants, despite being non-binding in nature (Ambagtsheer, 2021; De Jong, 2017:31). These principles were revised in 2010. Guiding Principle 5 confirms the prohibition of trade as a foundational principle.

---

12   Jessica de Jong "Human trafficking for the purpose of organ removal" (2017) PhD thesis, Utrecht University, p. 30.

13   Title 42 Chapter 6A Subchapter II Part H Section 274e.

14   Fortieth World Health Assembly "Developing guiding principles for human organ transplants" (Geneva, 4-15 May 1987) available at https://www.who.int/transplantation/en/WHA40.13.pdf; De Jong, p. 31.

It prohibits payment for organs since

> payment for cells, tissues and organs is likely to take unfair advantage of the poorest and most vulnerable groups, undermines altruistic donation and leads to profiteering and human trafficking. Such payment conveys the idea that some persons lack dignity, that they are mere objects to be used by others.

The principle, however, permits the compensation of a donor for reasonable and verifiable expenses.

The WHO Guiding Principles further encourage the maximum development of organ donation from deceased donors and stipulate that living donors should be genetically, legally, or emotionally related to the recipients of their organs.[15] It further emphasises the requirement of consent for removal of tissue or organs from a deceased donor,[16] the independent determination of death of a deceased donor,[17] and advocates for the prohibition of donations from living donors who are minors. Narrow exceptions to this prohibition are to be determined by national law.[18] The WHO Guiding Principles determine that decisions regarding transplantation should be guided by clinical criteria and ethical norms only[19] and that health professionals and insurance should not engage in transplantation of organs or tissue that have been obtained through exploitation, coercion, or payment to the donor or his/her next of kin.[20] Health professionals should further be prohibited from receiving any payment other than compensation for their professional services.[21] The long-term outcomes of transplantation for both donors and recipients must be monitored and measured to ensure quality and safety.[22] The organisation and execution of transplantation services and their clinical results must be transparent, while the anonymity of donors and recipients must be protected.[23]

---

15   Guiding Principle 3.
16   Guiding Principle 1.
17   Guiding Principle 2.
18   Guiding Principle 4. This also applies in respect of legally incompetent persons.
19   Guiding Principle 9.
20   Guiding Principle 7.
21   Guiding Principle 8.
22   Guiding Principle 10.
23   Guiding Principle 11.

7.2.2   The prohibition of human trafficking for organ removal: Binding international law

The United Nations Convention Against Transnational Organised Crime came into operation on 29 September 2003. This Convention is supplemented by, among others, the United Nations Protocol to Prevent, Suppress and Punish Trafficking in Persons, Especially Women and Children.[24] This Protocol is referred to as 'the Palermo Protocol'.

The Palermo Protocol recognises trafficking of persons for the purpose of organ removal as a specific form of exploitation that warrants criminalisation. Trafficking in persons is defined in broad terms and requires member states to criminalise trafficking in persons in national legislation. 'Trafficking in persons' means:

> the recruitment, transportation, transfer, harbouring or receipt of persons, by means of threat or the use of force or other forms of coercion, of abduction, of fraud, of deception, of the abuse of power or of a position of vulnerability or of the giving or receiving of payments or benefits to achieve the consent of a person having control over another person for the purpose of exploitation.[25]

Exploitation is then defined to include the removal of organs. Other forms of exploitation included in the open list of articles 3(a) are "the prostitution of others or other forms of sexual exploitation, forced labour or services, slavery or practices similar to slavery [and] servitude."

De Jong (2017) explains that the definition of trafficking in persons has three elements that must be proven in the event of a victim being an adult. Firstly, the definition requires an act (that which is done) which includes recruitment, transportation, transfer, etc.; secondly, a means (how the act is done) which could be through coercion, fraud, threat, abuse of power, etc.; and thirdly, the purpose of exploitation which in this instance is for the purposes of the removal of an organ (De Jong, 2017:33). Where the victim is a child, it is not necessary to establish a means because the vulnerability that necessarily comes with being a child is acknowledged.

Importantly, the Protocol stipulates that the consent of the victim of trafficking is irrelevant in the determination of whether a crime was committed.[26] Thus,

---

24   The text of the Protocol can be accessed at https://www.unodc.org/res/human-trafficking/2021the-protocol-tip_html/TIP.pdf

25   Article 3(a) of the Palermo Protocol.

26   Article 3(b).

where a would-be donor/seller agrees to the removal of his/her organ for payment, he/she is a victim of trafficking and the persons involved in arranging the recruitment, transportation, transfer, harbouring, or receipt of the victim for the purposes of organ removal are guilty of the crime of trafficking in persons, regardless of their ostensible consensus. It is important to note that the focus of the Protocol is on trafficking in persons for various exploitative purposes and in that way, it differs from the WHO Guidelines with their focus on prohibiting commercial trade in organs.

7.2.3   Non-commercialisation and altruism confirmed: The Istanbul Declaration

In 2008, the International Society for Nephrology and the Transplantation Society organised an international meeting in Istanbul, Turkey. That meeting, which was attended by representatives of more than 150 scientific and medical organisations, government officials, social scientists, and ethicists, adopted the Declaration of Istanbul on Organ Trafficking and Transplant Tourism. In 2010, the two societies established a custodian group, the Declaration of Istanbul Custodian Group, to oversee the dissemination of the Declaration to governments and professional organisations (Martin et al., 2019). The Group also oversaw the revision and updating of the Declaration. The 2018 version of the Declaration of Istanbul was released on 1 July 2018.[27]

The South African Renal Society and the Southern African Transplantation Society are two of the 128 societies, organisations, or governments which endorsed the non-binding declaration.[28]

The point of departure of the Istanbul Declaration is that of altruistic donation and non-commercialisation. The Declaration commences with definitions of "organ trafficking", "trafficking in persons for the purpose of organ removal", "travel for transplantation", and "transplant tourism". It defines organ trafficking widely. "Organ trafficking" includes the removal of organs without consent or authorisation from a living or deceased donor, or in exchange for financial gain or a similar advantage to the donor or a third person. The transportation, use and/or transplantation of such organs is included in the definition, as is payment or a request to another to enable such removal or transplantation, the recruitment of donors or recipients, and any attempt or aiding another to perform any of these acts.

---

27   The text of the Declaration is available at https://www.declarationofistanbul.org/the-declaration

28   See https://www.declarationofistanbul.org/endorsements

The definition of "trafficking in persons for the purposes of organ removal" as employed by the Declaration aligns with that of the Palermo Protocol and confirms that the consent of the person recruited, transported, or received for purposes of the removal of his/her organ is irrelevant.

"Travel for transplantation" is defined as the movement of persons across jurisdictional borders for purposes of transplantation. This includes movement across state or provincial lines. While "travel for transplantation" is not *per se* prohibited, "transplant tourism" is defined as unethical and involves trafficking in organs, trafficking in persons for purposes of organ removal, or the movement of resources, including organs, the professionals, and centres to provide transplantation to non-resident patients thus undermining the country's ability to provide transplantation services to its own population.

The Declaration advocates for adequate programmes within states to prevent organ failure.[29] The overall health and well-being of both donors and recipients should remain the primary goal of any transplantation programme.[30] It affirms the prohibition and criminalisation of trafficking in human organs or trafficking in persons for purposes of organ removal.[31] Commercial trade in organs and trafficking in persons exploit the vulnerable in society as it "targets the poor as a source of organs and stigmatizes donation". It justifies its opposition to commercialisation as the latter disincentivises altruistic donation and jeopardises the sustainability of donation and transplantation programmes which operate on that basis. The Declaration acknowledges that the costs relating to donations may be prohibitive and that authorities should legally permit recovery of expenses on the principle of financial neutrality, i.e., with no financial gain for either donor or recipient or their families.

The Declaration stipulates that each country should develop a legislative and regulatory framework to govern the organ transplantation from deceased and living donors in line with international standards.[32] Authorities overseeing the implementation of this regulatory framework must be accountable for donation, allocation of organs, and transplantations to ensure standardisation, traceability, transparency, quality, safety, fairness, and public trust.[33] Every resident in a country should have equitable access to donation and transplantation services

---

29   Principle 1.
30   Principle 2.
31   Principle 3.
32   Principle 5.
33   Principle 6.

and to organ allocation in their country of residence.[34] Significantly, and to curb transplant tourism, the Declaration sets as a standard that the allocation of organs are guided by clinical and ethical norms within a particular jurisdiction or country.[35] Similarly, governments and health care professionals are to play active roles in discouraging and preventing transplant tourism.[36]

7.2.4   International standards: Key points

In the absence of a comprehensive international convention, setting a binding standard to be adhered to by member states, the standards gleaned from the non-binding and binding international law documents provide guidance to states in formulating their national regulatory frameworks.

The Declaration of Istanbul focuses attention on national or jurisdictional self-sufficiency in respect of organ donation and transplantation to discourage transplant tourism. It shares with the WHO Guidelines and the Palermo Protocol the commitment to altruism in organ donation, the principle of non-commercialism, and the prohibition of human trafficking, all bolstered by criminal sanctions. The international standards further highlight the importance of national regulatory frameworks which require consent to donation, transparency in the regulation of donation, organ allocation, and transplantation and application of clinical and ethical norms in fairness to all citizens. Medical professionals carry a specific obligation to uphold the commitment to non-commercialism in organ transplantation.

While the congruence between the international law documents outlined above is attractive in its simplicity, it does not have universal support. Ambagtsheer and Weimar (2012:571) warn that international laws' identical treatment of commercialism (buying and selling of organs) and trafficking (coercion and exploitation of donors) fail to take account of the existing challenges of enforcement. It also fails to acknowledge that prohibition of trade necessarily creates a black market for organs which in turn encourages trafficking in persons. To curb exploitation, these authors suggest that the supply of organs must be increased. To achieve this, they recommend that living donations should be encouraged as a matter of principle, and that incentives to living donors should be permitted. Neither the WHO Guiding Principles nor the Declaration of Istanbul encourage living donations, leaving no guidance to states but the accepted truism that living donations encourage trade and exploitation.

---

34   Principle 7.
35   Principle 8.
36   Principles 9 and 10.

Against the background of the international framework and its contestation referred to above, I turn to outline the provisions of the South African law as it relates to organ trafficking and transplant tourism.

7.3 THE SOUTH AFRICAN LEGAL FRAMEWORK

7.3.1 The National Health Act and its regulation of organ transplanting

The National Health Act (hereinafter referred to as NHA) was enacted in 2003 to provide for a structured, uniform health system which takes account of the socio-economic disparities in South African society and the inequity in the provision of health services, the legacy of apartheid, and colonialism.[37]

It deals with tissue donation and use, including transplantation, from living and deceased donors, together with the donation and use of blood and gametes in a single chapter. Chapter 8 of the NHA brings these different aspects together but provides for differentiated regulations to deal with practical matters in relation to some of these. So, for example, specific regulations to regulate blood and blood products,[38] tissue banks,[39] stem cell banks,[40] and artificial fertilisation of people[41] were published separately. However, as far as organ donation and transplantation is concerned, the Regulations: General Control of Human Bodies, Tissue, Blood, Blood Products and Gametes, relating to the chapter of the NHA as a whole, provide the practical regulatory details.[42]

The Act defines "tissue" to include "an organ".[43] "An organ", in turn, is defined as a part of the human body "adapted by its structure to perform any particular vital function", including the eye.[44] In what follows, I refer to 'organ' where the Act uses the phrase "tissue, blood or gametes".

---

37   Preamble.

38   *Government Gazette*. Regulation Gazette No. 35099 of 2 March 2012. Vol. 561 No. 9699, Government Notice R179 under the NHA.

39   Ibid. Government Notice R182.

40   Ibid. Government Notice R183.

41   Ibid. Government Notice R175.

42   Ibid. Government Notice R180.

43   Section 1 defines tissue as "human tissue, and includes flesh, bone, a gland, an organ, skin, bone marrow or body fluid, but excludes blood or a gamete".

44   Section 1: organ is defined as "any part of the human body adapted by its structure to perform any particular vital function, including the eye and its accessories, but does not include the skin and appendages, flesh, bone, bone marrow, body fluid, blood or a gamete".

Section 55 of the NHA prohibits the removal of an organ from the body of a living person without the person's written consent and in accordance with pre-scribed conditions. Section 56 stipulates that the removal of an organ may only take place for medical (or dental) purposes as prescribed, which may include transplantation. The Minister is empowered to authorise the removal of an organ and may impose necessary conditions in respect of such removal. Section 56(2) further prohibits the removal of an organ from a person who is mentally ill as defined in the Mental Health Care Act 17 of 2002.

Similarly, it prohibits the removal of an organ which is not replaceable by natural processes or a gamete from a minor. Regulation 2(1)(a) of the General Control of Human Bodies regulations provides that a person older than 18 must consent in writing to the removal of an organ for purposes of transplantation into the body of another person for the production of a therapeutic, diagnostic, or prophylactic substance, as designated permitted purposes by regulation 3(1). A donation made for any other than the permitted purposes is of no force and effect.[45] Where the donor is under the age of 18, the written consent of his/her parents is required.[46] The requirement of written parental consent may seem to contradict section 129(3) of the Children's Act 38 of 2005 (Slabbert, 2018:75).

This section of the Children's Act provides that a child over the age of 12 may consent to surgery if he/she is of sufficient maturity and has the mental capacity to appreciate the benefits and risks and consequences of the operation, provided that he/she is assisted by his/her parent or guardian. A cursory reading of the health regulation may lead one to conclude that the regulation denies the child's right to consent to surgery. However, section 129(3) of the Children's Act requires that the child be assisted by parent or guardian. Thus, a harmonious reading of the consent requirements means that a minor donor above the age of 12 with sufficient maturity may consent to the removal of an organ for purposes of transplantation but that the assistance of the parents or guardian in such an instance must take the form of written consent.[47]

---

45   Regulation 7 of the Regulations: General Control of Human Bodies, Tissue, Blood, Blood Products and Gametes.

46   Ibid. Regulation 2(1)(b).

47   CJ Davel and A Skelton *Commentary on the Children's Act* (2007) Revision Service 13-2013 at 63: "The phrase 'duly assisted' seems to presuppose concurring parental acquiescence or agreement, if not actual 'consent' in the legal sense (i.e., a parental signature on the relevant authorisation form, the place of which can now be taken by the signature of the child)."

The removal of organs from living donors for purposes of transplantation may only be carried out in hospital or in an authorised institution.[48] The removal must be authorised in writing by the medical practitioner in charge of clinical services at the hospital or institution, or the medical practitioner designated by that person. Where a hospital or institution does not have a practitioner in charge of clinical services, the removal must be authorised by a medical practitioner authorised to do so by the person in charge of the hospital.[49] The medical practitioner who authorises the removal of an organ for purposes of transplantation may not participate in the transplant of that organ into another human being.[50] Only registered medical practitioners may remove an organ from a living person.[51]

While not included as a legal requirement in the Act or regulations, living donations from an unrelated donor must be approved by the Ministerial Advisory Committee on Organ Transplantation (Moosa, 2019:238).

Regulation 4 lists the institutions that may receive donations from living donors. A donor may donate an organ to a hospital, a university, an authorised institution, a medical practitioner or dentist or a tissue bank or person who requires therapy in which the organ can be used.

Organ donations of deceased donors may be made by the donor in his/her will or in a document or by an oral statement in the presence of two witnesses.[52] The donor may donate his/her body or specified tissue such as an organ to be used after his/her death as provided for in the NHA, and in the case of an organ for transplantation into another person. Regulation 14(3) permits a medical practitioner to act upon the will or a document in which the organ donation was made on the face of it as if valid.

The death of a deceased donor must be established by at least two medical practitioners. One of these practitioners must have been in practice for at least five years at the time of the certification of the person's death. Neither of the certifying practitioners may be involved in the transplantation of organs removed from the deceased into a living person.[53] Death is defined in the NHA as brain death.[54]

---

48   Section 58(1)(a).
49   Section 58(1)(b).
50   Section 58(2).
51   Section 59(1).
52   Section 62(1).
53   Regulation 9.
54   Section 1.

A recipient of a post-mortem donation of a specific organ has 24 hours after the death of the donor to remove the organ or to cause it to be removed. Should the recipient fail to have the organ removed within 24 hours, the body may be claimed for burial or cremation by the family of the deceased.[55] Authority shall not be granted to remove an organ unless the medical practitioner is satisfied that the organ was donated.[56]

A living donor may revoke his/her consent to the transplantation of his/her organ prior to the transplantation thereof. A will or document giving consent for the donation of a body or organ may be revoked by intentional destruction of the will or document.[57]

Section 60 of the NHA regulates payment of costs in connection to bring an organ to a hospital or authorised institution. It restricts this to compensations for costs reasonably incurred. Section 60(3) further permits remuneration of health care workers for professional services rendered.

Section 61(3) requires the written permission of the Minister of Health for the transplantation of an organ into a person who is not a South African citizen or permanent resident. A person who transplants an organ to a non-South African citizen or resident without the requisite permission, or who charges a fee for the organ is guilty of an offence. The penalty on conviction is a fine or imprisonment of up to five years, or both.

The sale of or trade in organs is explicitly criminalised by section 60(4)(a). Conviction on such a charge carries a penalty of a fine or a sentence of imprisonment of up to five years or both. Regulation 25 of the General Control Regulations under chapter 8 of the NHA similarly creates a criminal offence in that it provides that any person who, unless as permitted by the Act and these regulations or in terms of any other law acquires, uses, or supplies an organ of a living or deceased person in any other manner or for any other purpose than permitted by the Act and the regulations, commits an offence. Non-compliance with a demand or requirement of a health officer in relation to provisions of the NHA and regulations similarly constitutes an offence, as does hindering a person in the performance of his/her duties in terms of the Act and regulations. Conviction on these charges may result in a fine and/or imprisonment of up to 10 years.

---

55   Regulation 8.
56   Regulation 14(1).
57   Section 65.

Regulation 16 provides for recordkeeping by the medical practitioner who removed an organ from a deceased donor, including the nature of the donation and the details of the donor and the receiving authorised institution.

Chapter 8 of the NHA and its regulations set out clear consent requirements for living and deceased organ donation. In respect of the latter, it gives families the last say. This may limit the number of donations from deceased donors, as families may for religious, cultural, or other reasons refuse to disclose consent communicated to them by the deceased or refuse their permission for donation. To ensure optimum donations from deceased donors, a written donation signed by the donor and witnesses is thus advised (Etheredge, 2019).

The NHA casts its criminal net of prohibitions far wider than the Human Tissue Act. Buying and selling of organs, and the use of organs other than permitted in terms of NHA and its regulations are criminalised and those convicted face harsh penalties.

It is a concern that the regulatory framework for organ donation and transplantation is included in a general framework, rather than being dealt with separately and with greater specificity tailored particularly to the requirements of organ donation and transplantation. However, this seems to be by choice. A draft focused policy framework for organ transplantation was published in 2002 for comment, and a related focused draft set of regulations were published in 2008 for comment, but these focused frameworks fell by the wayside when the Minister published the General Control Regulations in 2012 (Slabbert, 2018:72-73).

7.3.2   The Prevention and Combating of Trafficking in Persons Act

As pointed out above, South Africa signed and ratified the United Nations Convention Against Transnational Organised Crime and its supplementing Protocol to Prevent, Suppress and Punish Trafficking in Persons, Especially Women and Children.[58] To give effect to the Protocol, the legislature passed the Prevention and Combating of Trafficking in Persons Act 7 of 2013 (hereinafter referred to as PCTPA). It came into operation on 9 August 2015.

---

58   South Africa signed and ratified the Protocol against the Smuggling of Migrants by Land, Sea and Air on the same dates. The third protocol to the Convention, the Protocol against the Illicit Manufacturing of and Trafficking in Firearms, their Parts and Components and Ammunition was signed on 14 October 2002 and ratified on 20 February 2004.

Section 4 of the PCPTA creates the offence of trafficking in persons in the following terms:

> *Trafficking in persons*
>
> (1) Any person who delivers, recruits, transports, transfers, harbours, sells, exchanges, leases, or receives another person within or across the borders of the Republic, by means of –
>
> > (a) a threat of harm;
> >
> > (b) the threat or use of force or other forms of coercion;
> >
> > (c) the abuse of vulnerability;
> >
> > (d) fraud;
> >
> > (e) deception;
> >
> > (f) abduction;
> >
> > (g) kidnapping;
> >
> > (h) the abuse of power;
> >
> > (i) the direct or indirect giving or receiving of payments or benefits to obtain the consent of a person having control or authority over another person; or
> >
> > (j) the direct or indirect giving or receiving of payments, compensation, rewards, benefits or any other advantage,
>
> aimed at either the person or an immediate family member of that person or any other person in a close relationship to that person, for the purpose of any form or manner of exploitation, is guilty of the offence of trafficking in persons.

"Exploitation", in turn, is defined to include "the removal of body parts".[59] The "removal of body parts" is explained to "mean the removal or trade in any body part in contravention of any law". It thus includes the removal of an organ for purposes of transplantation.

It is not a defence to a charge of trafficking that the victim has consented to the intended exploitation or that the person who has authority of the child who was trafficked has consented to the intended exploitation.[60]

---

59 The full definition reads: "exploitation includes, but is not limited to –
    (a) all forms of slavery and practices similar to slavery;
    (b) sexual exploitation;
    (c) servitude;
    (d) forced labour;
    (e) child labour as defined in section 1 of the Children's Act;
    (f) the removal of body parts;
    (g) the impregnation of a female person against her will for the purpose of selling her child when the child is born."

60 Section 11(1) of the PCPTA.

Section 4(2) of the PCPTA prohibits the adoption of a child, legally or illegally, and forced marriage of a person for purposes of exploitation and criminalises it. The offences created by section 4 carry harsh penalties. In addition to attracting a discretionary minimum sentence of imprisonment as provided for in section 51 of the Criminal Law Amendment Act 105 of 1997, a person convicted of trafficking in persons is liable on conviction to the payment of a fine of up to R100 million or imprisonment, including life imprisonment or both.[61] Conviction of the offence of adopting of a child or the forced marrying of person for purposes of exploitation may result in a fine of up to R100 million, imprisonment, including life imprisonment, or both.

The PCPTA also creates offences related to trafficking in persons by criminalising possession, destruction, confiscation, and concealment of or tampering with the identification, passport or travel documents of a victim.[62] A conviction of this offence carries a penalty of up to 15 years imprisonment without the option of a fine.[63] A person who intentionally benefits financially or otherwise from the services of a victim of trafficking is guilty of an offence and liable to a fine or a sentence of imprisonment of up to 15 years, or both.[64] The facilitation of trafficking by intentionally leasing premises enabling trafficking in persons and printing or advertising information to facilitate or promote trafficking and financing of trafficking are similarly criminalised.[65] Conviction on facilitation of person trafficking carries the penalty of a fine or imprisonment of up to 10 years, or both.[66] Electronic communications service providers are obliged to take reasonable steps to prevent the use of their services for advertisement or promotion of trafficking in persons. When such a service provider becomes aware of any communication aimed at the promotion of trafficking in persons, it must report such use to the police service, preserve any evidence it may have regarding the promotion of trafficking in persons, and prevent continued access to such information by its customers. A service provider's failure to comply with the provisions amounts to an offence,[67] and a service provider so convicted is liable to a sentence of imprisonment of up to 5 years or a fine, or both.[68]

---

61   Section 13(1)(a) and (b) of the PCPTA.
62   Section 6.
63   Section 13(1).
64   Section 7 read with section 13(1)(c).
65   Section 8(1).
66   Section 13(1)(d).
67   Section 8(3).
68   Section 13(1)(e).

The PCPTA prohibits human trafficking in wide terms. It criminalises trafficking of persons for the purposes of removing body parts which go beyond the prohibition of the Palermo Protocol to include the use of body parts in African traditional medicine or *muti* (see Labuschagne, 2004:19; Mswela, 2017:114).

7.3.3 Revisiting the Netcare scandal: An improved legal response compliant with international standard?

With the benefit of the current legal framework, prosecutors in the Netcare kidney trafficking matter would have had clarity on several issues that presented as challenges in their investigation and prosecution of the matter more than a decade ago. These include the explicit prohibition and criminalisation of trade in organs, the explicit criminalisation of transplanting an organ into non-citizens or non-permanent residents, and the prohibition and criminalisation of trafficking in persons and related activities which strike widely to include all the role-players in an organ trafficking and transplant tourism network. As such, the regulatory framework relevant to organ trafficking and transplant tourism has been adapted and provides legal certainty to meet the wide criminal prohibition required by the binding and non-binding international law.

7.4   CONCLUSION

The WHO Guidelines encourage states to maximise the donation of organs from deceased donors while the Declaration of Istanbul advocates for self-sustainability within states in respect of donations and transplantation to curb organ trade and transplant tourism respectively. In doing so, these international instruments address the need to increase the source of organs for transplantation in line with the Declaration's principled commitment to altruism and non-commercialism. While the South African legal framework reflects its commitment to the principles of altruism and non-commercialism in its clear criminal prohibition of trade and trafficking in organs, it lacks commitment to the principles of the Declaration in its encouragement for donations, particularly for donations from deceased donors.

Bibliography

Allain, J. 2011. Trafficking of persons for the removal of organs and the admission of guilt of a South African hospital. *Medical Law Review*, 19(1):117-122. https://doi.org/10.1093/medlaw/fwr001

Ambagtsheer, F. 2021. Understanding the challenges to investigating and prosecuting organ trafficking: a comparative analysis. *Trends in Organized Crime.* https://bit.ly/3i7eSyq [Accessed 20 February 2022].

Ambagtsheer, F. & Weimar, W. 2012. A criminological perspective: why prohibition of organ trade is not effective and how the Declaration of Istanbul can move forward. *American Journal of Transplantation*, 12(3): 571-575. https://doi.org/10.1111/j.1600-6143.2011.03864.x

Daily News Report. 2010. Netcare 'dismay' at charges. 16 September:1.

Davel, C.J. & Skelton, A. 2007. *Commentary on the Children's Act.* Cape Town: Juta.

De Jong, J. 2017. Human trafficking for the purpose of organ removal. PhD thesis. Utrecht: Utrecht University.

Etheredge, H. 2019. *The complex reasons for South Africa's organ shortage.* https://bit.ly/3gBDuyJ [Accessed 30 March 2022].

Labuschagne, G. 2004. Features and investigative implications of muti murder in South Africa. *Journal of Investigative Psychology and Offender Profiling*, 1:191-206. https://doi.org/10.1002/jip.15

Martin, D.E., Van Assche, K., Dominguez-Gil, B., Lopez-Fraga, M., Gallont, G., Muller, E. & Apron, A.M. 2019. Strengthening global efforts to combat organ trafficking and transplant tourism: implications of the 2018 edition of the Declaration of Istanbul. *Transplantation Direct*, 5(3). https://doi.org/10.1097/TXD.0000000000000872

Moosa, M.R. 2019. The state of kidney transplantation in South Africa. *South African Medical Journal*, 109(4):235-240. https://doi.org/10.7196/SAMJ.2019.v109i4.13548

Mswela, M. 2017. Violent attacks against persons with albinism in South Africa: a human rights perspective. *African Human Rights Law Journal*, 17(1):114-133. https://doi.org/10.17159/1996-2096/2017/v17n1a6

Scheper-Hughes, N. 2011. Mr Tati's holiday and João's safari: seeing the world through transplant tourism. *Body & Society*, 17(2-3):55-92. https://doi.org/10.1177/1357034X11402858

Slabbert, M. 2018. The law as an obstacle in solid organ donations and transplantations. *Journal of Contemporary Roman-Dutch Law*, 18:70-84.

Slabbert, M. & Oosthuizen, H. 2007. Establishing a market for human organs in South Africa Part 2: shortcomings in legislation and the current system of human procurement. *Obiter*, 28(2):304-323.

Slabbert, M. & Oosthuizen, H. 2011. The payment for an organ and the admission of guilt by a South African hospital: *The State v Netcare Kwa-Zulu Natal (Pty) Ltd* – Agreement in terms of section 105A (1) of the Criminal Procedure Act 51 of 1977, Netcare Kwa-Zulu (Pty) Ltd and the State, Commercial Crime Court, Regional Court of Kwa-Zulu Natal, Durban – Case No. 41/1804/2010. *Obiter*, 32:740-746. https://bit.ly/3F1ZMDm

International Law

Declaration of Istanbul Custodian Group, to oversee the dissemination of the Declaration to governments and professional organisations.

Declaration of Istanbul on Organ Trafficking and Transplant Tourism. International Summit on Transplant Tourism and Organ Trafficking convened by The Transplantation Society and International Society of Nephrology in Istanbul, Turkey, 30 April through 2 May 2008.

Protocol against the Illicit Manufacturing of and Trafficking in Firearms, their Parts and Components and Ammunition was signed on 14 October 2002 and ratified on 20 February 2004.

Protocol against the Smuggling of Migrants by Land, Sea and Air on 14 December 2000 and ratified these on 20 February 2004.

Protocol to Prevent, Suppress and Punish Trafficking in Persons, especially Women and Children.

United Nations Convention against Transnational Organized Crime and the Protocols Thereto. Adopted by the UN General Assembly, 15 November 2000, by resolution 55/25.

United Nations Protocol to Prevent, Suppress and Punish trafficking in Persons, especially Women and Children, supplementing the United Nations Convention against Transnational Organized Crime (New York, 15 November 2000).

WHO Fortieth World Health Assembly. Developing Guiding Principles for Human Organ Transplants (Geneva, 4-15 May 1987). https://bit.ly/3Vf4enG

South African Legislation: Acts

Children's Act 38 of 2005.

Criminal Law Amendment Act 105 of 1997.

Criminal Procedure Act 51 of 1977.

Human Tissue Act 65 of 1983.

Mental Health Care Act 17 of 2002.

National Health Act 61 of 2003.

Prevention and Combating of Trafficking in Persons Act 7 of 2013.

Prevention of Organised Crime Act 121 of 1998.

Legislation: Regulations

National Health Act Regulations:

Government Gazette. 2012. Regulation Gazette No. 35099 of 2 March. Vol. 561 No. 9699.

South African Case Law

Robbs and Five Others v Deputy Director for Public Prosecutions, KZN (case number 13510) KwaZulu-Natal High Court, Durban (14 December 2012) (unreported judgment).

The Ethics of Mental Health Service Delivery in a Multicultural Setting

Johannes R (Hanru) Niemand

Keywords: cultural competence; culture; ethics; language; logic; multiculturalism; psychology; psychotherapy

8.1   INTRODUCTION

The problems posed by multiculturalism are typically encountered and discussed in the political sphere. However, the harm pertinent to multicultural situations is primarily psychological in nature (which in no way diminishes such harm) and the inequalities that authors such as Will Kymlicka (1989:175) highlight are the result of expending energy and resources to avoid psychological harm. As such, it would be worth investigating to what extent the political dilemmas of multiculturalism translate to obligations/responsibilities of practitioners, particularly in mental health service delivery. In this chapter we discuss some of these obligations, all of which can be summarised under the heading of cultural competence. Cultural competence, however, comes in many shapes and sizes. We will discuss cultural competence in terms of: (1) the obligations of larger structures, including policymakers, educators, and selectors to create structures for cultural equality; and (2) the obligations of practitioners and theorists to practice an approach characterised by (a) an awareness of the cultural conditioning involved in their existing models and (b) a willingness to understand models with different cultural origins as if from the inside, and not as so-called neutral observers. In this regard, we also pay special attention to criticisms aimed at the scientific method as practiced by mainstream or 'Western' psychology.

The various challenges will be discussed with reference only to the Rules of Conduct Pertaining Specifically to the Profession of Psychology, henceforth refer to as the Rules of Conduct (RSA DoH, 2004:15-47), but the pertinent sections are present in other codes as well, such as the Ethical guidelines for Good Practice in Health Care Professions (HPCSA, 2008).

8.2 DEFINITION OF CULTURE

To gain a conceptual grasp on the challenges of mental health in a multicultural setting, the concept of culture requires a sharper definition. Culture is defined here as a system that is constituted by the communicative relationships between people. Communicative relationships are therefore the elements of the cultural system. In turn, a communicative relationship between two people may simply be defined as the pattern of agreement and disagreement between them, or put differently, which meanings they share and which they do not. These communicative relationships shape the way people process meanings (and are in turn shaped by the meanings people continually process). Because they play a part in our processing of meaning, they are involved in how we fundamentally make sense of the world. They therefore make significant contributions to the norms and values we hold.

It is important to note that, so far, our definition of culture requires us to think of it as a broad and amorphous system that is shared (in principle) by all of humanity (and one could plausibly claim that there is strictly speaking only one 'culture' as opposed to various different 'cultures'). Conversely, the communicative relationships that any given person has been embedded in during his lifetime is unique to that person (so that one could plausibly claim that there are as many 'cultures' as there are people). This poses a problem, as it is exactly this idea of 'cultures' as discrete entities or groups of people that is referred to in the Rules of Conduct (RSA DoH, 2004:15-47).

This problem can be solved if we conceive of distinct cultures as being delineated by historical conflicts (Niemand, 2015:255).[1] In multicultural society, we see that the minority groups or, more pertinent to the South African context, previously disadvantaged groups, ceded their sovereignty involuntarily, through conquest or colonisation. These conflicts create a delineation between the conquerors and the conquered, so that a definition of the group can take the form of 'those people who were forced to cede sovereignty' in various conflicts, avoiding formulations

---

[1]   The notion of delineation through conflict relies to some extent on Henri Tajfel's Social Identity Theory, which has considerable empirical, experimental support (Tajfel, Billig, Bundy & Flament, 1971:149; Diehl, 1990:263, 292; Tajfel, 1982:39).

that require that they share certain characteristics. In this regard, one can also think of various 'colonisations' and conquests, a group need not have been involved in only one conflict and could also have been the conqueror in some of them.

The *internal* disunities between the group's members prior to that moment of conflict do not disappear but are moved thoroughly to the background. One could compare this to the respective supporters of two opposing *provincial* sport teams defining themselves in terms of their common *national* team when the contest is with an international competitor. Furthermore, unlike the sports allegory we just used, societal conflicts have long-term or even permanent effects when they continue to maintain the conquered group's marginalisation, thereby arresting an otherwise fluid and dynamic group identification. As such, defining cultures in terms of historical conflicts allows delineation of the culture without needing to claim a common essence that characterises the whole culture or all of its members.

Assuming such homogeneity is, of course, inaccurate. A wide variety of different beliefs, values, and practices may occur inside a so-called culture. Nevertheless, the delineation via historical conflict allows one to think of cultural differences as occurring where two people or two parties differ; where the difference appears to be related to the different communicative relationships they have been imbedded in, and the difference is characterised by originating from opposing sides of a historical conflict to which cultural difference is a shorthand reference.

8.3 MULTICULTURAL ISSUES

The aforementioned conflicts also plot the landscape of what we would refer to as multicultural or intercultural issues. The first relates to multicultural or inter-cultural inequalities. These issues can be characterised by concerns or conflicts about the fair distribution of goods. Where the members of the dominant culture can pursue their goals without needing to expend any energy or resources to maintain that culture, members of a previously disadvantaged culture have to expend effort and resources to maintain their culture, leaving them little energy or few resources to pursue the life goals they would want to (cf. Kymlicka, 1989:189). They are thus disadvantaged, not as a result of their choices, but as a result of something they had no control over, e.g., having been born into that culture. Furthermore, if members from a previously disadvantaged culture then choose to relinquish their culture, and assimilate into the dominant culture, this comes at an expense, at least of energy and resources and at worst at the loss of an important attachment, as Kymlicka argues (1989:175). The examples we discuss below of what we term 'simple multicultural issues' mainly pertain to addressing these inequalities.

A second pertinent aspect of multicultural issues relates to the imposition of Western values or norms onto other cultures. In political matters, this leads to particularly tricky dilemmas, due to the question whether the liberal response to cultural differences may in itself represent Western norms that are unfairly applied to other cultures. Accordingly, the neutrality of the public sphere becomes a problematic notion in multicultural affairs (Niemand, 2013:23-32).

In the field of mental health, the problem is not so much with classical liberal ideas such as those pertaining to tolerance, procedural rights, and autonomy. Rather, the imposition would be in the form of Western theories imposing their world view on patients from other cultures. Psychology as a discipline fundamentally deals with meanings. All the phenomena we usually term 'psychological' can be understood in terms of meaning. For instance, all our thoughts about the world carry with them the relevance these facts may have in our lives. The same is true of our experience of emotions. Emotions are always already *interpreted* emotion. If not, they are merely instinctive, bodily reactions. Furthermore, emotions serve to orientate us in the world, they prime us for what we need to do next and as such, they are answers to the question of meaning (Niemand, 2013:84). In dealing with meanings, as opposed to objective fact (in as much as that is ever possible), psychological theories would always reflect, or be suspected of reflecting, the cultural background or their authors'. As such, they may not be applicable to people of other cultures.

One may object that this may not represent such a tricky dilemma. One can for instance say: "let us be careful to validate our theories on other cultures before we assume them to be universally valid." However, the problem potentially runs deeper. Some critics we discuss below even reject the very method of studying psychological phenomena, including such fundamental notions as requiring theories to be based on empirical evidence and avoiding metaphysical explanations for (psychological) phenomena. With these criticisms, we arrive at an impasse similar to the ones we encounter in political matters.

It is important to note that in these multicultural issues, some values, beliefs, principles, and practices two parties may disagree on are so basic that they are to be considered *axiomatic*. They cannot be proven by reason or science, because they are the suppositions from which we reason and that underlie our scientific endeavours. They themselves cannot be proven; we can only believe in them. This means that any two people could have been embedded in communicative relationships that are so different that they have differences that are axiomatic and upon which they cannot agree, despite their utmost willingness and ability to reason.

In this regard, the challenges we outline below may be divided into two types of problems. The first we will call simple multicultural challenges, which do not pose difficult theoretical conundrums and do not represent any real clash between different sets of values. Rather, the differences at play represent the unfamiliarity that different cultures may have with regard to each other. Furthermore, they may also pertain to certain intercultural inequalities, created by the historical conflicts that simultaneously served to delineate the cultures in question. Though these problems may not involve insurmountable or axiomatic differences, they are nonetheless very important to address. They set goals that may be very difficult to achieve practically and would also require the political will to take multiculturalism seriously.

The second type of problem we will call complex multicultural problems. In these cases, axiomatic differences may be at play, where no neutral Archimedean point is possible. We will address these below.

We discuss these different types of problems with reference to the Rules of Conduct (RSA DoH, 2004:15-47). Furthermore, the rules we discuss may all be regarded as extensions of a master requirement, in Rule 12 (RSA DoH, 2004:20), that prohibits unfair discrimination based on race, gender, and religious belief. Discrimination based on cultural beliefs is also not allowed and the practitioner may not force his opinions/beliefs on the patient.

8.3.1 Language and multiculturalism

According to rule 9 of the Rules of Conduct (RSA DoH, 2004:18), practitioners are to make sure that, where language is an issue, suitable interpreters are used. These should be suitably qualified, maintain confidentiality, and should not be in multiple relationships with the patient. The content of this rule does not appear problematic at first glance. However, it glosses over an important challenge for intercultural fairness we face due to the linguistic landscape of the country. We face an important question: how do we assure non-discrimination based on linguistic background in the delivery of mental health services? Rule 9 stipulates requirements for the use of interpreters, but anyone who has ever been in a psychotherapy session requiring an interpreter would attest to the extreme frustration involved in the process. Sessions such as these are at best suboptimal in quality. In this regard, the more general stipulation in rule 12(3) (RSA DoH, 2004:20), which requires appropriate services to be made available and appropriate standards of language proficiency to be met, is more suitable.

Psychotherapy requires a human response when revealing, for example, an intimate fear. Revealing an intimate fear and then having to wait to see your therapist's response, diminishes the human quality of the interaction.[2] Building rapport and containing emotions require interaction, uninterrupted, even when some pauses may be tense.

The optimal solution to the challenges posed by the reality of language differences in South Africa lies with greater linguistic competence among mental health practitioners. We need therapists who can speak to their patients in their mother tongue, be able to do so fluently, and be able to convey sometimes quite complex ideas in that language. While some patients may be able to express themselves in their second language, nevertheless, one's most intimate thoughts and feelings often require the safety of one's mother tongue.

In this context, therapists who are practically monolingual are simply not acceptable. This would mean that the roughly 10% of English mother tongue speakers in the country have full access to therapy in their first language, while the remainder of the population, the majority of which would be considered previously disadvantaged, do not. This situation clearly represents an unfair distribution of goods, and the skew distribution is based entirely on the language group a person has been born into. This clearly does not pass the test of non-discrimination. Accordingly, the selection of monolingual therapists is already an act of discrimination perpetrated by selection panels. Conversely, bilingual or multilingual abilities should be considered an *operational requirement*, not just a nice-to-have. Likewise, therapists posted in areas where the population is predominantly non-English speaking should be required to be fluent in at least the dominant language of that region. Moreover, if certain linguistic groups are found to be underrepresented in the pool from which selected, progressive steps need to be taken to correct the under-representation.

8.4   CULTURALLY FAIR ASSESSMENTS

Next, we turn to rule 48 (RSA DoH, 2004:31). This rule pertains to the administration of culturally fair assessments. Practitioners are to make sure that assessment methods are valid and reliable for the designated population and should make sure that the assessments used are culturally fair. As with the case of language differences discussed above, the contravention of this rule is a clear case of discrimination and poses no theoretical dilemma.

---

2   Many people have by now experienced something similar to this due to the Covid-19 pandemic and concomitant lockdown regulations, where psychotherapy sessions are conducted online with poor Wi-Fi connections. The same lack of fluency described above applies here.

Accordingly, personality tests should at least be validated on local populations. Ideally, local personality tests should be developed from the ground up using local data (as opposed to using international, possibly Western concepts and dichotomies that may not apply to the local populations.) In this regard, recent developments in the South African Personality Inventory are promising, but also indicate that full cultural validation has not yet been achieved (Hill, Hlahleni & Legodi, 2021).

Aptitude and cognitive tests should naturally be available in all local languages. Moreover, certain items and subtests of existing tests can be considered unfair as they rely on background knowledge a person not born into Western culture may not have. The true aim of these assessments should be to assess intellectual capacity, not cultural knowledge. Intellectual capacity, in turn, should be thought of as the ability to master cognitive tasks on exposure to them. Maintaining a cultural disadvantage would have the effect of excluding intellectual gifted, potentially good candidates from competition for no reason other than the cultural group they were born into. This is the opposite of meritocracy and clearly a form of discrimination. In this regard, learning potential assessments such as the APIL ([Conceptual] Ability, Processing of Information, and Learning), TRAM-2 and TRAM-1 (Transfer, Automatisation, and Memory) appear to hold promise in that they purposefully avoid measuring already acquired knowledge, which may be cultural in origin (Taylor, 2013:166-168).

While the challenges outlined above do not pose particularly thorny theoretical dilemmas, they nonetheless pose practical challenges. Consequently, because they are difficult to achieve in practice, they result in dilemmas on ground level. How does one, for instance, do an assessment if, perhaps due to lack of resources, the required culture fair assessment is not available, or the necessary linguistic capacities are not present? In the case of assessments, one may consider not administering the assessment at all, as the results may simply not be valid. In contrast, practising psychotherapy in suboptimal linguistic conditions may be necessary. In this regard, one may spare a thought for the under-resourced practitioner, who, most often through no fault of their own, may be required to render suboptimal services. The true failing in such cases lie not with the practitioner, but with the larger structures that shape mental health service delivery in South Africa.

8.5   DIAGNOSIS

Diagnosis is complex in multicultural environments due to the fact that the practitioner must be able to discern between (a) universal pathology that is just expressed differently – e.g., somatisation of depression in certain societies (cf.

Swartz, 1998:121-139), (b) culture specific illnesses, and (c) normal cultural practices. Of course, the correct diagnosis has a very important bearing on treatment. Moreover, especially in serious cases, the practitioner's assessment can lead to suspend the person's right to autonomy (e.g., in cases of involuntary admission), which the practitioner will need to justify.

Now, part of the problem is already adequately covered by the Rules of Conduct's prescription against cultural discrimination (RSA DoH, 2004:20) and training on cultural illnesses is already part of most curricula. However, this does not yet go far enough. Recall from our earlier definition of culture that it resists any essentialist definitions. This means that our competence needs to be practised in *particular cases*. The practitioner can expand his ability with knowledge from comparative studies, but, crucially, these rely on the construct of 'cultures' that does not do justice to the full diversity one might possibly find in practice. This requires one to choose a *hermeneutical approach* as supplement to one's existing knowledge. This means that one has to justify one's diagnosis based on existing knowledge and supplement it with considering what the symptoms/signs would *mean* for this *particular* person, within his/her *particular* background.

8.6   BEST PRACTICE

Where the previous rules we discussed may by typified as simple (but nonetheless challenging) multicultural problems, the issue of best practice has aspects to it that are decidedly complex. Where issues around diagnosis may still be regarded as simple (but difficult) problems, requiring great competence in cultural matters, the questions around treatment introduce some complex issues.

The concept of best practice has been intimately connected with evidence-based treatment and more specifically to quantitative empirical studies. What complicates the matter is the centrality of meaning in psychology, as discussed above. While other fields medicine can agree on, for instance, a virus under the microscope, even while justifiably situating their fields within biopsychosocial model, the problem to be addressed in psychotherapy cannot be conceptualised at all without reference to some idea of the good life or some orientations to the world. Moreover, the value system thus constituted to understand and address problems in psychology is culturally conditioned. It has been arrived at via the communicative relationships within which the authors of the various theories are situated. Likewise, within any practitioner's cultural framework, their clinical judgement about whether some behaviour is interpretable, that is, whether it constitutes a sign of some underlying pathology, may be culturally conditioned.

What is considered assertive from one vantage point may be considered aggressive, even anti-social, from another. Even fundamental concepts, like psyche, are not free from cultural conditioning. For instance, Baloyi and Ramose (2016) argue for the use of the term *moya* instead of *psyche* when creating African theories of psychology. They also show convincingly what is lost in translation between the two terms.

What is the psychological damage caused by being incorrectly pathologised? Incorrect judgements such as these can most accurately be understood as a form of violence because they are not supported by evidence and reason, but represent the suppositions from which evidence was gathered, and from which deductions and inferences are made. They are judgements that therefore are not strictly speaking rational, that need to be *enforced* either by convention, tradition, or the authority bestowed upon a medical professional. Furthermore, it goes without saying that patients in a mental health service setting tend to be emotionally vulnerable and a message conveying that certain thoughts and behaviours are signs of insanity (to put it harshly) – while they themselves have not been convinced properly of this judgement – can cause considerable emotional distress and may have a lasting impact on their self-image. Given the power dynamic between a professional and lay person, a professional opinion may be especially damaging, as it tends to be harder to shrug off as 'just someone's opinion'.

It is for this reason that the inappropriate application of Western concepts may be regarded as offensive. Moreover, one should be wary of generalising from gold-standard treatment efficacy studies. They still only present evidence that a certain treatment does well on average, compared either to other treatments or to placebos. It simply does not follow that such treatments are universally applicable to all mental health patients in all situations.

Once again, as with linguistic capacity and culturally fair assessments, practitioners can become more skilled in adopting an approach in which they collaborate with their patients and humbly gain understanding from an initial point of ignorance, instead of going in guns blazing, armed with their existing conceptual framework. Yet, the aforementioned ignorance can of course never be a blank slate. Practitioners have been trained in models that explain, at least to some extent, human behaviour and psychopathology. In this regard, the skill required would involve being well versed in as many models as possible (for no model offers a complete understanding of the human condition) and to be open to the possibility that the patient may introduce new perspectives that may require the practitioner to adapt and/or refute some of their current understandings of psychology.

It is worth noting that not all psychotherapy necessarily requires confrontations about conceptual *content*. On the contrary, many psychotherapy approaches can be of great benefit in addressing the problems with *form* of thought, such as over-generalisations, attribution errors, miscounting positive evidence, etc. Further-more, many behavioural approaches also aim to address operant and classical conditioning that led to distress or psychopathology, and therefore avoid to a large extent the biases associated with ideas, beliefs, values, and norms that could be culturally conditioned. Therefore, in practice, cross cultural psychotherapy is less of an intercultural conflict than one might expect, notwithstanding that there are pitfalls that are to be avoided, as discussed above.

A theoretically interesting, but perhaps practically less pertinent question, is whether the openness and collaborative approach required from a practitioner in a multicultural setting itself represents a Western norm that is being imposed on patients from other cultures. We would argue that, if it is indeed Western in origin, it nevertheless does not represent an imposition. A value like openness, when practised in a situation, may threaten other values, but has the benefit of doing so not by use of force, but by being convincing. It therefore represents an exit possibility. An exit possibility in multicultural settings refers to arranging the situation in such a way that members of a cultural group can freely relinquish a cultural value, so that, if they continue to adhere to that value, they do so not due to force, but due to conviction (Niemand, 2013:191). Put differently, being exposed to openness does not force anyone to become a convert to Western values.

Perhaps a more difficult problem arises when critics of Western psychology take issue with the scientific method it uses in studying psychological phenomena. Nwoye (2015) for instance, takes issue with Western psychology's insistence on using only empirical evidence in its theories. Likewise, she argues that the Aristotelian logic typically employed in Western thought, where a statement is either true or false, with no third option, excludes other possible logics, where contradictions are more acceptable. She argues that "under the Aristotelian binary logic of the excluded middle, one is either tall or short; and not tall AND short at the same time" and that "we can call somebody 'mom' even-though she is not directly our mom but is related to our mom or plays the role of mom in our lives" (Nwoye, 2015:108). Similarly, Adésínà (2002) argues for the use of Ti'bi-t'ire logic, where contradictory forces are allowed to cohere and where these are understood to already have their contradictions embedded in them.

If these criticisms hold, they represent a deeper problem than merely navigating different conceptual frameworks. Rather, they would explode any notion of common preconceptions and rules of engagement by which consensus about an argument or a state of affairs may be achieved. We do not, however, think these criticisms are fully tenable. Firstly, the inclusion of evidence other than empirical evidence is problematic. We would agree that metaphysics may be valuable, perhaps even indispensable in providing *meaning* to phenomena, and as such, *understanding* a patient may very well require one to understand their metaphysical framework. However, when *researchers* use metaphysics to *explain* behaviour or other psychological phenomena (e.g., "this mystical force caused him to do x"), it becomes problematic. What happens in a case where two people do not share the same metaphysical conceptions? Can only researchers who share the metaphysics of those they study be engaged in a psychology of those people? If so, to what extent can one still call it science? We would argue that the possibility of criticism and refutation is central to the scientific endeavour, and as such, being able to confirm or disconfirm something is crucial to the scientific process. Likewise, theory must go further than tradition – as valuable as tradition may be in terms of providing insight into the human condition – in that it should be able to revise, question, and even refute some of what is held in that tradition.

As is often the case with multicultural matters, the manner or process in which something is refuted is important. For instance, the Freudian approach to religions[3] is condescending and offensive, mainly because it does not take religion seriously *ab initio* and consequently forces its concepts onto something that is not understood from the inside. This is similar to an anthropologist simply judging a different society from their own colonial perspective. In contrast, when the revision comes from *within* the perspective of another culture, taking experiences and concepts seriously and then proceeding from there, the revisions are less easily dismissed as condescending and arrogant.

We therefore hold that psychologists and theorists in the field should not be dismissive of others' beliefs. Moreover, these beliefs should not be rejected as irrational and indiscriminately (and often condescendingly) be reduced to materialist explanations. However, one can take such beliefs seriously *and* study empirically the results of those beliefs among people. Put differently, while the objects of belief may not be accessible to empirical study, these beliefs are held by certain people and the role those beliefs play, among other things in providing meaning to those who hold them, are phenomena that are empirically observable. Furthermore, given the cultural conditioning inherent in psychological theorising and the clear overrepresentation of European and Anglo-American theorists in

---

3   In these examples, religion is also considered cultural. This does not represent a
     reductionist view of religion. However, the aspect of religion pertinent to a conflict is
     that which it shares with culture. In this regard, it is a system of beliefs and concepts
     that to some extent demands collective observance and action (Niemand, 2013:13).

mainstream curricula, calls for representation of a wider variety of theorists are clearly justified.

The second type of criticism, aimed at Aristotelian logic, is not tenable. Firstly, the examples Nwoye (2015) mentions do not pose a serious challenge to the excluded middle, as is alleged. To say that John is tall (with the added context: "for a 9-year-old") and saying John is not tall (with the added context: "for a rugby player") clearly does not constitute a contradiction and in a real-world situation, the context would clearly be added if one ever needed to *argue from that premise*. Likewise, that somebody can be both a mother and an aunt to the same person can easily be non-contradictory, if one admits varying definitions of motherhood. If the definition is stricter, e.g., the person who was pregnant with you and who raised you after birth, the aunt is clearly excluded. Furthermore, in cases where a continuum between two poles exists, another logic complementary to Aristotelian logic (e.g., fuzzy logic) exists and implicitly assumes that contradiction is not allowed (cf. Pelletier, 2004). If contradictions were allowed, it would render the logic worthless, as one would not be able to move forward and make inferences from premises, given that any conclusion, even a flat-out contradiction, is permitted. In making an argument with concepts that have degrees, one would, for instance, need to be able to say definitively that x is taller than y.

Furthermore, Adésínà (2002), in arguing for the use of Ti'bi-t'ire logic, where contradictions cohere and statements have their opposites embedded in them, then goes to great lengths to position this type of logic as the opposite of Aristotelian logic, the former being valid while the latter is not. This of course at once confirms and refutes his argument. However, we would argue that the opposition of the two (and the paradox it creates) is already unnecessary. The two modes of thinking are clearly complementary, and the full weight and clarity of insight gained by understanding how contradictory concepts are embedded in each other is only fully understood on the basis of understanding their binary opposition.

In other examples of logics that permit other options beyond a statement being true or false, such as the tetralemma in Buddhist thought, the concepts involved all aim to denote the ineffable, a limit of thought as it were.[4] These concepts are perhaps best elucidated by poetry, symbolism and/or ritual, and the result of engagement in these activities is not *knowledge* but *meaning*. In sum, for all except the ineffable concepts, rules exist to which all interlocutors can agree,

---

4   Being confronted with a limit of thought may in turn be very valuable in psychotherapy. It may for instance, signify that the patient is asking the wrong type of questions, barking up the wrong tree, so to speak. It is useful in this manner precisely because it does not permit an argument to proceed from there onwards.

and those from different cultural background need not withdraw themselves into windowless monads from which no dialogue is possible. The aim of such a dialogue would indeed be to widen the array of perspectives involved in our growing understanding of psychological phenomena. The criticisms often laid against Western perspectives, e.g., that they are not holistic enough or that they do not give enough weight to context (Nwoye, 2015), should all be taken seriously and should be addressed by gathering evidence from a wider variety of sources and making sound inferences from these findings, not by discarding logic and evidence in one fell swoop.

The possibility of *dialogue* has interesting implications for psychotherapy in a multicultural situation. Given that dialogue does not equate with either a mere repetition of traditional understanding, or a simple imposition of existing models on new phenomena and given that any meaningful dialogue (with the possibility of transcending existing understandings of phenomena) would always require some difference in perspectives, we suggest that a true blank slate for practitioners is not simply unattainable, but a logical impossibility. Some threat to the patient's cultural perspective is always present. Unlike the case of simple multicultural problems, which at least have a more or less objective end state to be striven for, which is at least achievable in theory, the dilemma attached to best practice does not have a satisfactory end state. Instead of being obligated to solve this problem, the obligation that rests with practitioners lies in their attitude, in the manner in which they approach these matters.

8.6.1 Children: An added complication

The case of treatment for children adds further complexity to the above dilemma. In the case of treatment for adults, their consent acts as a type of escape from what the patient may perceive as a discriminatory or offensive practice. This means that continuing something like psychotherapy is also tacit consent for the difficult process of putting one's cultural framework – indeed many of one's central meanings – on the table, with the risk of having to let go of some of it. However, as we argued above, the therapeutic setting does represent an imbalance of power and as such consent is not always as perfectly free as one would like. Evening out this power balance requires some innovative thinking. Perhaps one option would be to have more traditional options available to the patient, to which they can escape without foregoing treatment altogether.

However difficult it would be to achieve a free consent with an adult patient, the case becomes markedly more difficult with children. In cases with minors, their assent is sought, as well as the consent of the parents, and yet South African law requires practitioners to act in the best interest of the child and not allow cultural norms to interfere with what would be the best interest (RSA, 2005). How would the best interest be determined? By existing scientific knowledge. And so, we return to the above dilemma, only this time, parents would not technically be able to withdraw their consent if, e.g., non-treatment is not in the best interest of the child.

8.7   PROCESS MODEL OF JUSTIFICATION

The great difficulty with a multicultural setting is that it casts profound doubt on any form of alleged neutral or objective judgement, especially in matters where meaning is involved. As argued above, practitioners and theorists may not be able to achieve such neutrality in mental health service delivery. Instead, they would have to justify their judgement on the process by which they arrived at it. How would such a process look? The practitioner/theorist would need to display self-reflectivity: they would need to show that they have reflected on their own background and how it may colour their perceptions of a case. They would also need to try actively to understand the other culture's values from *within* and not as if they are a neutral observer, studying rituals in a far-off tribe as if it were a lab experiment. If the practitioner then, after this process of self-reference, still holds their view, it has the character of an authentic decision: they have not followed their cultural background blindly, but have argued from axiomatic fundamentals, knowing that they could be wrong, but believing, as a leap of faith, that they hold those fundamentals true not because they were culturally socialised into it, but because it does in fact represent a valuable idea.

While not escaping the charges of discrimination, decisions that have a self-referential quality serve to diminish the offence. Where enforcing one's culture on others implies an arrogant approach, which constitutes most of the offence caused by ethnocentrism, self-referential decisions represent an authentic response. We would argue that this serves to draw attention away from a response's cultural origin and may instead draw attention to the claim regarding the value of an idea, regardless of its cultural origin. This is the basis upon which dialogue can continue with the aim of a mutual understanding. One may point out, of course, that this process could also be construed as carrying certain values/norms. This is a valid point. We would point out, however, that rejecting it simply due to its origin does very little to advance dialogue. One may, of course, reject it on other grounds, which would be a very valuable conversation in search of the optimal way to deal with differences in norms. However, such criticism would be aimed at the ideas, not their origin.

8.8 CONCLUSION

In this chapter, we have set out some of the obligations of institutions like the Department of Health, training institutions, selection panels, as well as the obligations of practitioners and academics. The progressive equality to be striven for, particularly by larger structures, represents a solution to simple (but practically difficult to achieve) multicultural problems. In contrast, the freedom from bias that is to be achieved, particularly by practitioners and academics, is a logical impossibility. The obligation that rests with practitioners and academics lies in their attitude, in the process in which they approach these matters.

In both the simple and complex cases, what lies at the heart of cultural competence is a healthy doubt, by politicians, academics, and practitioners alike, of anything that appears to be neutral. It is through this healthy doubt that dialogue becomes possible and a retreat to impenetrable laagers avoided.

Bibliography

Adésínà, J.O. 2002. Sociology and Yorùbá studies: epistemic intervention or doing sociologyin the 'vernacular'? *African Sociological Review*, 6(1):91-114. https://doi.org/10.4314/asr.v6i1.23204

Baloyi, L. & Ramose, M. 2016. Psychology and psychotherapy redefined from the viewpoint of the African experience. *Alternation Journal*, 18:12-35. https://bit.ly/3Vjsgh8

Diehl, M. 1990. The minimal group paradigm: theoretical explanations and empirical findings. *European Review of Social Psychology*, 1:263-292. https://doi.org/10.1080/14792779108401864

Hill, C., Hlahleni, M. & Legodi, L. 2021. Validating indigenous versions of the South African Personality Inventory. *Frontiers in Psychology*, 20 May:1-13. https://doi.org/10.3389/fpsyg.2021.556565

HPCSA (Health Professions Council of South Africa). 2008. *Ethical guidelines for good practice in the health care professions*. Pretoria: HPCSA. https://bit.ly/3U2M0V2 [Accessed 5 May 2022].

Kymlicka, W. 1989. *Liberalism, community and culture*. Oxford: Clarendon Press.

Niemand, J.R. 2013. The autonomy of culture: a cultural-philosophical analysis. PhD thesis. Stellenbosch: Stellenbosch University.

Niemand, J.R. 2015. 'Cultures' and cultural protection. *Human Affairs*, 25:251-260. https://doi.org/10.1515/humaff-2015-0021

Nwoye, A. 2015. What is African Psychology the psychology of? *Theory & Psychology*, 25(1):96-116. https://doi.org/10.1177/0959354314565116

Pelletier, F.J. 2004. On some alleged misconceptions about fuzzy logic. *Artificial Intelligence Review*, 22:71-82. https://doi.org/10.1023/B:AIRE.0000044308.48654.c1

RSA (Republic of South Africa). 1996. *Constitution of the Republic of South Africa*. Pretoria: Government Printing Works.

RSA (Republic of South Africa). 2005. *Children's Act 38 of 2005*. Pretoria: Government Printing Works.

RSA DoH (Republic of South Africa. Department of Health). 2006. Rules of conduct pertaining specifically to the profession of psychology. *Government Gazette*, No. 29079 of 4 August. https://bit.ly/3ia2ihW

Swartz, L. 1998. *Culture and mental health: A southern African view*. Oxford: Oxford University Press. https://doi.org/10.4102/hsag.v4i1.7

Tajfel, H. 1982. Social psychology of intergroup relations. *Annual Review of Social Psychology*, 33:1-39. https://doi.org/10.1146/annurev.ps.33.020182.000245

Tajfel, H., Billig, M., Bundy, R.P. & Flament, C. 1971. Social categorisation and intergroup behaviour. *European Journal of Social Psychology*, 1:149-177. https://doi.org/10.1002/ejsp.2420010202

Taylor, T. 2013. APIL and TRAM learning potential assessment instruments. In: S. Laher, K. Cockcroft, Z. Amod, K. Bain, F. Bhabha, M. Brink, et al. *Psychological assessment in South Africa: research and applications*. Johannesburg: Wits University Press. 158-168. https://doi.org/10.18772/22013015782.16

9

Towards a More Globally Inclusive and Relevant Neuroethics

Considerations for developing the field in Africa

Andrea Palk

Keywords: equity; ethics of neuroscience; global mental health; inclusivity; neuroethics; neuroethics activism; neuroethics in Africa; neuroscience of ethics; solidarity

9.1 INTRODUCTION

Neuroethics is an interdisciplinary field, encompassing the full array of ethical, legal, and social implications (ELSI) of our study, understanding and deepening knowledge of the human brain, as afforded by the neurosciences, including our ability to increasingly and potentially alter or enhance our brains, by way of neurotechnologies. Neuroethics, as a distinct field of focus, originated in 2002 following various conferences held in the United States and Canada, all of which focused explicitly on the ELSI of developments in neuroscience.[1] These developments, and increased ethical interest, followed progress made during the 'decade of the Brain' in the 1990s, a movement initiated by the Library of Congress and the National Institute of Mental Health in the United States, and subsequently embraced across the globe (Buniak, Darragh & Giordano, 2014; Tandon, 2000). The aim of declaring the decade of the brain was twofold: to provide more impetus and funding for research of the neurobiological basis of

---

1   Most notedly, the Dana Foundation's (2002) *Mapping of the Field* conference which included many of the thinkers who have subsequently become renowned in the field. For more information about the participants in this conference see: https://www.dana. org/article/neuroethics-mapping-the-field/

various disorders, with implications for improved treatment, and to improve public understanding of the human brain.[2] The scope of the field of neuroethics has grown significantly in subsequent decades, as neuroscience itself advances, and increasingly includes non-medical applications, as well as more philosophical and speculative areas of interest.

While the field of neuroethics is broad in scope, its conceptualisation and domi-nant areas of interest have been largely shaped by the input of those situated in high income countries (HICs), with less participation from ethicists working in low-resourced contexts (Lombera & Illes, 2009). In particular, participation of African scientists and ethicists in neuroethics discussions has been lacking, although this seems to be gradually changing, given recent contributions.[3] There are various possible reasons for these low levels of participation, but it is likely due, in part, to the specialised nature of the field, coupled with the fact that there are fewer trained bioethicists in resource strained contexts, like Africa (Andoh, 2013). It may also be that some of the concerns that have dominated the field of neuroethics are regarded as less pressing in contexts where neuroscience is not established to the extent that it is in HICs (Maina et al., 2021), or where more urgent concerns compete for ethicists' attention. Given that neuroethics responds to developments in neuroscience, it is likely that interest will grow as neuroscience becomes more established in African contexts.

The reasons for this underrepresentation aside, it has been argued that the field of neuroethics suffers from a lack of global diversity (Buller, 2020; Matshabane, 2021) and that a "more inclusive ... 'cross cultural', 'global' or 'international' neuroethics is needed" (Lanzilao et al., 2013; Salles, Herrera-Ferra & Cabeta, 2018). However, it is not self-evident what would constitute a more globally inclusive and diverse neuroethics, or what would suffice as having made inroads in this regard (Lanzilao et al., 2013; Salles et al., 2018). At the very least, it would firstly necessitate more equitable participation and collaboration between scientists and neuroethicists from different contexts, thereby ensuring that the

---

2   This focus has continued in the United States with the establishing of the National Institute of Health's Brain Initiative in 2013, which includes a neuroethics working group. The International Brain Initiative (IBI) was formed in 2017 and includes members from Japan, China, Korea, Europe, the US, Canada and Australia. The IBI also includes a neuroethics working group.

3   See various chapters in the recent volume *Global Mental Health and Neuroethics* (Stein & Singh, 2020) and Cordeiro-Rodrigues and Ewuoso (2021) which explores an *Afro-Communitarian Relational Approach to Brain Surrogates Research*. There is also a strong interest in the philosophical and ethical implications of cognitive enhancement in South Africa, for example, see Beyer, Staunton and Moodley (2014), and Verster and Van Niekerk (2012).

field considers an array of perspectives, methodologies, and concerns. Secondly, it would also likely entail paying more attention from an ethical perspective to gaps in the availability of neuroscience technologies, resources, and research capabilities between HICs and low-resourced countries, and the medical and scientific priorities pertaining to brain and mental health in these latter contexts. Thirdly, an evidence-base can be built comprising the perspectives of underrepresented populations on established neuroethics concerns, so that findings applicable to HICs are not erroneously generalised to other contexts. Fourthly, there is also the more ambitious task of reconfiguring the normative foundations, or underlying moral framework of the field, to encompass a more global focus and relevance (Shook & Giordano, 2014). These are just four potential ways in which the field of neuroethics stands to be enriched and diversified that will be considered in the second half of this chapter, but there are likely to be many more options.

In light of these observations, the point of departure in this chapter is that there is a need to critically engage with neuroethics, with the aim of working towards a field that is more globally informed and inclusive of a range of concerns and perspectives. Given that neuroethics is not well established in South Africa, in the first half of this chapter I provide an overview of the field, including an outline of its traditional conceptualisation, with examples of the areas in neuroscience that are typically identified as ethically concerning or interesting.[4] In the second half of the chapter, based on the four possibilities mentioned above, I provide four suggestions for developing the field in African contexts, thus working towards increasing its global relevance. My suggestions include: building neuroethics capacity through the growth of neuroscience research collaborations across the African continent; exploring congruence with the global mental health movement to engage in neuroethics activism to address brain and mental health research and treatment priorities in Africa; drawing on the strong tradition of empirical ethics research on the continent to establish an evidence-base comprising the perspectives of underrepresented populations on established neuroethics concerns; and finally, engaging with the underlying moral framework of neuroethics by drawing on African moral frameworks.

While developing neuroethics in Africa will benefit those who are impacted by its reach in African contexts, the field itself also stands to benefit, insofar as it is recognised that any field or area of focus is improved by including a plurality of perspectives, concerns, and input.

---

4   Given the vast terrain of the field of neuroethics, I will not attempt to be exhaustive in this overview.

9.2   DEFINING THE FOCUS OF THE FIELD

While there are various definitions that may give us an idea of the focus and scope of neuroethics, one has been particularly influential. Based, in part, on the input of participants in attendance at one of the seminal conferences which marked the formal start of the field of neuroethics in 2002, Adina Roskies offered two distinct areas of focus the field should concern itself with: "the ethics of neuroscience" and "the neuroscience of ethics" (2002). This clever distinction has largely informed the conceptualisation of the field going forward and will be discussed next.[5]

9.2.1   The ethics of neuroscience

The ethics of neuroscience encompasses two subdivisions. The first focuses on the ethical concerns associated with neuroscience-related research, or more specifically, ethical research design of studies of the brain, including translational and clinical studies. This includes a focus on cross-cutting ethical issues such as minimising risk for research participants, feedback of incidental findings (Illes et al., 2006), ensuring the privacy of participants in the context of data sharing, given the sensitivity of information about the brain (Fothergill et al., 2019; White, Blok & Calhoun, 2022), and challenges with securing informed consent, particularly in cases where participants may have impaired decisional capacity due to neuropsychiatric disorders (Vaishnav & Chiong, 2018), among others. In this area there is much overlap with traditional research ethics, and in particular, with the ethics of genetic studies (Tairyan & Illes, 2009). This practically-oriented domain of neuroethics also includes ethical issues arising from clinical care and practice in the fields of neurology, neurosurgery, psychiatry, and their paediatric specialisations (Chatterjee & Farah, 2013).

The second subdivision of the ethics of neuroscience is vast in its scope and focuses on the ELSI of the findings and applications of neuroscience-related

---

5   While this distinction has been extremely influential, it should not be taken as implying that these two areas bear no impact on each other, or that one is descriptive whilst the other is normative (Shook & Giordano, 2014). In fact, there is much interplay between the two domains and the belief in a 'purely descriptive' neuroscience of ethics vs a normative ethics of neuroscience belies the fact the normative underpinnings of the former are simply better hidden, but nevertheless reflect a particular perspective on morality (Shook & Giordano, 2014). As posited by Shook and Giordano, even the assumption that neuroscience can inform or alter our self-understanding is a normative one.

research and neurotechnologies.[6] There is consensus that this area of neuroethics elicits unique ethical concerns due to the inextricable relationship between the mind and the brain,[7] so that information about the brain tends to deeply impact our sense of self, and concomitantly, our conceptions of identity, personhood, and agency, with various implications. One of these implications is a more "mechanistic understanding of brain function" and the self (Roskies, 2002:21). In this regard, there is a strong focus on the communication and interpretation of information about the human brain in public contexts and the way in which this increased knowledge could, and should, impact our social and legal institutions (Illes & Racine, 2005).[8] To ascertain how information about the brain is interpreted by laypersons, this area of the ethics of neuroscience includes an emphasis on the importance of qualitative studies, also known as empirical ethics, to investigate the interpretations and views of populations in different socio-cultural contexts with implications for health outcomes and addressing stigma, among others. It is not only the implications of public interpretations – and misinterpretations – of this increasingly sensitive and improved knowledge of the brain that is a topic of focus, but also the uses this knowledge could be put to that is of ethical interest. In what follows, I provide a few examples of the kinds of topics that have dominated the terrain of the ethics of neuroscience.

An area of considerable interest is the ELSI of neuroimaging studies, and in particular, functional magnetic resonance imaging (fMRI) correlation studies, which measure and map brain activity while a participant performs a particular mental operation of interest. While there is a strong focus on ethical issues elicited by the potential of imaging modalities for improved screening, diagnosis, and prediction of risk for neurological and psychiatric disorders (Illes et al., 2007; Lane, Hunter & Lawrie, 2020), what is of particular interest to many neuroethicists is the use of fMRI to identify the neural correlates of certain non-medical mental states, socially-oriented dispositions, and behavioural traits. For example, studies have detected the neural correlates of mental states and traits ranging from implicit racial bias, sexual preference, deception, risk aversion,

---

6   See Martin et al. (2016) and Becker et al. (2017) for a systematic survey of the literature pertaining to the two subdivisions of the ethics of neuroscience.

7   While it is unlikely that there will ever be agreement about the mind-body problem, referring to the question of how conscious, immaterial, mental states arise from the brain, which is physical in nature, it is undeniable, at least in terms of current capabilities, that without a brain there can be no mind. In this way, it is uncontroversial to describe the mind and the brain as inextricably related.

8   The belief that advances in our understanding of brain structure and function can add to our understanding of complex behaviour, and transform our institutions, is evidenced by newly formed fields such as "neurolaw, neuroeconomics, neurophilosophy, neuromarketing, and neurofinance" (Schultz, 2018).

trustworthiness, cooperativeness, and religious experience, to predisposition for certain behaviours, such as criminality or likelihood of recidivism (Racine, Bar-Ilan & Illes, 2006). Of course, fMRI requires a high degree of interpretation and inference (Roskies, 2008), and is not yet sufficiently robust to be used outside of research contexts.

However, as these technologies improve and concomitantly, our ability to monitor, identify, and predict mental states and behaviours such as the aforementioned, this may have significant future implications for mental privacy and a potential for misuse in insurance or employment contexts. Should these findings become sufficiently robust in the future, some of the issues that will have to be addressed will be: how, to what extent, and in which contexts imaging findings should be used and when, if ever, should we act upon risk or susceptibility information (Fitzpatrick, 2006).

At an even more fundamental level, evidence of processes in the brain, over which there seems to be minimal control, implies a need to reconsider certain assumptions regarding agency and possibly free will (Levy, 2012). Of course, the challenge posed by these findings may be a case of 'old wine in new bottles' insofar as our existing frameworks of free will are able to accommodate them without significant disruption.[9] However, newly established fields such as neurolaw and neurocriminology imply that many think the legal system stands to be impacted, in some way, by neuroscience study findings, indicating the neurobiological underpinnings of criminal behaviour (Glenn & Raine, 2014; Straiton & Lake, 2021). Difference does not imply dysfunction, and the causes of criminal behaviour are undoubtedly complex, however, the question of whether, and to what extent, our notions of moral responsibility and concomitantly, culpability and blameworthiness, should be reconfigured to account for these differences in some way, remains a valid area of discussion.

Other philosophical concepts stand to be challenged due to the implications of the use and effects of certain psychopharmacological interventions and neuro-technologies for both treatment and enhancement purposes. In terms of the former, much has been written about the perceived impact, on personal or narrative identity, of interventions like deep brain stimulation (DBS), which is

---

9   The main challenge for accounts of free will has been to provide a theory that preserves it, given the recognition of determinism. Compatiblism is the view that free will exists despite determinism and there have been effective arguments in support of this view, which is the dominant view in analytic philosophy. As pointed out by Wassermann and Johnson (2014), the question that requires answering in neuroethics is whether "neuroimaging pose[s] new challenges to the compatibilist views that have predominated in moral and legal thinking for the past fifty years."

generally used to treat severe motor dysfunction associated with conditions such as Parkinson's disease and other movement disorders, as well as treatment resistant psychiatric disorders.[10] Impacts on identity are attributable to the sometimes significant and abrupt personality and behavioural changes that follow from DBS (Jotterand & Giordano, 2011). While it has been argued that the threat to identity posed by DBS has been overstated and applies to a static and thin conception of identity (Baylis, 2013), the personality changes associated with DBS undoubtedly provide us with opportunities to advance our understanding of the neurobiological basis of identity and our metaphysical notions of free will and agency (Lipsman & Glannon, 2013).

The ethical implications of neuroenhancement, not only through off label use of medications, but in the future, through various neural devices and technologies, currently in development for treatment purposes, is also another area that has received considerable attention.[11] Bioenhancement is generally defined as using biomedical interventions to improve species' typical or 'normal' functioning and capacities. This is contrasted with the treatment of disease, disorder, or dysfunction to restore functioning to such levels (Boorse, 1975; Daniels, 2000). This distinction has, however, been subject to extensive contestation, given conceptual challenges in establishing what constitutes normal mental functioning as opposed to dysfunction in the face of considerable human variation and the inescapably normative component of such a distinction (Bostrom & Roache, 2008; Buchanan et al., 2009; Harris, 2007; Kass, 1998; Savulescu, Sandberg & Kahane, 2011).

These challenges aside, areas of neuroenhancement that have been discussed, in terms of their ethical implications, include various aspects of cognition, including memory and attention (Racine, Sattler & Boehlen, 2021), wakefulness (Ravelingien & Sandberg, 2008), mood (Palk & Stein, 2020a), and even pro social attitudes like empathy, referred to as moral bioenhancement (Persson & Savulescu, 2012). Cognitive enhancement, however, receives significant attention in discussions of neuroenhancement. Arguments in support of neuroenhancement generally invoke a right to cognitive liberty, referring to the view that the decision of whether or not to enhance is an individual one that should be made without external interference. Arguments against enhancement encompass a range of both practical, consequentialist concerns, which hold in common the view that, in some way, enhancements will render us worse off, and in-principle

---

10   See Martin et al. (2016) for a list of papers on this issue.

11   See Becker et al. (2017) for a comprehensive list of publications that have focused on the ethics of various forms of neuroenhancement.

concerns,[12] which draw on non-consequentialist approaches such as concerns about inauthenticity or the unnaturalness of biomedical enhancements (Fukuyama, 2002; Kass, 2003; Sandal, 2007).

9.2.2 The neuroscience of ethics

The above examples are just a few areas of focus within the vast domain of the ethics of neuroscience. The second distinction identified by Roskies (2002:22), the neuroscience of ethics, and morality itself is narrower and more specialised in its focus.[13] This area aligns with the fields of neurophilosophy or experimental philosophy (Klar, 2021). Studies in this domain aim to identify the neurobiological underpinnings of moral cognition and emotion, and to deepen our understanding of how this informs our moral judgements and social behaviours.[14] As Giordano, Becker and Shook (2016) put it: "mapping the 'moral brain'". However, this description should not be taken as indicating that there are mechanisms and processes in the brain dedicated solely to moral deliberation. Rather, what seems to be the case is that the neural bases of moral judgements are largely the same as those involved with the deliberation of matters deemed salient to individuals and which require them to assess the advantages and disadvantages associated with particular courses of action (Giordano et al., 2016).

Of particular interest is the relationship between this potential 'neuromorality' and our approaches to ethical decision-making, which have traditionally fallen with the domain of moral philosophy. The various moral theories which have dominated the field of ethics are themselves informed by widely held moral intuitions and assumptions regarding the appropriate basis for moral decision-making. However, these approaches presuppose certain metaphysical notions such as the freedom of the will to form intentions which can be deliberated and acted upon in a rational and relatively straightforward manner. They also presuppose a relatively strict delineation between cognitive and affective processes in moral decision-making. These assumptions, and in particular the reliability of the moral

---

12 The distinction between in-practice and in-principle ethical concerns is a useful one suggested by Agar (2015). While in-practice concerns are consequentialist in nature, in-principle objections draw on non-consequentialist approaches and generally provide arguments to support the position that neuroenhancement is ethically undesirable, regardless of any practical benefits or avoidance of harms that it may produce.

13 See Darragh, Buniak and Giordano (2015) for a systematic survey of the literature addressing the neuroscience of ethics and Racine et al. (2017) for a critical discussion of the kinds of studies that comprise the field.

14 This focus ties in with that of the recently formed, and wider, field of social neuroscience which investigates the relationship between brain structure and function and social behaviour and interactions.

intuitions that inform certain theories, have been challenged by neuroscience study findings (Cushman, Young & Greene, 2010). The neuroscience of ethics thus includes both the empirical study of moral decision-making processes and behaviour, including studies of neurological conditions and damage that impact these processes and behaviour (Damasio, 2007) and the often controversial, normative interpretations, inferences, and discussions of these study findings (Churchland, 2013).

While there is optimism regarding the potential of the neuroscience of ethics to contribute to our understanding of morality, these studies, and the conclusions drawn from them, have not been without criticism (Berker, 2009; Racine et al., 2017). In this regard, we should not overstate what such studies can tell us. As pointed out by Damasio (2007), such studies have primarily focused on "reveal[ing] patterns of neurobiological activity in response to, and involved in certain types of situations, dilemmas, and activities that are construed to be moral and/or ethical".[15] However, criticisms aside, the neuroscience of ethics arguably remains an area of potential long-term significance and interest.

---

15   Joshua Greene's research is frequently cited as it was the first of its kind in what came to be known as the neuroscience of ethics, but also due to the controversial normative inferences that Greene makes elsewhere (Greene, 2008). Since 2001, Greene has used fMRI to study the brain activity of research participants when responding to moral dilemmas, with preliminary findings indicating that both cognitive and affective responses play a pivotal role in moral judgements (Greene et al., 2001). More specifically, Greene posits that his studies show that differences in participants' responses to dilemmas, such as the two famous variations of the Trolley problem, are informed by the strength of participants' emotional responses to the dilemma, rather than the reasons which are typically offered. The more personal or direct the involvement of the participant with the dilemma that is sketched out, the stronger the emotional response and vice versa. Greene posits that certain moral judgements, particularly those which involve the violation of deontological restrictions, typically associated with Kantian style, "higher order" reasoning, are, in fact, a product of the strength of the emotional response which is then rationalised post hoc. But, he points out that imaging indicates that "typically consequentialist", utilitarian judgements indicate the presence of the kind of cognitive processes typically associated with deontological approaches. Greene then argues that these findings have normative implications for the suitability of deontology as an approach to morality. Insofar as automatic emotional responses are the product of biases, social conditioning, and various other factors, the argument is that an approach such as consequentialism which is characterised by more cognitive processing and slower reactions to the moral situation in question would be a preferable form of ethical decision-making in contemporary contexts (Greene, 2008).

9.3   CONSIDERING A GLOBALLY INCLUSIVE AND DIVERSE NEUROETHICS FROM AN AFRICAN PERSPECTIVE

As mentioned above, with the field of neuroethics entering its third decade, there have been increasing calls advocating for a more internationally or globally relevant neuroethics. It is likely that this internationalisation of the field will progress in a piecemeal manner as awareness of this important goal grows and more contributions are made. In terms of the potential trajectory of an increased neuroethics engagement in African contexts, two points of meaningful entry into debates seem appropriate.

Firstly, given resource scarcities that significantly impact access to treatment and research of mental disorders on the continent (Sankoh, Sevalie & Weston, 2018), neuroethics engagement that is responsive to these more immediate and practical concerns seems fitting. This would include neuroscience research ethics issues related to mental health studies in African contexts as well as establishing an evidence-base through conducting empirical studies to assess the beliefs and attitudes of populations regarding neurological and psychiatric disorders, and their interpretations of such study findings, which stand to have implications for health outcomes.

Secondly, the rich variety of African moral frameworks and theories which respond to ethical challenges from a more communitarian or relational perspective offer an appropriate foundation for engaging with neuroethics concerns in these contexts. However, there is also a significant contribution to be made conceptually, and foundationally, in terms of articulating the principles and values prevalent in African contexts that could enrich the dominant bioethics paradigm itself, which has largely relied on Beauchamp and Childress' principlism (2019), and which informs neuroethics, as part of bioethics. The above areas of focus are likely to be followed by engagement with the wider societal implications of neuroscience study findings and neurotechnology applications in various areas, including their impact on notions like personhood and identity in these contexts.

In what follows, I provide suggestions for establishing more of a neuroethics presence in African contexts, as well as some potential areas in which local bio-ethicists could make significant contributions, thus enriching the field of neuro-ethics. I have grouped my suggestions in accordance with the four possible approaches to developing a more globally relevant neuroethics, mentioned in the introduction.

9.3.1 Building neuroethics capacity through the growth of neuroscience research collaborations across the continent

Working towards a more globally relevant and diverse neuroethics, inclusive of an array of perspectives, methodologies, and concerns, requires, first and foremost, focusing on the practical goal of increased and meaningful participation of bioethicists and neuroscientists (with an interest in neuroethics) from underrepresented contexts, such as Africa. As mentioned above, a growth in engagement with themes in neuroethics in Africa is likely to be proportionate to the growth of neuroscience on the continent.[16] Neuroscience research in Africa, however, remains comparatively minimal[17] due to various factors, including a lack of resources, funding, infrastructure, and scientists specialising in the requisite areas (Maina et al., 2021). Despite this, there have been concerted efforts to address the African neuroscience research gap in recent years (Yusuf, Baden & Prieto-Godino, 2014; Karikari, Cobham & Ndams, 2016; Balogan et al., 2018; Baden et al., 2020),[18] with cause for optimism given indications of a decisive increase in publications of studies led by African scientists in recent years (Maina et al., 2021).[19]

International research collaborations involving multiple study sites and partners, not only globally but also across the African continent, are another effective way of fostering neuroscience networks and research capacity as well as cultivating

---

16 The recently inaugurated Neuroscience Institute at the University of Cape Town and the subsequent establishing of an arm within the associated Brain Behaviour Unit, focused on advancing neuroethics in Africa, provides support for this assumption.

17 A recent survey of the neuroscience-related literature between 1996 to 2017 identified 5 219 publications led by African scientists, with 77% of these publications produced by only five African countries (Egypt, South Africa, Nigeria, Morocco, and Tunisia) (Maina et al., 2021). The predominant focus of these studies is on neurodegeneration and brain injury, which is appropriate, given figures indicating that by 2050 just under three-quarters of persons living with dementia-related conditions will reside in LMICs (Baden et al., 2020).

18 An example is the formation of the UK-led non-profit organisation, TReND in Africa (Teaching and Research in Natural Sciences for Development in Africa) in 2011. This organisation comprising volunteers from various universities across the globe and partners from African universities, focuses on capacity building of scientists (including neuroscientists) from Africa with the goal of promoting independence, empowerment, and scientific exchange as well as public and policy engagement on neuroscience-related issues (Baden et al., 2020).

19 Evidence of the growth of neuroscience on the continent is also indicated by increased attendance at conferences presented by the Society of Neuroscientists of Africa (SONA) which operates as an overarching organisation for various neuroscience groups throughout Africa, as well as increases in applications for neurosciences study programmes in African institutions (Maina et al., 2021).

an interest in neuroethics on the continent. As mentioned above, developing research ethics capacity related to neuroscience studies of this kind would be an obvious point of meaningful entry into the field for local ethicists, given the urgency of the psychiatric and neurological disease burden on the continent. Global neuroimaging genetics networks such as ENIGMA (Enhancing Neuroimaging Genetics through Meta-Analysis), comprising scientists from over 45 countries, are an example of such a collaborative endeavour (Palk et al., 2020).[20] While international collaborations of this kind hold great benefits in terms of collectively addressing global mental health inequities and fostering science diplomacy insofar as they are led and funded by HICs, attention must be paid to issues such as equitable data sharing, among others (Palk et al., 2020). However, with over 50 working groups focusing on various neurological and psychiatric disorders, consortia such as ENIGMA are in a good position to contribute towards neuroethics capacity building in underrepresented contexts (Palk et al., 2020).

Exemplars in the field of neuropsychiatric genetics that can provide a model for capacity building of neuroethics in Africa are the Human Heredity and Health in Africa (H3Africa) Initiative comprising genomic studies at multiple sites across Africa, focusing on various disorders and diseases, including mental disorders (Mulder et al., 2018) and the Neuropsychiatric Genetics of African Populations Consortium (NeuroGAP) which investigated psychotic and neurodevelopmental disorders with sites in four African countries (Stevenson et al., 2019). While both consortia are led and funded by institutions from HICs, what is significant for the topic at hand is that both formed dedicated ethics working groups, comprising bioethicists from across the African continent. These groups have focused on ethical and regulatory issues arising from the studies they are attached to, using ethical frameworks that are sensitive to the socio-cultural context, as well as conducting related empirical ethics research to ascertain the attitudes and beliefs of different populations about genetic information, particular explanatory models of disease, the stigmatising of certain disorders, and views about feedback of study findings, among others (De Vries, Landouré & Wonkam, 2020; Matimba et al., 2022; Ralefala et al., 2021). Along with the ethics and regulatory working group, H3Africa includes working groups focused on outreach and communication as well as ethics and community engagement (Tindana et al., 2015).

---

20 Imaging genetics combines imaging modalities with neuropsychiatric genetics study findings to decipher the role of genetic variation on brain structure and function, thus deepening our understanding of neuropsychiatric disorders. Such collaborations, in which brain imaging data is pooled and compared, and study findings can be replicated, are crucial given the significant costs associated with imaging studies, which restrict sample sizes, resulting in underpowered study findings (Thompson et al., 2020).

The NeuroGAP consortium includes the Africa Ethics Working Group (AEWG) which focuses explicitly on issues arising from neuropsychiatric genetic studies and findings in African contexts. Membership involves access to funding and training opportunities, establishing meaningful bioethics networks with colleagues in other African countries and globally, as well as capacity building of junior colleagues entering the field of bioethics.[21] Establishing these kinds of working groups for neuroethics in Africa is arguably one of the most effective ways of encouraging the growth of the field on the continent in the same way that the ethics of genetic studies and practice, commonly described as 'genethics', has become a significant area of focus in this context.

9.3.2 Exploring congruence with the global mental health movement to engage in neuroethics activism to address brain and mental health research and treatment priorities in Africa

As mentioned above, the urgency of addressing inequities in brain and mental health research and treatment in Africa requires neuroethics engagement that is responsive to these medical and research priorities. The second suggestion therefore includes approaching the development of neuroethics on the continent using the tools of bioethics activism. Drawing from the related field of global mental health could also be useful in this regard and in particular, recent work which has explored the intersection between neuroethics and global mental health, including an entire volume dedicated to the topic (Stein & Giordano, 2015; Stein & Singh, 2020).

Global mental health has recently emerged both as an independent field and an increasing organised social movement, informed by the recognition of an ethical obligation to rectify unjust mental health inequities between nations, insofar as they were caused by exploitative conditions in the colonial era (Patel, 2012; Patel et al., 2018). The overarching aim of the field is thus to cultivate equity in access to mental health in low resourced contexts by means of "efficient, innovative, cost-effective approaches that are context-sensitive and evidence-based" (Palk & Stein, 2020b). Given congruence between this aim of global mental health and the need for a neuroethics engagement in Africa that is responsive to such needs, a "neuroethics of global mental health" (Stein & Giordano, 2015) is a fitting potentially fruitful domain within which ethicists working in these contexts could situate themselves. Moreover, this domain would include not only a focus on fleshing out this potential domain from the perspective of ethicists working

---

21 See Kamuya et al. (2021) for a discussion of the Africa Ethics Working Group (AEWG) as a model of collaboration for psychiatric genomic research in Africa.

in African contexts but equally important, it would benefit from neuroethics advocacy or activism.

As argued by Rogers and Scully (2021), insofar as it is directed at normative ends, "bioethics is inescapably partisan … [w]here disagreement arises is over the degree to which bioethicists should be activists". In certain areas, however, an activist approach is clearly justified and needed. Neuroethics activism may take many different forms, at various levels. Meyers (2021) considers activism in bioethics at "micro, meso, and macro" levels whilst Draper (2019) provides a taxonomy to identify what can be considered activism in bioethics. An obvious form of advocacy would be to create awareness in the public realm and the academic literature of the kinds of concerns that would occupy a neuroethics of global mental health and the need to develop the field in Africa.

Other options that have been suggested would be advocating for more international funding for collaborative neuroethics studies and projects led by researchers from underrepresented contexts and for increased participation and leadership roles in international neuroethics working groups, conferences, organisations, and programmes by researchers from these contexts (Matshabane, 2021). Bioethicists interested in developing more of a neuroethics presence in Africa should also put efforts into driving their own collaborations and developing their own positions within the field, from an African perspective.

9.3.3 Drawing on the strong tradition of empirical ethics research on the continent to establish an evidence-base comprising the perspectives of underrepresented populations on established neuroethics concerns

An area of focus that has received much attention in neuroethics debates is the nature of public interpretations of study findings about the brain, including widespread interpretations of information about the neural bases of neurological and psychiatric disorders. As mentioned above, these interpretations have various implications ranging from their impact on self-understanding, and other related philosophical concepts, to ensuring optimal clinical outcomes. However, as far as can be ascertained, no studies of this kind have been conducted in African contexts, with the result that assumptions informed by studies conducted in Western contexts are uncritically generalised to other contexts where they may not hold. The third important point of entry to establishing a truly global neuroethics, inclusive of African concerns and perspectives, is therefore building an evidence-base of the views and beliefs of local populations by means of qualitative studies. Given the strong presence in African contexts of bioethicists who engage in empirical ethics and conduct qualitative studies of this kind, there is an abundance of researchers who could be enlisted in this important task, thereby contributing to developing the field in Africa. Studies of this kind would help to ensure that neuroscience-related study protocols are contextually sensitive and appropriate, and findings are communicated based on accurate information. Moreover, conducting studies in local contexts that gather evidence of views about the brain and notions of personhood, identity, agency, and morality itself will shed light on the extent to which certain ideas are subject to cultural variation, and impacted by more communitarian world views, and which are more universally held.

Tversky and Kahneman (1974) famously wrote about the fact that human beings are generally prone to certain cognitive biases or heuristics, referring to short cuts in our thinking that simplify complexity. The implications of these (mis)interpretations of complex information have been widely studied and discussed in subsequent decades, particularly in terms of their impact on how genetic information is understood. However, this is even more pertinent in the case of how information about the brain is interpreted, given the fact that the causal pathways between genes and phenotypes is more diluted and distal in comparison to brain physiology and phenotypes. In this regard, qualitative neuroethics studies have found that information about the brain is generally interpreted in essentialist ways. Neuroessentialism is the view that "for all intents and purposes, we are our brains" (Schultz, 2018), or put differently, that our psychological experiences are best explained with reference to, or are caused solely by, our brains. When essentialist interpretations hold sway there is a tendency to downplay or disregard the influence of environmental factors on mental and physical health, and behaviour in general (Schultz, 2018).

Essentialism may also inform neuroreductionism which is the "tendency to reduce complex mental phenomena to brain states, [often] confusing correlation for physical causation" (Savulescu & Earp, 2014). For example, as neuroimaging modalities become increasingly sensitive and improved, enabling the identification of the neural correlates of various mental states and traits, this information can be interpreted as indicating that certain experiences and feelings are reducible to, or nothing more than, brain chemistry or function. Reductionism is problematic, not only to the extent that it is incorrect, but particularly insofar as it disregards the fact that phenomena have multiple explanatory levels, and the biological level is only one possible way of understanding ourselves.

Neuroessentialism may also inform neurodeterminism which generally refers to the view that findings about the brain challenge our belief in our own agency or control over our health and behaviours (Schultz, 2018). For example, while imaging genetics studies have deepened our understanding of how genetic variation influences brain structure and function, with implications for improving the understanding, diagnosis, and treatment of mental disorders, attention must be paid to the implications of how this information is interpreted by study participants and the public when it is communicated via the media. Given that neurological and mental disorders sometimes impact behaviour in significant and variable ways, such disorders are subject to a wide array of problematic, and possibly stigmatising, causal ascriptions (Ngui et al., 2010; Palk & Stein, 2021).

Initially, it was hoped that information about the neurobiological basis of certain mental disorders might decrease stigma. Some early studies gave cause for optimism in this regard insofar as they indicated that, in the case of disorders of addiction, this information seemingly correlated with increased tolerance and understanding, with subsequent decreases in stigma (Haslam & Kvaale, 2015). This was attributed to the fact that this information might support the view that it is unfair to blame individuals for their behaviours, if they had little choice in the matter, implying that agency is comprised or eradicated if the disorder has a neurobiological basis. The validity of such findings has however been increasingly contested by more recent studies which indicate that the opposite may be the case (Canadian Health Services Research Foundation, 2013; Hammer et al., 2013; Lebowitz & Ahn, 2014).[22] These findings are congruent with other studies that have shown that information about the neural basis of other disorders, such as schizophrenia, is frequently interpreted in essentialist ways, which increase levels of stigma directed at such disorders, manifesting as the desire to avoid or distance oneself from the person in question (Loughman & Haslam, 2018; Schomerus, Matschinger & Angermeyer, 2014). Here the interpretation is that insofar as a disorder is "biologically" based, it is essential to the person in question and marks them as different or "other". Importantly, insofar as information about the neurobiological basis of such disorders tends to be interpreted in essentialist ways, thereby increasing stigma, studies are needed in African contexts to ascertain the impact this information may have on the high levels of stigma associated with many such disorders in these contexts (Palk & Stein, 2021).

A further problem associated with these kinds of essentialist or deterministic interpretations is that they can lead to prognostic pessimism, which is the view that if a disorder or disease has a neurobiological basis, it is a fixed and unchangeable part of the person in question and will not be amenable to treatment or improvement (Lebowitz & Appelbaum, 2019). Again, given that the presence

---

22   See Heather (2017) for an interesting discussion of this issue in the context of models of addiction.

and influence of such neuroessentialist thinking is taken as self-evident in neuro-ethics discussions, based on study findings from HICs, it is crucial that similar studies are conducted in African contexts.

9.3.4 Engaging with the underlying moral framework of neuroethics by drawing on African moral frameworks

Ethical issues and concerns arising in biomedical research and health care are typically addressed in terms of the framework of principlism which has dominated globally since its inception in 1979 in the now famous *Principles of Biomedical Ethics* by Beauchamp and Childress, currently in its 8th edition. The principles of respect for autonomy, non-maleficence, beneficence, and justice are typically framed as informed by a common morality, thus carrying universal weight. This assumption has however been contested and principlism has been extensively criticised for its Western liberal individualistic foundations. Given the fact that a significant proportion of the world's population subscribe to a more communitarian and relational world view, the perceived overemphasis on respect for individual autonomy has received the bulk of critical engagement (Behrens, 2018). Beauchamp and Childress (2019) have paid attention to these criticisms and have provided comprehensive and nuanced responses in subsequent editions of their work, including engagement with relational conceptions of autonomy and emphasising that the four principles are equal. However, the ideal conception of principlism, as articulated by its authors, does not necessarily equate with how it is applied in practice across the globe, and in this regard, the principlist framework has become an entity that is independent of its authors. This point aside, any normative framework is, by definition, reflective of a particular perspective, and the dominance of principlism in bioethics, and its perceived association with a particular worldview, has stimulated thinkers in African contexts to make interesting and important contributions to the literature.[23]

Engaging with such foundational concerns from the perspective of bioethics on the African continent can take many forms. It may include accepting principlism but applying it in a contextually sensitive manner to bioethical challenges in Africa (Kamaara, Kong & Campbell, 2020); developing a substantive moral theory or framework informed by insights and values prevalent in sub-Saharan Africa, as an alternative to principlism, which may be more appropriate for responding to bioethical challenges arising in African contexts (e.g., Metz, 2007 & 2010; Tangwa, 1996); or, articulating principles or values which could be used to adapt and enhance the principlist framework (e.g., Behrens, 2013; Rakotsoane

---

23   See Coleman (2017) for a review of some of these contributions.

& Van Niekerk, 2017). As part of the wider field of bioethics, neuroethics is also informed and founded on the principlist framework. Therefore, given that foundational level engagement is an established area of focus within bioethics in Africa, this is both an obvious point of entry into the field of neuroethics and an area where such a focus stands to enrich the field itself.

This aim is responsive to calls for engagement with the foundational assumptions and framework of the field to ensure its global relevance (Lanzilao et al., 2013; Shook & Giordano, 2014).[24] In this regard, the principle of solidarity has received attention in the international bioethics' literature (Prainsack & Buyx, 2012). The notion of solidarity is inherently relational and proactive insofar as it is understood as comprising "manifestations of the willingness to carry costs to assist others with whom a person recognises sameness of similarity in a least one relevant respect" (Prainsack & Buyx, 2012:346). Solidarity also occupies a central position in African moral world views, implying the value of acting with "good will" and "pro-attitudes" or care; "[b]eing invested in [the well-being of] others" (Metz, 2010). Moreover, from a global health perspective, solidarity has been recognised as a way of grounding a "united force against global health challenges" (Tosam et al., 2018) and an effective way of justifying the rectificatory obligation to redress health inequities – based on previous injustices – across the globe, in a more effective way than the dominant paradigm (e.g., see Benatar, Daibes & Tomsons, 2016). While the notion of solidarity requires more substantive work, it is but one example of a more relational principle that could enhance the dominant paradigm and could also be an area of focus in terms of articulating how it could inform a more globally relevant neuroethics.

9.4   CONCLUSION

In this chapter, I have attempted to provide some suggestions for developing the field of neuroethics on the African continent and examples of meaningful points of entry into the field in which local bioethicists could make significant contributions. This goal ties in with the broader task of cultivating a neuroethics that is more inclusive of diverse perspectives from a range of contexts and is thus more globally relevant. As neuroethics is not established in Africa, to the extent that it is elsewhere, I provided an introductory overview of the field with some illustrative examples, followed by four possible ways of increasing its presence on the continent.

---

24   Lanzilao et al. (2013) argue for a reframing of principlism to assist in advancing a more "internationally-relevant neuroethics" and develop an account of autonomy as self-creativity, beneficence as empowerment, non-maleficence as non-obsolescence, and justice as citizenship.

My suggestions included firstly, drawing on the 'ethics working group model' used by several international collaborative genetics studies to build interest, capacity, and participation in neuroethics, in the same way that this model has supported the development of 'genethics' expertise in Africa. Secondly, exploring congruence between the field of global mental health and neuroethics to address urgent medical and scientific mental health priorities in Africa as a form of neuroethics activism. Thirdly, harnessing the strong tradition of empirical ethics research in Africa to encourage studies that can build an evidence-base of the views of African populations on established neuroethics issues. Finally, utilising the work of thinkers in African contexts who have focused on improving and reconfiguring the normative foundations of bioethics to engage with the foundational assumptions of neuroethics.

In conclusion, as interest in neuroethics grows on the continent, it is likely that this will be beneficial not only for those participating in the field and those affected by its impact in Africa, but also for the field of neuroethics itself, insofar as the inclusion of a diverse array of perspectives and concerns increases the relevance and value of any discipline.

Bibliography

Agar, N. 2015. Moral bioenhancement and the utilitarian catastrophe. *Cambridge Quarterly of Health Care Ethics*, 24(1):37-47. https://doi.org/10.1017/S0963180114000280

Andoh, C. 2013. Bioethics education in Africa: still complex challenges. *Open Journal of Philosophy*, (3):507-516. https://doi.org/10.4236/ojpp.2013.34073

Baden, T., Maina, M.B., Maia Chagas, A., Mohammed, Y.G., Auer, T.O., Silbering, A., Von Tobel, L., Pertin, M., Hartig, R., Aleksic, J., Akinrinade, I., Awadelkareem, M.A., Koumoundourou, A., Jones, A., Arieti, F., Beale, A., Münch, D., Salek, S.C., Yusuf, S. & Prieto-Godino, L.L. 2020. TReND in Africa: toward a truly global (neuro)science community. *Neuron*, 107(3):412-416. https://doi.org/10.1016/j.neuron.2020.06.026

Balogun, W.G., Cobham, A.E., Amin, A. & Seeni, A. 2018. Advancing neuroscience research in Africa: invertebrate species to the rescue. *Neuroscience*, 374:323-325. https://doi.org/10.1016/j.neuroscience.2018.01.062

Baylis, F. 2013. I am who I am: on the perceived threats to personal identity from deep brain stimulation. *Neuroethics*, 6(3):513-526. https://doi.org/10.1007/s12152-011-9137-1

Beauchamp, T.L. & Childress, J.F. 2019. *Principles of biomedical ethics* (8th edition). New York: Oxford University Press.

Becker, K., Shook, J.R., Darragh, M. & Giordano, J. 2017. A four-part working bibliography of neuroethics: Part 4 – ethical issues in clinical and social applications of neuroscience. *Philosophy, Ethics, and Humanities in Medicine*, 12(1). https://doi.org/10.1186/s13010-017-043-y

Behrens, K.G. 2013. Towards an indigenous African bioethics. *South African Journal of Bioethics and Law*, 6(10):32-35. https://doi.org/10.7196/sajbl.255

Behrens, K.G. 2018. A critique of the principle of 'respect for autonomy', grounded in African thought. *Developing World Bioethics*, 18(2):126-134. https://doi.org/10.1111/dewb.12145

Benatar, S., Daibes, I. & Tomsons, S. 2016. Inter-philosophies dialogue: creating a paradigm for global health ethics. *Kennedy Institute of Ethics Journal*, 26(3):323-346. https://doi.org/10.1353/ken.2016.0027

Berker, S. 2009. The normative insignificance of neuroscience. *Philosophy & Public Affairs*, 37(4):293-329. https://doi.org/10.1111/j.1088-4963.2009.01164.x

Beyer, C., Staunton, C. & Moodley, K. 2014. The implications of methylphenidate use by healthy medical students and doctors in South Africa. *BMC Medical Ethics*, 15(20). https://doi.org/10.1186/1472-6939-15-20

Boorse, C. 1975. On the distinction between disease and illness. *Philosophy & Public Affairs*, 5(1):49-68. http://www.jstor.org/stable/2265020

Bostrom, N. & Roache, R. 2008. Ethical issues in human enhancement. In: J. Ryberg, T. Petersen & C. Wolf (eds.). *New waves in applied ethics*. London: Palgrave Macmillan. 120-152.

Buchanan, A., Brock, D.W., Daniels, N. & Wikler, D. (eds.). 2009. *From chance to choice: genetics and justice*. New York: Cambridge University Press.

Buller, T. 2020. *Diversity and inclusion in neuroethics*. The Neuroethics Blog: Emory University Centre for Ethics. https://bit.ly/3tOBh6g [Accessed 25 April 2022].

Buniak, L., Darragh, M. & Giordano, J. 2014. A four-part working bibliography of neuroethics: Part 1 – overview and reviews: defining and describing the field and its practices. *Philosophy, Ethics, and Humanities in Medicine*, 9(9). https://doi.org/10.1186/1747-5341-9-9

Canadian Health Services Research Foundation. 2013. Myth: reframing mental illness as a 'brain disease' reduces stigma. *Journal of Health Services Research & Policy*, (18)3:190-192. https://doi.org/10.1177/1355819613485853

Chatterjee, A. & Farah, M.J. 2013. Neuroethics in practice. *Oxford Scholarship*

Online. https://doi.org/10.1093/acprof:o
so/9780195389784.001.0001

Churchland, P.S. 2013. *Touching a nerve: the self as brain.* New York: W.W. Norton & Co.

Coleman, A.M.E. 2017. What is "African bioethics" as used by sub-Saharan African authors: an argumentative literature review of articles on African bioethics. *Open Journal of Philosophy,* 7:31-47. https://doi.org/10.4236/ojpp.2017.71003

Cordeiro-Rodrigues, L. & Ewuoso, C. 2021. An Afro-communitarian relational approach to brain surrogates research. *Neuroethics,* 14(3):561-574. https://doi.org/10.1007/s12152-021-09475-7

Cushman, F., Young, L. & Greene, J.D. 2010. Multi-system moral psychology. In: J.M. Doris (ed.). *The moral psychology handbook.* Oxford: Oxford University Press. 47-71. https://doi.org/10.1093/acprof:oso/9780199582143.003.0003

Damasio, A. 2007. Neuroscience and ethics: intersections. *The American Journal of Bioethics,* 7(1):3-7. https://doi.org/10.1080/15265160601063910

Dana Foundation. 2002. *Neuroethics: mapping the field.* https://bit.ly/3OlUmpO [Accessed 25 April 2022].

Daniels, N. 2000. Normal functioning and the treatment-enhancement distinction. *Cambridge Quarterly of Health Care Ethics,* 9(3):309-322. https://doi.org/10.1017/S0963180100903037

Darragh, M., Buniak, L. & Giordano, J. 2015. A four-part working bibliography of neuroethics: Part 2 – neuroscientific studies of morality and ethics. *Philosophy, Ethics, and Humanities in Medicine,* 10(2). https://doi.org/10.1186/s13010-015-0022-0

De Vries, J., Landouré, G. & Wonkam, A. 2020. Stigma in African genomics research: gendered blame, polygamy, ancestry and disease causal beliefs impact on the risk of harm. *Social Science & Medicine,* 258(113091). https://doi.org/10.1016/j.socscimed.2020.113091

Draper, H. 2019. Activism, bioethics and academic research. *Bioethics,* 33(8):861-871. https://doi.org/10.1111/bioe.12574

Fitzpatrick, T.E. 2006. Are we in need of a neuromorality? *Science and Environment,* Fall. https://bit.ly/3gldJCI

Foot, P. 1967. The problem of abortion and the doctrine of double effect. *Oxford Review,* 5:5-15.

Fothergill, B.T., Knight, W., Carsten Stahl, B. & Ulnicane, I. 2019. Responsible data governance of neuroscience big data. *Frontiers in Neuroinformatics,* 13(28). https://doi.org/10.3389/fninf.2019.00028

Fukuyama, F. 2002. *Our posthuman future: consequences of the biotechnology revolution.* New York: Picador.

Giordano, J., Becker, K. & Shook, J.R. 2016. On the "neuroscience of ethics": approaching the neuroethical literature as a rational discourse on putative neural processes of moral cognition and behavior. *Journal of Neurology & Neuromedicine,* 1(6):32-36. https://doi.org/10.29245/2572.942X/2016/6.1062

Glenn, A.L. & Raine, A. 2014. Neurocriminology: implications for the punishment, prediction and prevention of criminal behaviour. *Nature Reviews Neuroscience,* 15(1):54-63. https://doi.org/10.1038/nrn3640

Greene, J.D. 2008. The secret joke of Kant's soul. In: W. Sinnott-Armstrong (ed.). *Moral psychology, Vol. 3. The neuroscience of morality: emotion, brain disorders, and development.* Cambridge: MIT Press. 35-80.

Greene, J.D., Sommerville, R.B., Nystrom, L.E., Darley, J.M. & Cohen, J.D. 2001. An fMRI investigation of emotional engagement in moral judgment. *Science,* 293(5537):2105-2108. https://doi.org/10.1126/science.1062872

Hammer, R., Dingel, M., Ostergren, J., Partridge, B., McCormick, J. & Koenig, B.A. 2013. Addiction: current criticism of the brain disease paradigm. *AJOB Neuroscience,* 4(3):27-32. https://doi.org/10.1080/21507740.2013.796328

Harris, J. 2007. *Enhancing evolution: the ethical case for making better people*. Princeton, NJ: Princeton University Press.

Haslam, N. & Kvaale, E.P. 2015. Biogenetic explanations of mental disorder: the mixed-blessings model. *Current Directions in Psychological Science*, 24(5):399-404. https://doi.org/10.1177/0963721415588082

Heather, N. 2017. Q: Is addiction a brain disease or a moral failing? A: Neither. *Neuroethics*, 10:115-124. https://doi.org/10.1007/s12152-016-9289-0

Holtug, N. 1998. Creating and patenting new life forms. In: H. Kuhse & P. Singer (eds.). *A companion to bioethics*. Oxford: Blackwell Publishers. 206-214.

Illes, J., Kirschen, M.P., Edwards, E., Stanford, L.R., Bandettini, P., Cho, M.K., Ford, P.J., Glover, G.H., Kulynych, J., Macklin, R., Michael, D.B., Wolf, S.M. & Working Group on Incidental Findings in Brain Imaging Research. 2006. Incidental findings in brain imaging research. *Science*, 311(5762): 783-784. https://doi.org/10.1126/science.1124665

Illes, J. & Racine, E. 2005. Imaging or imagining? A neuroethics challenge informed by genetics. *Amercian Journal of Bioethics*, 5(2):5-18. https://doi.org/10.1080/15265160590923358

Illes, J., Rosen, A., Greicius, M. & Racine, E. 2007. Prospects for prediction: ethics analysis of neuroimaging in Alzheimer's disease. *Annals of the New York Academy of Sciences*, 1097:278-295. https://doi.org/10.1196/annals.1379.030

Jotterand, F. & Giordano, J. 2011. Transcranial magnetic stimulation, deep brain stimulation and personal identity: ethical questions, and neuroethical approaches for medical practice. *International Review of Psychiatry*, 23(5):476-485. https://doi.org/10.3109/09540261.2011.616189

Kamaara, E., Kong, C. & Campbell, M. 2020. Prioritising African perspectives in psychiatric genomics research: issues of translation and informed consent. *Developing World Bioethics*, 20(3):139-149. https://doi.org/10.1111/dewb.12248

Kamuya, D., Bitta, M.A., Addissie, A., Naanyu, V., Palk, A.C., Mwaka, E., Kamaara, E., Tadele, G., Teka, T., Nakigudde, J., Manku, K., Musesengwa, R. & Singh, I. 2021. The Africa Ethics Working Group (AEWG): a model of collaboration for psychiatric genomic research in Africa. *Wellcome Open Research*, 6:190. https://doi.org/10.12688/wellcomeopenres.16772.1

Karikari, T.K., Cobham, A.E. & Ndams, I.S. 2016. Building sustainable neuroscience capacity in Africa: the role of non-profit organisations. *Metabolic Brain Disease*, 31:3-9. https://doi.org/10.1007/s11011-015-9687-8

Kass, L.R. 1998. The wisdom of repugnance: why we should ban the cloning of humans. *Valparaiso University Law Review*, 32(2): 679-705. https://bit.ly/3H8xSH6

Kass, L.R. 2003. Ageless bodies, happy souls: biotechnology and the pursuit of perfection. *The New Atlantis*, 1:9-28.

Klar, P. 2021. What is neurophilosophy: do we need a non-reductive form? *Synthese*, 199:2701-2725. https://doi.org/10.1007/s11229-020-02907-6

Lane, N.M., Hunter, S.A. & Lawrie, S.M. 2020. The benefit of foresight? An ethical evaluation of predictive testing for psychosis in clinical practice. *NeuroImage Clinical*, 26(102228). https://doi.org/10.1016/j.nicl.2020.102228

Lanzilao, E., Shook, J., Benedikter, R. & Giordano, J. 2013. Advancing neuroscience on the 21st-century world stage: the need for and a proposed structure of an internationally relevant neuroethics. *Ethics in Biology, Engineering and Medicine: An International Journal*, 4:211-229. https://doi.org/10.1615/EthicsBiologyEngMed.2014010710

Lebowitz, M.S. & Ahn, W.K. 2014. Effects of biological explanations for mental disorders on clinicians' empathy. *PNAS*, 111:17786-17790. https://doi.org/10.1073/pnas.1414058111

Lebowitz, M.S. & Appelbaum, P.S. 2019. Biomedical explanations of psychopathology and their implications for attitudes and beliefs about mental disorders. *Annual Review of Clinical Psychology*, 15:555-577. https://doi.org/10.1146/annurev-clinpsy-050718-095416

Levy, N. 2012. Neuroethics. *Wiley Interdisciplinary Reviews Cognitive Science*, 3:143-151. https://doi.org/10.1002/wcs.1157

Lipsman, N. & Glannon, W. 2013. Brain, mind and machine: what are the implications of deep brain stimulation for perceptions of personal identity, agency and free will? *Bioethics*, 27(9):465-470. https://doi.org/10.1111/j.1467-8519.2012.01978.x

Lombera, S. & Illes, J. 2009. The international dimensions of neuroethics. *Developing World Bioethics*, 9(2):57-64. https://doi.org/10.1111/j.1471-8847.2008.00235.x

Loughman, A. & Haslam, N. 2018. Neuroscientific explanations and the stigma of mental disorder: a meta-analytic study. *Cognitive Research: Principles and Implications*, 3:a43. https://doi.org/10.1186/s41235-018-0136-1

Maina, M.B., Ahmad, U., Ibrahim, H.A., Nasr, F.E., Salihu, A.T., Abushouk, A.I., Abdurrazak, M., Awadelkareem, M.A., Amin, A., Imam, A., Akinrinade, I.D., Yakubu, A.H., Azeez, I.A., Mohammed, Y.G., Adamu, A.A., Ibrahim, H.B., Bukar, A.M., Yaro, A.U., Goni, B.W., Prieto-Godino, L.L. & Baden, T. 2021. Two decades of neuroscience publication trends in Africa. *Nature Communications*, 12:a3429. https://doi.org/10.1038/s41467-021-23784-8

Martin, A., Becker, K., Darragh, M. & Giordano, J. 2016. A four-part working bibliography of neuroethics: Part 3 – "second tradition neuroethics" – ethical issues in neuroscience. *Philosophy, Ethics, and Humanities in Medicine*, 11(7). https://doi.org/10.1186/s13010-016-0037-1

Matimba, A., Ali, S., Littler, K., Madden, E., Marshall, P., McCurdy, S., Nembaware, V., Rodriguez, L., Seeley, J., Tindana, P., Yakubu, A. & De Vries, J. on behalf of the H3Africa Ethics and Community Engagement Working Group. 2022. Guideline for feedback of individual genetic research findings for genomics research in Africa. *BMJ Global Health*, 7:e007184. https://doi.org/10.1136/bmjgh-2021-007184

Matshabane, O.P. 2021. Promoting diversity and inclusion in neuroscience and neuroethics. *EBioMedicine*, 67(103359). https://doi.org/10.1016/j.ebiom.2021.103359

Metz, T. 2007. Toward an African moral theory. *Journal of Political Philosophy*, 15(3):321-341. https://doi.org/10.1111/j.1467-9760.2007.00280.x

Metz, T. 2010. African and Western moral theories in a bioethical context. *Developing World Bioethics*, 10(1):49-58. https://doi.org/10.1111/j.1471-8847.2009.00273.x

Meyers, C. 2021. Activism and the clinical ethicist. *Hastings Center Report*, 51(4):22-31. https://doi.org/10.1002/hast.1269

Mulder, N., Abimiku, A., Adebamowo, S.N., De Vries, J., Matimba, A., Olowoyo, P., Ramsay, M., Skelton, M. & Stein, D.J. 2018. H3Africa: current perspectives. *Pharmacogenomics and Personalized Medicine*, 11:59-66. https://doi.org/10.2147/PGPM.S141546

Ngui, E.M., Khasakhala, L., Ndetei, D. & Roberts, L.W. 2010. Mental disorders, health inequalities and ethics: a global perspective. *International Review of Psychiatry*, 22(3):235-244. https://doi.org/10.3109/09540261.2010.485273

Palk, A.C., Illes, J., Thompson, P.M. & Stein, D.J. 2020. Ethical issues in global neuroimaging genetics collaborations. *NeuroImage*, 221(117208). https://doi.org/10.1016/j.neuroimage.2020.117208

Palk, A.C. & Stein, D.J. 2020a. Ethical issues in global mental health. In: D. Stein & I. Singh (eds.), *Global mental health and neuroethics*. Elsevier. 265-285. https://doi.org/10.1016/B978-0-12-815063-4.00016-2

Palk, A.C. & Stein, D.J. 2020b. Cosmetic psychopharmacology in a global context. In: D. Stein & I. Singh (eds.), *Global mental health and neuroethics*. Elsevier:

95-115. https://doi.org/10.1016/B978-0-12-815063-4.00007-1

Palk, A.C. & Stein, D.J. 2021. Ethical implications of genomic research on dementia in sub-Saharan Africa: Addressing the risk of stigma. In: V. Dubljević & F. Bottenberg (eds.), *Living with dementia. Advances in neuroethics*. The University of Edenburgh, Scotland: Springer, Cham. 199-221. https://doi.org/10.1007/978-3-030-62073-8_12

Patel, V. 2012. Global mental health: from science to action. *Harvard Review of Psychiatry*, 20(1):6-12. https://doi.org/10.3109/10673229.2012.649108

Patel, V., Saxena, S., Lund, C., Thornicroft, G., Baingana, F. et al. 2018. The *Lancet* Commission on global mental health and sustainable development. *The Lancet*, 392(10157):P1553-P1598. https://doi.org/10.1016/S0140-6736(18)31612-X

Persson, I. & Savulescu, J. 2012. *Unfit for the future: the need for moral enhancement*. Oxford: Oxford University Press. https://doi.org/10.1093/acprof:oso/9780199653645.001.0001

Prainsack, B. & Buyx, A. 2012. Solidarity in contemporary bioethics: towards a new approach. *Bioethics*, 26(7):343-350. https://doi.org/10.1111/j.1467-8519.2012.01987.x

Racine, E., Bar-Ilan, O. & Illes, J. 2006. Brain imaging: a decade of coverage in the print media. *Science Communication*, 28(1):122-142. https://doi.org/10.1177/1075547006291990

Racine, E., Dubljević, V., Jox, R.J., Baertschi, B., Christensen, J.F., Farisco, M., Jotterand, F., Kahane, G. & Müller, S. 2017. Can neuroscience contribute to practical ethics? A critical review and discussion of the methodological and translational challenges of the neuroscience of ethics. *Bioethics*, 31(5):328-337. https://doi.org/10.1111/bioe.12357

Racine, E., Sattler, S. & Boehlen, W. 2021. Cognitive enhancement: unanswered questions about human psychology and social behavior. *Science and Engineering*

Ethics, 27(2):a19 (25 pages). https://doi.org/10.1007/s11948-021-00294-w

Rakotsoane, F.C.L. & Van Niekerk, A.A. 2017. Human life invaluableness: an emerging African bioethical principle. *South African Journal of Philosophy*, 36(2):252-262. https://doi.org/10.1080/02580136.2016.1223983

Ralefala, D., Kasule, M., Matshabane, O.P., Wonkam, A., Matshaba, M. & De Vries, J. 2021. Participants' preferences and reasons for wanting feedback of individual genetic research results from an HIV-TB genomic study: a case study from Botswana. *Journal of Empirical Research on Human Research Ethics*, 16(5):525-536. https://doi.org/10.1177/15562646211043985

Ravelingien, A. & Sandberg, A. 2008. Sleep better than medicine? Ethical issues related to "wake enhancement". *Journal of Medical Ethics*, 34(9). https://doi.org/10.1136/jme.2007.022590

Rogers, W.A. & Scully, J.L. 2021. Activism and bioethics: taking a stand on things that matter. *The Hastings Center Report*, 51(4):32-33. https://doi.org/10.1002/hast.1270

Roskies, A. 2002. Neuroethics for the new millennium. *Neuron*, 35(1):21-23. https://doi.org/10.1016/S0896-6273(02)00763-8

Roskies, A. 2008. Neuroimaging and inferential distance. *Neuroethics*, 1:19-30. https://doi.org/10.1007/s12152-007-9003-3

Salles, A., Herrera-Ferra, K. & Cabrera, L. 2018. *Global neuroethics and cultural diversity: some challenges to consider*. The Neuroethics Blog: Emory University Centre for Ethics. https://bit.ly/2JzV1ly [Accessed 30 March 2022].

Sandel, M. 2007. *The case against perfection: ethics in the age of genetic engineering*. Cambridge: Harvard University Press. https://doi.org/10.4159/9780674043060

Sankoh, O., Sevalie, S. & Weston, M. 2018. Mental health in Africa. *The Lancet: Global Health*, 6(9):E954-E955. https://doi.org/10.1016/S2214-109X(18)30303-6

Savulescu, J. & Earp, B.D. 2014. Neuroreductionism about sex and love. *Think*, 13(38):7-12. https://doi.org/10.1017/S1477175614000128

Savulescu, J., Sandberg, A. & Kahane, G. 2011. Well-being and enhancement. In: J. Savulescu, R. Ter Meulen & G. Kahane (eds.). *Enhancing human capacities*. Oxford: Wiley-Blackwell. 3-18. https://doi.org/10.1002/9781444393552

Schomerus, G., Matschinger, H. & Angermeyer, M.C. 2014. Causal beliefs of the public and social acceptance of persons with mental illness: a comparative analysis of schizophrenia, depression and alcohol dependence. *Psychological Medicine*, 44(2):303-314. https://doi.org/10.1017/S003329171300072X

Schultz, W. 2018. Neuroessentialism: theoretical and clinical considerations. *Journal of Humanistic Psychology*, 58(6): 607-639. https://doi.org/10.1177/0022167815617296

Shook, J.R. & Giordano, J. 2014. A principled and cosmopolitan neuroethics: considerations for international relevance. *Philosophy, Ethics, and Humanities in Medicine*, 9(1): 1-13. https://doi.org/10.1186/1747-5341-9-1

Stein, D.J. & Giordano, J. 2015. Global mental health and neuroethics. *BMC Medicine*, 13(44). https://doi.org/10.1186/s12916-015-0274-y

Stein, D.J. & Singh, I. (eds.). 2020. *Global mental health and neuroethics*. London: Elsevier. https://doi.org/10.1016/C2017-0-02033-5

Straiton, J. & Lake, F. 2021. Inside the brain of a killer: the ethics of neuroimaging in a criminal conviction. *BioTechniques*, 70(2):69-71. https://doi.org/10.2144/btn-2020-0171

Stevenson, A., Akena, D., Stroud, R.E., Atwoli, L., Campbell, M.M., Chibnik, L.B., Kwobah, E., Kariuki, S.M., Martin, A.R., De Menil, V., Newton, C.R.J.C., Sibeko, G., Stein, D.J., Teferra, S., Zingel, Z. & Koenen, K.C. 2019. Neuropsychiatric genetics of African populations-psychosis (NeuroGAP-Psychosis): a case-control study protocol and GWAS in Ethiopia, Kenya, South Africa and Uganda. *BMJ Open*, 9(2): e025469. https://doi.org/10.1136/bmjopen-2018-025469

Tairyan, K. & Illes, J. 2009. Imaging genetics and the power of combined technologies: a perspective from neuroethics. *Neuroscience*, 164(1):7-15. https://doi.org/10.1016/j.neuroscience.2009.01.052

Tandon, P.N. 2000. The decade of the brain: a brief review. *Neurology India*, 48:199-207.

Tangwa, G.B. 1996. Bioethics: an African perspective. *Bioethics*, 10(3):183-200. https://doi.org/10.1111/j.1467-8519.1996.tb00118.x

Thompson, P.M., Jahanshad, N., Ching, C.R.K., Salminen, L.E., Thomopoulos, S.I., Bright, J. & The Enigma consortium. 2020. ENIGMA and global neuroscience: a decade of large-scale studies of the brain in health and disease across more than 40 countries. *Translational Psychiatry*, 10(100). https://doi.org/10.1038/s41398-020-0705-1

Tindana, P., De Vries, J., Campbell, M., Littler, K., Seeley, J., Marshall, P., Troyer, J., Ogundipe, M., Alibu, V.P., Yakubu, A. & Parker, M. 2015. Community engagement strategies for genomic studies in Africa: a review of the literature. *BMC Medical Ethics*, 6(24). https://doi.org/10.1186/s12910-015-0014-z

Tosam, M.J., Chi, P.C., Munung, N.S., Oukem-Boyer, O.O.M. & Tangwa, G.B. 2018. Global health inequalities and the need for solidarity: a view from the global south. *Developing World Bioethics*, 18(3):241-249. https://doi.org/10.1111/dewb.12182

Tversky, A. & Kahneman, D. 1974. Judgment under uncertainty: heuristics and biases. *Science*, 185(4157):1124-1131. https://doi.org/10.1126/science.185.4157.1124

Vaishnav, N.H. & Chiong, W. 2018. Informed consent for the human research subject with a neurologic disorder. *Seminars in Neurology*, 38(5):539-547. https://doi.org/10.1055/s-0038-1668077

181

Verster, G.C. & Van Niekerk, A.A. 2012. Moral perspectives on stimulant use by healthy students. *South African Medical Journal*, 102(12):909-911. https://doi.org/10.7196/SAMJ.6090

Wasserman, D. & Johnston, J. 2014. Seeing responsibility: can neuroimaging teach us anything about moral and legal responsibility? *The Hastings Center Report*, March-April:S37-S49. https://doi.org/10.1002/hast.297

White, T., Blok, E. & Calhoun, V.D. 2022. Data sharing and privacy issues in neuroimaging research: opportunities, obstacles, challenges, and monsters under the bed. *Human Brain Mapping*, 43:278-291.https://doi.org/10.1002/hbm.25120

Yusuf, S., Baden, T. & Prieto-Godino, L.L. 2014. Bridging the gap: establishing the necessary infrastructure and knowledge for teaching and research in neuroscience in Africa. *Metabolic Brain Disease*, 29:217-220. https://doi.org/10.1007/s11011-013-9443-x

Significantly Increased Longevity

Does it make sense?

Anton van Niekerk

Keywords: Aubrey de Grey; boredom; death; disease; ethics of responsibility; life expectancy; longevity; Yoval Noah Harari

10.1 INTRODUCTION

More and more are nowadays written about ageing, old age, and longevity than previously. Ageing is a serious topic, particularly for those who are lucky (or unlucky!) to grow old themselves. For the latter, ageing and longevity is no mere intellectual interest, but an existential interest – one is concerned with ageing because ageing is the portal to death (that awaits us all).

It does help a little to take recourse to a sense of humour when we reflect on old age and longevity. Julie Andrews, star of the 1965 film *The Sound of Music*, has recently drawn attention to a quite funny adaptation of one of the hit songs in the film, "My favourite things". It goes as follows:

> *Botox and nose drops and needles for knitting,*
> *Walkers and handrails and new dental fittings.*
> *Bundles of magazines tied up in strings,*
> *These are a few of my favourite things.*
>
> *Cadillacs and cataracts, hearing aids and glasses,*
> *Polydent and Fixodent and false teeth in glasses.*
> *Pacemakers, golf carts and porches with swings,*
> *These are a few of my favourite things.*

When the pipes leak, when the bones creak,
When the knees go bad,
I simply remember my favourite things,
And then I don't feel so bad.[1]

10.2   INCREASED LONGEVITY AS THE FUNDAMENTAL AGENDA OF THE 21ST CENTURY

The Israeli historian, Yuval Noah Harari, in a relatively recent book, titled *Homo Deus* (2016), allots the book the striking sub-title: "A brief history of tomorrow". What is particularly notable in Harari's work is his claim that longevity – indeed, possibly even immortality – is set to become the central agenda of the 21st century.[2] We have all been brought up with the conviction that the only complete unavoidables in life are death and taxes. The enormity of the upheaval that the Fourth Industrial Revolution is to bring to our way of life is, according to Harari (as well as gerontologists such as Aubrey de Grey), no less than a definitive end to the fear of death.

Let me quote Harari (2016:31) in this respect:

> Hence, even if we don't achieve immortality in our lifetime, the war against death is still likely to be the flagship project of the coming century. When you take into account our belief in the sanctity of human life, add the dynamics of the scientific establishment, and top it all with the needs of the capitalist economy, a relentless war against death seems to be inevitable. Our ideological commitment to human life will never allow us simply to accept human death. As long as people die of something, we will strive to overcome it.

Harari (2016:32-33) continues on the next page:

> If all that is not enough, the fear of death ingrained in most humans will give the war against death an irresistible momentum. As long as people assumed that death is inevitable, they trained themselves from an early age to suppress the desire to live for ever, or harnessed it in favour of substitute goals. People want to live forever, so they compose an 'immortal' symphony, they strive for 'glory' in some war or even sacrifice their lives so that their souls will 'enjoy everlasting bliss in paradise'. A large part of our artistic creativity, our political commitment and our religious piety is

---

1   To instantly recognise this (albeit adapted) song, of course, reveals the age of the reader/listener. I was 12 when the record-setting film was released, and I probably saw the film at least three times!

2   See also Harari (2018).

> fuelled by the fear of death … Once people think (with or without good
> reason) that they have a serious chance of escaping death, the desire for life
> will refuse to go on pulling the rickety wagon of art, ideology and religion,
> and will sweep forward like an avalanche.

It is, of course, one thing to strive for immortality or significantly increased longevity. It is something else to master the means of conquering the wide variety of
ways that might succeed with such an enterprise.

10.3   GROWING OLD WITHOUT BECOMING AGED: ENTER AUBREY DE GREY

One of the intellectuals who unwaveringly believes that death does not have
the final word, is Aubrey de Grey from Cambridge. While Harari is still quite
modest in his projections of expected longevity, De Grey has recently drawn
much attention with the considerably bolder claims he makes in this regard.
He identifies himself as a 'biogerontologist' and is currently chief science officer
of the Strategies for Engineered Negligible Senescence (SENS) Foundation in
Cambridge. He claims that "[ageing] is no more than a widespread, extremely
destructive, yet avoidable cluster of diseases that could all be reversed or cured in
view of extending our lifespan almost indefinitely" (De Grey, 2008:103). *We can
grow old without becoming aged.* To quote De Grey (2008:67-68) himself:

> Recent biotechnological progress indicates that many aspects of ageing
> may indeed be effectively treatable by regenerative medicine in the
> foreseeable future. We cannot yet know whether all aspects will be curable,
> but extensive scrutiny has failed to identify any definite exceptions.
> Therefore, at this point there is a significant chance that such therapies
> would postpone age-related decline by several years, if not more, which
> constitutes a clear case for allocating significant resources to the attempt
> to develop those therapies.

Just about every disease or degeneration of the human body associated with the
process of ageing can, according to De Grey, be 'reverse-engineered'. The big
challenge is to arrest the process of ageing, not at the equivalent of the bodily
prowess of a 90-year-old, but rather at that of a 40-year-old. De Grey is confident
that the first person to reach the age of 1 000 has already been born, and he has
high hopes that it will indeed be himself.

This chapter deals with the question as to the fleeting nature of youth as well
as whether death can be postponed indefinitely, as is increasingly argued by
scientists and intellectuals under the impression of our species' ability to take our
own evolution to hand.

These questions are also the outcome of the fact that human beings are capable of attaining control over their own evolution, rather than to simply continue our traditional submittance to changes in the process of evolution that occur beyond our knowledge or control. This issue is important because it contains the potential to transform our complete understanding of the meaning of our lives. If we do, in principle, have to fear death, or if we can bargain on 'eternal youth', all our normal life priorities are indeed submitted to a definitive transformation. As we currently live in the face of our mortality, life does indeed receive its seriousness and urgency from the reality of death.

It is of value to, in this respect, refer to the work of the Russian philosopher, Nicolas Berdyaev. He writes (1948:250):

> Heidegger is right in saying that the herd-mentality (das Man) is insensitive to the anguish of death. It feels merely a low fear of death as of that which makes life meaningless. But there is another half of the truth, concealed from the ordinary point of view. Death not merely makes life senseless and corruptible: it is also a sign coming.

10.4   OLD AGE AND THE FEAR OF DEATH

When people are asked for their reasons for fearing old age, the answer is normally quite straightforward and self-evident. None of us wishes (except maybe for very personal reasons) to become ugly, obese, overly skinny, constrained, stiff or immobile, forgetful, or (heaven forbid) incontinent. I once heard someone (on in years) say: "Life might start at 60, but my experience is that everything else then also starts to either wear out, implode or to spread sidewards!"

All the latter 'old age traits' are symptoms of a disease of one kind or another (heart disease, cancer, diabetes, stroke, arthritis, etc.). We fundamentally fear old age since old age is one of the most notable risk factors for (serious) disease. Many of the mentioned diseases cause death in a majority of cases (i.e., if death is not brought on by something else).

If that is the case, i.e., if old age is the most significant risk-factor for all these diseases, would it not be better to 'attack' old age itself and avoid death, rather than to attack (by treatments, medications, etc.) all these other 'causes of death' in the sense of bodily disease? Put differently: Is our fear of death not better overcome by interventions that slow down, halt, or repair those parts of the body that are hurt or dysfunctional? In this regard, again be reminded of the claim of Aubrey de Grey that biogerontology is making rapid progress towards 'reverse engineering' every body part that loses function or use.

We are seemingly not built or 'designed' to live forever. I will later deal with general longevity information. What is striking, nevertheless, is that while life expectancy is at the moment growing all over the world (i.e., more people are growing older than before, but also – significantly fewer infants are dying), this does not seem to have a notable effect on longevity. Many more people exceed the ages of 70, 80, and 90 than was the case a century or two earlier. But living individuals seem to have a kind of ceiling in terms of the age that they attain.

10.5   LIFE EXPECTANCY AND LONGEVITY

Let us illustrate this latter claim. Until recently, a French woman by the name of Jeanne Calment was the oldest human person recorded – 122 years and 164 days. She died on 4 August 1997 (*Wikipedia*, accessed 13 October 2022). Currently, the oldest person alive is Lucille Randon who also lives in France at the age of 118 years and 244 days. It is insightful that she was born in the year after the Wright brothers flew for the first time.

Kane Tanaka was a Japanese woman who lived for 119 years and 107 days. She died on 19 April 2022. It is told that, until she died, she had a crush on chocolates and soda drinks. She also loved board games and she thrived on building puzzles. The past did not interest her much – she was mainly focused on the future. The *Guinness Book of Records* recognised her as the oldest person while alive. She got married at the age of 19. Her family ran a noodle store since 1937, when her husband and son left to fight the Japanese war.

Demographers inform us that in 2040, Spain will overtake Japan as the world's population with the greatest average longevity. Average life expectancy in Spain at that time will be 86.

According to the Japanese Ministry of Health, in 2021 there were 86510 people alive at the age of 100 or more in Japan – 6060 more than the previous year. Yet, no one has up to now ever lived longer than the 122 years that Jeanne Calment lived. We might therefore wonder how regularly people in future will exceed the ages of 130 or 140, let alone 150. While it certainly is possible that that kind of age will be reached without dramatic technological innovations, it has not been achieved and there are no clear-cut signs that it is due to happen.

In general, there is no consensus among scientists on how long people are likely to live under ideal (e.g., pandemic-free) circumstances. A 2016 study found the upper limit to be more or less an age of 115, but another Italian study preferred to not impose a limit (Olshansky & Carnes, 2019). While it is a fact that a growing number of people surpass the age of 80, that in itself is not so remarkable. Steven

Pinker rightfully points out that there also were centenarians at the beginning of the 20th century (Pinker, 2011). Again: while life expectancy is rising all over the world, individual centenarians are not increasing significantly.

10.6   WHAT CAUSES DEATH?

Scientists today better understand the cellular and molecular processes that cause old age. A recent *JAMA*[3] study (2017) classified the most prevalent causes into four groups:

- Chronic inflammation;
- Cell disfunction;
- Changes in stem cells that prevent these cells from regenerating tissue; and
- Cellular ageing, the accumulation of cells that accompany disease.

Young people apparently have relatively few of these ageing cells. However, they start accumulating in the body after the age of 60 has been reached. The more these cells accumulate, it is striking that their growing number correlate with the disabilities of old age.

Would it be possible to replace these ageing cells with new, young cells? This is the topic of much research currently taking place. One study has shown that the old cells of mice have reacted quite favourably to two drugs: the one is Dasatinib (normally used as a cancer drug) and the other is Quercetin (Hickson, Prata, Bobart & Evans, 2019), normally a plant flavonoid. Flavonoids are a group of plant metabolites thought to provide health benefits through cell signalling pathways and antioxidant effects. These molecules are found in a variety of fruits and vegetables. Flavonoids are polyphenolic molecules containing 15 carbon atoms and are soluble in water.

10.7   IS OLD AGE A DISEASE?

This brings us to question of whether old age itself ought to be looked upon as some kind of disease. The opposing participants in this debate are Aubrey de Grey, to whom I have referred earlier, and Nir Barzilai, founding director of the Institute for Aging Research, the Nathan Schock Centre of Excellence in the Basic Biology of Aging, and the Paul F Glen Center for the Biology of Human

---

3   *JAMA* is the acronym for *Journal of the American Association of Medicine*, widely regarded as one of the best accredited medical journals in the world.

Aging Research at Albert Einstein College of Medicine of Yeshiva University in New York City, USA.

Barzilai is adamant that old age is not a disease. His main claim is that his research in this respect is only related to an assembly of age-related diseases that will, eventually, affect mortality.

Aubrey de Grey takes the opposite view. For him, ageing is indeed a disease. I quote again: "Age is no more than a wide-spread, extremely destructive, yet avoidable cluster of diseases that could all be reversed or cured in view of extending our lifespan almost indefinitely" (2008:103).

De Grey is a protagonist of so-called 'regenerative medicine' that facilitates the 'reverse-engineering' of worn-out body parts. All of the techniques or means to accomplish the latter are not yet available, but there is, according to De Grey, no reason why they cannot or should not be developed in the future. His biggest problem as of yet was to find the resources for this kind of research. Quite impressive laboratories where this kind of research is and can be done already have been erected at the universities of Cambridge, Harvard, and California (Berkeley).

One of the biggest challenges in this kind of work is to 'arrest' the process of ageing, not at the ages of 80 or 90 (that are normally associated with old age), but at the ages of 35 to 45, when people are normally 'at their physical and emotional best'. De Grey detests (the thought of) death. He is unpersuaded by the argument that death can indeed be a huge relief in our efforts to be safeguarded against monsters like Hitler, Stalin, or Mugabe and the extreme damage that they have brought upon (Western) civilisation.

In that respect, I surmise that De Grey will also be unpersuaded by Roald Dahl's gripping short story titled, "Genesis and catastrophe: A true story", from his short story volume *Tales of the Unexpected*. This is the (true!) story of the birth of Hitler, whose mother is inconsolable because of his unlikelihood of survival – he will be the third child she has to bury. Her husband is no consolation either. He is even more convinced that the weakly-developed little creature will eventually not survive. But, as we now know, the little creature did in the end survive. How much better and more hospitable might the world not have been if the young Adolf (named after his father Alois) did in fact not survive? Death can indeed often time be a salvation if we think of the havoc that moral monsters can cause. Yet even such a counterargument does not persuade De Grey – death is the all-time enemy that we ideally ought to avoid at all costs.

10.8   NOT LONGER BUT MORE HEALTHY LIVES

De Grey and Barzilai are, of course, not the only participants in these debates. A more conservative, yet internationally recognised researcher such as Prof. S. Jay Olshansky of the University of Illinois claims that there is an upper limit for our normal ageing process, viz. 85. Olshansky and his colleagues Carnes (2019:9,21) write in this regard: "Parts of the body, including the brain, are not designed for long-term use. We are seeing the consequences of pushing the limits of survival: the rise of Alzheimer's disease, dementias, joint and hip problems, loss of muscle mass."

We tend to think of these disease phenomena as instances of the failure of both body and mind to survive indefinitely. But Olshansky argues that these phenomena are not indicative of too much/early failure of the body, but rather of too much success in our efforts to make people live longer. We are making entities survive that have indeed long passed their shelf life. What we ought to try and accomplish in the expectation of death, is not a *longer* life, but indeed a *healthier* life. Olshansky and Carnes (2019:8,21) write in this respect:

> If the goal of aging science and modern medicine shifts from its historical emphasis on trying to make us live longer, to a new goal of extending the period of healthy life, we no longer have to fight the uphill battle against life table entropy.

10.9   IS A LONG LIFE DESIRABLE?

Do we really want to live indefinitely? On the basis of personal experience, I cannot say that I have ever come across someone with a clear and articulated desire to live longer than 90 or 100 years.[4] A recent survey among USA citizens showed that 38% of Americans wish to use life-prolonging drugs, against 56% who do not (the remaining 6% are non-committal). Of those polled, only 4% are of the opinion that the average age for humans ought to be 120. Interestingly enough, religious people are not more opposed to life-prolonging actions than non-religious people.

Another pivotal question remains: do we really want to live that long? In this respect, De Grey really seems to be an exception. I find the idea of living a couple

---

4   My own mother is a notable exception in this regard. She became quite old (95), and her final decade was marred by consistently decreasing quality of life. Yet neither I nor my siblings ever heard her express the desire to die. For a more complete discussion, see Van Niekerk (2017:39-43).

of hundred or even a thousand years quite unattractive. In a book published in the early 1970s, the English philosopher-ethicist Brian Williams correctly pointed out that the thing to fear most from an indefinitely prolonged life is sustained boredom (Williams, 1973). Suppose a 'normal' human life stretches out to 1 000 years ahead in time. It is safe to surmise that a career in the lives that we normally lead lasts for 40 or 50 years – let's make it 80 years in order to accommodate the exceptions among us. Someone who was a doctor in the first 80 years of living can hardly be conceived to proceed with his/her 'second stint' as a doctor with another 80 years awaiting. Careers could indeed be changed – but how often? Twice? Four times? Six? Imagine a person, having lived 600 years, and 'looking forward' to another 400! Apart from the medico-scientific-technological challenge of bringing this off, it seems to me like nothing but a sure formula for the utmost form of boredom. What is also unclear is the nature and quality of the interaction and communication that a 'mere spring chicken of 68' (my current age) might have with a person who lives into his/her three or seven hundreds.

I cannot imagine that such a life might amount to anything other than boredom and loneliness. Imagine the living memories of someone who has been around for a couple of hundred years! (For further aspects of this argument, see Nicolas Agar (2010:112-113).)

10.10   SOME FURTHER ISSUES

The argument above does not exhaust the array of ethical questions that are provoked by the prospect of unlimited longevity. The first of these questions asks who is to benefit most by research of this nature. Will it be credible that the party with the most interest in this research will indeed be future Aubrey de Greys whose only interest in life is to prolong it? It is indeed quite conceivable that a lot of money is probably to be made on this research, or that this whole enterprise amounts to an overt lucrative initiative emanating from Big Pharma.

A second question relates to the question of distributive justice in terms of who will benefit. Will there be justice in the distribution of the benefits emanating from this work?

Even if the justice of the production of the end-results could be demonstrated, the question of possible over-population remains. We are at the moment in the vicinity of 8 billion people inhabiting this planet. Are we seriously going to throw the best that science, technology, and big capital can offer to an enterprise such as (in principle) unlimited longevity and dramatic increases in life expectancy?

Therefore, while there are quite serious questions to raise about the scientific, economic, and technological viability of a project such as this, we ought, thirdly, to make sure that our attitudes with respect to either the embracing or the rejection of this practice are morally justifiable. We have noted concerns that question the desirability of these practices. We should, however, not reject a desire for longevity and life expectancy purely on the basis of the argument that such a desire amounts to a morally unjustifiable desire to biomedically enhance ourselves and/or our children.

If the argument amounts to no more than that medico-technological means are used to prolong longevity, it is fundamentally unclear as to why there is any sustainable moral objection to that. We have, as a species, enhanced ourselves for thousands of years. Furthermore, we are facilitating our life quality with a range of technological devices, ranging from wheelchairs to radios to television sets to renal dialysis machines – in each case to enhance the way we live, at both a young and old age. The reader who regards drastic life prolonging measures as an instance of doubtful human enhancement is invited to do a simple thought experiment: Imagine someone who died 400 years ago and gets 'resurrected' in our current-day world. The world in which we live would, for that person, hardly be recognisable. The world's appearance would by and large be the outcome of sustained 'enhancement' over four centuries.[5]

The objection to human enhancement cannot either be that we are departing from the canons of 'human nature'. It is a risky and sometimes inconsistent idea that 'human nature' should constitute a norm to which we should all adhere. If we are serious about such an idea, we ought to realise that if we decide for the normativity of 'human nature', that cannot only mean that we work with an idealised format of human nature. If 'human nature' becomes normative for all of us, we must be happy to take that idea on board – 'warts and all', as we say. 'Human nature' is not only represented by Mandela and Ghandi and Shakespeare. It is unfortunately sometimes also represented by Hitler and Stalin and Jack the Ripper. Embracing 'human nature' as that we ought to pursue in the process of enhancement is sure to land us with a character set that is not always desirable. It is not for nothing that the crime and mystery novelist Agatha Christie so often ascribes the reason for the crime being investigated in a certain book to the fact that the criminal is bound to act according to the dictates of 'human nature'. In her living room in St Mary's Meade, Christie's Miss Marple is regularly able to solve some crime on the basis of her knowledge of 'human nature'.

---

5   For a substantive debate about these issues, see Van Niekerk (2014) and (2016), and Penrose (2016).

What, then, remains to be said of Harari's prediction that the quest for significantly enhanced longevity, paired with significantly increased average life expectancy, will be the main technologically and scientifically mediated agenda of the 21st century?

I personally am not very attracted to this idea. For reasons that have been spelled out, I find the idea of radically enhanced longevity both boring and undesirable. I would much rather opt for the idea that human existence is best circumscribed, not as the indefinite survival of a small number of individuals who continue to live for little other reason than the fact that their current existence is the outcome of remarkable and unforeseen technological achievements. (A possible exception to this eventuality could be the situation of geniuses like Einstein and Darwin whose continued existence could significantly contribute to scientific, technological, and even political progress.)

However, both the literature on the matter as well as anecdotal evidence strongly suggest that a more prudent interpretation of a life that approaches old age is to regard it in terms of an organism which exists with and in terms of a history. Tirosh-Samuelson (2011:41) writes in this regard:

> Since the human being is an organism, rather than a mechanical device, human beings undergo the cycle of life, maturation, aging and death, which exemplifies the rhythm of creation and the gift of life. An organism has a beginning, a life cycle (or a history) and, eventually, a process of termination.

In the next paragraph, I translate and quote a passage written in this regard by the South African-Dutch philosopher, Vincent Brümmer, shortly before his own death in 2021:

> The lives of all people [excluding those that die young], with its limits of birth and death, pass through four phases. The phase between birth and roundabout 21 years is the phase in which a person grows up and attains maturity. The second phase stretches from attained maturity to retirement. This is the phase of one's life during which you work and start building a career and a family. This is the phase of life characterised by what Van Niekerk calls a 'life strategy': a network of shorter- and longer-term ideals or goals that bestow direction to what one does and what you strive for. This life strategy is not unchangeably fixed. It is regularly adapted in view of changed circumstances, obstacles on one's way and (often unforeseen) chances and opportunities that come your way unexpectedly. In this sense a person can, during this phase, be called 'modernist'. The third phase stretches from the time of retirement until you start requiring special care. People in this phase are often called 'yep's', the acronym for 'young elderly people'. Ideally people will be able to tighten loose ends during this

> phase, i.e., to complete undertakings that one could not tackle or complete during one's working life. The fourth phase is when one becomes entirely dependent on other people – a phase that leads to one's death. In this phase one lives from day to day. You do no longer aspire to attain short- or long-term ideals. This is the phase that Van Niekerk calls 'postmodern'. (Brümmer, in Jones, 2022:29)

This is, to my mind, a prudent and enlightening representation of how to gene-rally make sense of the totality of the lives that most of us lead.

10.11   CONCLUSION

I want to conclude by emphasising two aspects of this general metaphor. The first is that this way of thinking about life as we know it (i.e., not life as significantly prolonged), represents an organistic image of human life – that image which I find particularly helpful. An organism is a life form with a history – a history that typically undergoes the phases identified by Brümmer above. The life that an organism leads does not appear or disappear instantly. It is the outcome of a process – what I would like to call, a history.

Let me quote Alasdair MacIntyre (1981:197) on his enlightening discussion of the nature and scope of the "narrative quest" that we all embody in the process of growing old.

> Narrative is not the work of poets, dramatists and novelists reflecting upon events which had no narrative before one was imposed by the singer or the writer; narrative form is neither disguise nor decoration … It is now becoming clear that we render the actions of others intelligible in this way because action in itself has a basically historical character. It is because we all live out narratives in our lives and because we understand our own lives in terms of the narratives that we live out that the form of the narrative is appropriate for understanding the actions of others. Stories are lived before they are told – except in the case of fiction.

This then brings us, in conclusion, back to the question in the heading of this book chapter: "Significantly increased longevity: Does it make sense"? Consi-dering all the arguments that have been brought forward, and particularly bearing in mind what I argued about the organistic character of human beings and the narrative quest that accompanies all meaningful lives – but also reckoning with the boredom that will in all probability be part and parcel of indefinitely prolonged human lives, my answer to the question is in the negative.

Bibliography

Agar, N. 2010. *Humanity's end*. London: MIT Press. https://doi.org/10.7551/mitpress/9780262014625.001.0001

Ahmad, J. 2021. *Journal of the American Medical Association*, 325(18). https://bit.ly/3i25vzL

Berdyaev, N. 1948. *The destiny of man*. London: Geofrey Bless.

Berlinger, N., De Medeiros, K. & Girling, L. 2021. Bioethics and gerontology: the value of thinking together. *The Gerontologist*, 62(8):1097-1103. https://doi.org/10.1093/geront/gnab186

De Grey, A. 2008. *Ending aging*. Cambridge: Cambridge University Press.

Harari, Y.N. 2016. *Homo Deus*. London: Vintage. https://doi.org/10.17104/9783406704024

Harari, Y.N. 2018. *21 Lessons for the 21st century*. London: Jonathan Cape.

Hickson, L.T.J., Prata, L.G.P.L., Bobart, S.A. & Evans, T.K. 2019. Senolytics decrease senescent cells in humans: Preliminary report from a clinical trial of Dasatinib plus Quercetin in individuals with diabetic kidney disease. *eBioMedicine*. Elsevier.

Jones, C. 2022. 'n Filosofiese gesprek oor die dood en die sin van die lewe. *Tydskrif vir Geesteswetenskappe*, 62(1).

MacIntyre, A. 1981. *After virtue*. London: Duckworth.

Olshansky, S.J. & Carnes, A.C. 2019. Inconvenient truths about human longevity. *The Journals of Gerontology*: Series A, vol. 74. Issue Supplement 1, December, pp. S7-S12. https://doi.org/10.1093/gerona/glz098

Pinker, S. 2011. *The better angels of our nature*. London: Routledge.

Tirosh-Samuelson, H. 2011. Engaging transhumanism. In: G.R. Hansell & W. Grassie (eds.). *Transhumanism and its critics*. Philadelphia, PA: Metanexus.

Van Niekerk, A.A. 2014. Biomedical enhancement and the pursuit of mastery and perfection: a critique of the views of Michael Sandel. *South African Journal of Philosophy*, 33(2):155-165. https://doi.org/10.1080/02580136.2014.923697

Van Niekerk, A.A. 2016. A response to Penrose's "Sandel on enhancement: a response to Van Niekerk". *South African Journal of Philosophy*, 35(2):164-170. https://doi.org/10.1080/02580136.2016.1174814

Van Niekerk, A.A. 2017. *Die dood en die sin van die lewe*. Cape Town: Tafelberg.

Williams, B. 1973. *The Makropulos case: reflections on the tedium of immortality*. Cambridge: Cambridge University Press. https://bit.ly/3EQJPjc

11

End-of-Life Choices

Willem Landman

Keywords: advance directive; assisted dying; assisted suicide; constitutional rights; health care power of attorney; living will; right to bodily and psychological integrity; right to dignity; right to freedom and security of the person; right to security of and control over one's body; surrogacy; terminal pain management; voluntary euthanasia

11.1 INTRODUCTION

For some, dying is a peaceful and dignified process or event, without much suffering, perhaps even serene, and at the end of a completed life.

Others are less fortunate. For them, dying is a protracted process, a *via dolorosa* suffused with uncertainty, fear, suffering, and loss of dignity, in which a once fully human life is agonisingly dismantled. However, should this be our destiny, we are not entirely delivered to the inevitable. We have choices and can take some control.

End-of-life choices can be divided into four categories (Landman, 2001, 2012):

- End-of-life pain management that hastens death;
- Refusal of and refraining from life-sustaining treatment;
- Advance directives; and
- Assisted dying – assisted suicide and voluntary euthanasia.

In South Africa, unfortunately, each one of these options poses unresolved legal issues. Both end-of-life pain management and refraining from life-sustaining treatment that ought to be standard-of-care medical practices are mired in uncertainties. The legal status of advance directives, such as a living will, is unclear. Assisting with suicide and practising voluntary euthanasia constitute the common-law crime of murder.

What exactly is at issue in these end-of-life practices, and how could each of them assist to make dying gentler, more compassionate, and more dignified?

11.2   END-OF-LIFE PAIN MANAGEMENT THAT HASTENS DEATH

First, end-of-life pain management that hastens death seeks to ease suffering during the dying process. Suffering is a complex, intensely personal experience induced by physical pain, mental distress, or both. At the end of life, suffering may be unbearable and intractable. It may become so all-consuming that continued life becomes increasingly undesirable and devoid of meaning and purpose.

Throughout our lives, we seek to remove or alleviate others' suffering as far as it is within our power to do so. It should be no different at the end of life. Adequate end-of-life pain management, however, may have the foreseen, unintended, yet inevitable, secondary *consequence* of hastening death.

But then such terminal pain management resulting in inevitable death would appear to be indistinguishable from voluntary euthanasia that terminates life *in order to* terminate pain. Or, at the very least, any distinction would appear to be tenuous. After all, both result in ending pain as well as life. So, the difference between the lawful and the unlawful would appear to hinge precariously on the description of the exact mental content – the intention – of the medical practitioner without there necessarily being any overt or perceivable behavioural difference.

Unfortunately, perceived legal risk associated with terminal pain management is a factor in under-treatment of pain. Ideally, end-of-life pain management should be located in a comprehensive palliative care setting, based on clinical judgement, and informed by consultation with patient and family. And the law should create an enabling and protective environment for medicine to do what it should.

In its final report on end-of-life choices, the South African Law Commission (SALC) (RSA, 1998:59)[1] appended a draft bill – the "End of Life Decisions Act" – stating that if pain medication proves to be inadequate, then a medical practitioner or nurse may increase the dosage with the object of relieving pain even if the secondary effect is the shortening of the patient's life. This report was shelved by Parliament, which means that uncertainty about legal liability, and therefore unnecessary suffering, persist. This lost opportunity compromises responsible medicine in an increasingly litigious environment. Standard-of-care

---

1   At the time of the report's publication, the South African Law Reform Commission (SALRC) was known as the South African Law Commission (SALC).

medical practice, unlike medical malpractice, should not be the domain of the courts (Landman, 2012:38-39).

The Supreme Court of Appeal (SCA) stepped into this partial legal void when a full bench of five SCA judges held the following in the Stransham-Ford case (2016:Para 34):

> [...] a medical practitioner commits no offence by prescribing drugs by way of palliative treatment for pain that the doctor knows will have the effect of hastening the patient's death. This is referred to as the 'double effect', where the drugs serve the purpose for which they were prescribed, but have potentially detrimental [secondary, foreseen, but unavoidable] side effects.

Thus the SCA confirms the common law and goes some way towards addressing ignorance and fear of litigation.

However, explicit legislation – along the lines proposed by the SALC (RSA, 1998:59) – is required to communicate unambiguously the common-law position, thus allaying unfounded fear of legal risk and creating a more enabling and comforting legal environment for all concerned – patient, family, and medical practitioner.

11.3   REFUSAL OF AND REFRAINING FROM LIFE-SUSTAINING TREATMENT

Modern medicine can extend biological life to the point where it is no longer good, desired, or dignified. When would a medical practitioner be legally justified to refrain from life-sustaining treatment (medication, procedures, life-support machines, and the like) by withholding (before it commences) or withdrawing (once commenced) such treatment (Landman, 2012:41-62)? And whose choice should it be?

Decisions to refuse and refrain from[2] life-sustaining treatment – a second category of end-of-life choices – involve both competent and incompetent individuals.

---

2   Referring to refraining from, withholding, or withdrawing life-sustaining treatment as 'passive euthanasia' attracts unnecessary controversy towards a routine medical practice by dint of mere terminological association with 'active euthanasia'. Other things being equal, 'active' and 'passive' euthanasia are morally equivalent (Landman, 1982). Whether one's action is an act (active) or an omission (passive), one can be held morally and legally accountable for either, so nothing of moral or legal substance hinges on the active-passive distinction *in itself*.

11.3.1 Competent persons

The National Health Act (RSA, 1996:Sec 7(1)(e)) prohibits the provision of "a health service" without a person's informed consent, that is, *any* medical treatment, routine or life-sustaining, regardless of the person's health status. Thus, competent[3] persons are legally entitled to *refuse* contemporaneously life-sustaining treatment – while continuing to receive palliative care – and medical professionals should accordingly *refrain* from such treatment.

There are, of course, recognised exceptions to the general requirement of informed consent, such as a medical or public-health emergency.

The SALC (RSA, 1998:43) confirmed our common law's "unambiguous recognition and acceptance of the right of the patient, who need not be terminal, to refuse life-saving medical intervention". This is consistent with the constitutional right to bodily integrity (RSA, 1996:Sec 12(2)), which includes the right to control over one's body (RSA, 1996:Sec 12(2)(b)).

The SCA (Stransham-Ford, 2016:Para 31. Emphasis added.) stated the ethical and legal principles regarding refusal of and refraining from life-sustaining treatment as follows:

> A person may refuse treatment that would otherwise prolong life. This is an aspect of *personal autonomy* that is constitutionally protected and would not ordinarily be regarded as suicide. Medical treatment without the patient's consent is regarded as *assault* so that the patient is *always* entitled to refuse medical treatment.

Thus, by refusing life-sustaining treatment – which may include artificial nutrition and hydration – the patient allows natural processes to take their course so that the underlying illness becomes the proximate cause of death (Stransham-Ford, 2016:Para 31).

Manipulating information to obtain informed consent undermines patient autonomy. Medical practitioners might do this for several reasons, such as managing perceived risk, ignorance of the law, traditional views of professional authority, personal religious persuasions, or monetary gain.

---

3   In a health care context, 'competence' refers to the capacity of persons to understand, reason about, make decisions, and communicate about their health care. Competence is task-specific. Thus, one may be competent to choose chocolate rather than vanilla ice cream, but incompetent to make an irreversible, life-changing decision (Landman, 2012:42).

11.3.2 Incompetent individuals without advance directives

Incompetent[4] individuals lack the necessary mental competence and legal capacity to make decisions about their continued health care, including life-sustaining treatment. They could be *formerly* competent individuals or individuals who have *never* been, and will never become, competent, for example seriously defective newly born infants.

How should we make decisions about continued life for incompetent individuals?

Some jurisdictions have dedicated legislation creating the *right to a natural death*, free from intrusive medical interventions. Thus, North Carolina (NC, 1977: 90-320 to 90-322) provides for refraining from (withholding or withdrawing) life-sustaining treatment, including artificial nutrition and hydration, for incompetent patients, that is, patients who are:

- Comatose without any reasonable possibility of returning to cognitive function *or* mentally incompetent; *and*

- Either terminal and incurable *or* in a permanent vegetative state (PVS – see footnote 4); *and*

- Sustained by extraordinary means *or* artificial nutrition and hydration.

Should all these clinical conditions obtain – mental, physical, and dependence – then the incompetent individual's attending physician may refrain from life-sustaining treatment, with the concurrence of the surrogate.

South Africa has no equivalent legislation regulating refraining from life-sustaining treatment. The effort by the SALC (RSA, 1998) was fruitless expenditure. But we have developed relevant common-law principles.

In the Clarke (1992) case, the court ruled that discontinuing medical treatment would not be unlawful. The patient, Dr Clarke, became deeply comatose and went into a PVS and remained so for several years. Having approached the court, his wife was appointed curatrix to her husband with the power to authorise withholding or discontinuance of any life-sustaining treatment. Significantly, the court held that, in cases such as these, it would not be contrary to public policy if a court would make an evaluation of the quality of life of the patient to determine whether life-sustaining measures should be discontinued. This recognises that

---

4   Incompetence may be due to (1) being clinically dead in the sense of whole-brain death; (2) being in a permanent vegetative state (PVS), that is, totally and irreversibly non-conscious while the brain stem still functions; or (3) irreversibly lacking higher brain (cortical) function necessary for rational choice (being mentally incompetent) while still capable of awareness, discomfort, or pain (Landman, 2012:57-62).

medical treatment is not about merely extending biological life in the total and irreversible absence of conscious life.

So, refraining from life-sustaining treatment of an incompetent individual is lawful provided the necessary clinical conditions obtain. This would include switching off machines; withholding or withdrawal of medication, procedures, or artificial nutrition and hydration; and issuing do-not-resuscitate (DNR) orders.

A decision about the continued life of an irreversibly incompetent individual involves judging the value of a life. If a medical intervention is unable to attain any worthwhile goal beyond mere biological functioning, then life-sustaining treatment is futile or pointless. Maintaining vital functions without the possibility of any conscious or subjective life – biology without biography – does not enable a life that is worth living, given the lives normal human beings live.

In sum, a doctor who ceases treatment of an incompetent patient, or any other medical intervention, that serves no therapeutic or palliative purpose does not commit an offence (Stransham-Ford, 2016:Para 33).

11.3.3 Surrogate decision-making

Crucial for end-of-life choices on behalf of incompetent individuals is a duly authorised surrogate, proxy, or substitute decision-maker who decides for the incompetent individual according to legally prescribed provisions. Surrogacy is also a key notion in advance directives (discussed in the next section). Medical practitioners and health care facilities are legally obliged to respect a surrogate's decision *as if* it is the incompetent patient's own competent expression of will. The surrogate *fully* assumes the decisional capacity of the patient. This is of great significance since some doctors all too often ignore – sometimes with poor communication and even arrogance – the legitimate pleas by surrogates, mostly close family, to cease treatment.

The National Health Act (RSA, 2003) explicitly recognises the legal authority of a surrogate decision-maker for an incompetent individual. Likewise, the SCA (Stransham-Ford, 2016:Para 31) confirmed the principle that treatment against one's will, or a substitute's will – treatment without informed consent – constitutes assault. Thus, medical practitioners should draw comfort from this protection against legal liability, even if a surrogate decides against life-sustaining treatment for a patient. In fact, on the contrary, overruling the surrogate may invite legal liability.

Ideally, a medical practitioner and surrogate should be *ad idem* about appropriate end-of-life treatment in the incompetent patient's best interest. Disagreements originate in inadequate understanding of their respective authority and powers, and this is in no small measure attributable to lack of dedicated legislation.

Should efforts at constructive communication and persuasion be unsuccessful, and a medical practitioner continues treatment against the surrogate's wishes, the surrogate can have their authority confirmed by means of a court order (Clarke, 1992). The SALC report (RSA, 1998:235) affirms the legal position that a medical practitioner shall not act in a manner that "would be contrary to the wishes of the interested family members of the patient, unless authorised by a court to do so".

Conversely, should a surrogate insist on futile treatment serving neither a therapeutic nor palliative purpose (Stransham-Ford, 2016:Para 33), while merely extending biological life in the irreversible absence of consciousness, the medical practitioner, after good-faith attempts at persuading the surrogate, would have the full backing of the law to override unilaterally the surrogate's decision.

The SCA (Stransham-Ford, 2016:Para 31) points out that all these common-law principles regarding refusal of life-sustaining treatment are recognised in the right to dignity given by section 10 of the Constitution (RSA, 1996) and the right to bodily integrity given by Section 12(2)(b). The only condition that refusal of treatment needs to meet is the required level of mental competence and legal capacity of the decsion-maker (principal or surrogate) (Stransham-Ford, 2016:Para 32). One should add that the person's decision should be made autonomously, free from coercion, pressure, or undue influence, and in terms of a stable set of personal values.

11.4   ADVANCE DIRECTIVES

A third category of end-of-life choices is advance directives, that is, instruments designed to assist medical practitioners and surrogates to decide for incompetent individuals. They are advance expressions of a competent person's preferences regarding future medical treatment should they ever become incapable of making their own decisions. They are documents drawn up, signed, attested by witnesses, and deposited for safekeeping in places where they can be accessed when needed. Still, verbal instructions may also constitute valid advance directives.

Although enjoying increasing popularity, advance directives have a precarious legal status in South Africa which undermines their credibility and effectiveness. They raise questions of interpretation, for example: What standards should guide a surrogate's decisions? For what reasons, if any, may a medical practitioner dishonour an advance directive? Is a medical practitioner immunised against criminal or civil liability for honouring an advance directive? What formalities, if any, do advance directives require?

The two kinds of advance directives recognised in dedicated legislation of other jurisdictions are a health care power of attorney and a living will.

11.4.1 Health care power of attorney

A health care power of attorney is a *substitute directive* where a competent person appoints or mandates a designated individual as their surrogate to make health care decisions on their behalf should they become incapacitated (Landman, 2012:64, 67-69). It confers *general* decision-making powers on the surrogate to make all health care decisions, including decisions about life-sustaining treatment. It may also contain *specific* instructions for prescribed circumstances, for example a DNR order, medication, procedures, nutrition and hydration, or any other form of life support.

A health care power of attorney is *durable* – it endures for life, unless revoked by its issuer while still competent. The surrogate (agent) fully steps into the patient's (principal's) shoes and makes *all* health care decisions on their behalf.

The term 'health care power of attorney' or a cognate does not appear in the National Health Act (RSA, 2003), but the Act provides for a person to *mandate in writing* another person of their choice to grant consent on their behalf should they become unable to do so (RSA, 2003:Sec 7(1)(a)). Such a mandate constitutes a health care power of attorney.

In the absence of a mandate, the Act (RSA, 2003:Sec 7(1)(b)) provides for a *family member* – such as a parent, spouse, sibling, or child – to *automatically* become the incompetent patient's surrogate, empowered to make all health care decisions on their behalf on the basis of recognised decision-making standards.[5]

The Act (RSA, 2003:Sec 7(1)(c)) also provides for the appointment of a surrogate by *court order*. This may be necessary in adverserial circumstances, for example when a medical practitioner refuses to act on a surrogate's instructions.

---

5   There is a descending hierarchy of decision-making standards applied according to a surrogate's familiarity with an incompetent patient's preferences while still competent: (1) The subjective standard is what a patient *actually* would have wanted; (2) the substituted-judgment standard is what a patient *probably* would have wanted, and (3) the best-interest standard calculates which option would have the *highest net benefit* for the patient. The SCA (Stransham-Ford, 2016:Para 32) refers to justifications for court orders regarding patients who are not clinically brain dead, but on a ventilator and unaware of their surroundings, ranging from "the concept of substituted judgment to the best interest of the patient".

Should the surrogate be unavailable or uncontactable, the attending medical practitioner is legally entitled to decide about instituting or discontinuing life-sustaining treatment.

Although our legislation provides for issuing a health care power of attorney – in the form of a "mandate" – it lacks detail. Since the SALC report's draft bill on end-of-life decisions (RSA, 1998:224-237) was shelved, questions such as the following have been left hanging in the air: Would the "health service" (RSA, 2003:Sec 7(1)), about which the substitute can decide, include withholding or withdrawal of life-sustaining treatment? Is anyone – a medical practitioner or family member – empowered to override a surrogate's decision? If so, in what circumstances and on what grounds? What is to be done if the application of the Act means that there are two substitute decision-makers – for example, two children – insisting on different treatment pathways for their parent?

11.4.2 Living will

The living will is an advance directive that is increasingly embraced as people better understand what is at stake in end-of-life choices (Landman, 2012:63-64, 66-67). It is an *instruction directive* – a signed document attested by witnesses – with a *very specific focus* in which a competent person instructs medical practitioners and all others to *refrain* from life-sustaining interventions – which may be listed in the document – should they become irreversibly incompetent and thus unable to make their own choices.

In South Africa, the legal status or enforceability of a living will is unclear. This is extremely unsatisfactory, since so many people, often with the assistance of lawyers, draft living wills in good faith but only have a nebulous legal assurance that their wishes, as expressed in their living will, would be honoured.

A case could be made for a living will being implicit or embedded in the National Health Act (RSA, 2003:Sec 7(1)(e)), given the Act's insistence on informed consent as a requirement for medical treatment, even though a living will is not mentioned by name. This is not good enough. A living will should be explicitly legislated and issues surrounding it clarified – such as its purpose and scope, its format and minimum formalities, whether it may in any circumstances be overridden by family or medical practitioners, and whether someone acting in good faith in accordance with it is immune from criminal and civil liability.

Despite its legal hiatus, it would be cynical to disregard a living will's evidentiary value in ascertaining the wishes of an incompetent individual. Medical practitioners ignore a living will at their peril since a strong legal argument can be mustered, on the basis of recognised principles in our law, for taking a living will seriously.

The SALC report's (RSA, 1998:233-235) proposed draft legislation on advance directives – both "a written power of attorney" (a health care power of attorney) and "a written directive" (living will) – has been shelved for 24 years.

Significantly, the SCA (Stransham-Ford, 2016:Para 32, footnote 30. Emphasis added.) says the following about "a living will or similar document or expression of wishes": "There is however much to be said for the position that *any* such prior instructions clearly expressed *should be heeded*." The SCA then backs this up with reference to legislation in the United Kingdom and the United States of America.

Indeed, several other jurisdictions have living-will legislation. There is no valid reason why we should lag behind (Landman & Henley, 2000). So, in 2018, an initiative by DignitySA and Ms Deidre Carter, MP, of the Congress of the People (Cope), assisted by Parliament's legal team, resulted in a private member's draft bill, the "National Health Amendment Bill" (RSA, 2018). It was an amendment to the National Health Act (RSA, 2003), explicitly recognising and regulating both forms of advance directives. The election of a new parliament and Covid-19 buried this initiative.

In sum, end-of-life choices involve (1) pain management that hastens death, (2) refusal of and refraining from life-sustaining treatment, and (3) advance directives. But in South Africa, lack of an unambiguous legal affirmation and protection of these legitimate medical practices encumber them with ignorance, misunderstanding, fear of legal liability, and even wilful dismissal. This has been an egregious neglect of moral obligation and legal duty by Parliament since 1998.

11.5 ASSISTED DYING : ASSISTED SUICIDE AND VOLUNTARY EUTHANASIA

Assisted dying – the fourth category of end-of-life choices – is a controversial option that evokes strong emotions and heated arguments. It occurs when a competent, terminally ill,[6] and suffering but autonomous person dies with the assistance, help, or aid of another person, at their voluntary request and for their own good. In the circumstances, the person who seeks assistance with dying considers death as desirable and preferable to continued life.

---

6   It could be argued persuasively that illness need not be terminal, for example, mental illness with competence intact, quadriplegia, or a 'completed' life. Thus, future legislation will have to consider whether terminal illness should be a necessary condition for assisted dying, in the process considering the constitutional equality rights of non-terminal persons, for example, quadriplegics.

Assisted dying is an umbrella term for assisted suicide and voluntary euthanasia. With *assisted suicide*, the helper supplies the patient with means to commit suicide which the patient then self-administers, resulting in death. With *voluntary euthanasia*, the helper supplies as well as administers the means that leads to the patient's death.[7]

The theoretical debate about the *ethics of* assisted dying, important as it is, is interminable and unlikely to lead to moral consensus (Landman, 1997, 1998, 2022a). The more pressing societal debate, however, concerns the *ethics of decriminalising or legalising* assisted dying, that is, the ethics of public policy (Landman, 2000). It remains an ethical debate, though, since law is ultimately rooted in ethics. Earl Warren (1962), a former American chief justice, put it elegantly: "In civilized society, law floats in a sea of ethics". In South Africa, the Constitution's Bill of Rights (RSA, 1996:Ch 2) is an ethical document setting out the moral values and moral rights upon which we agreed to build a good and just society. So, it is an ethical imperative that our legal position on assisted dying should reflect the Constitution's Bill of Rights.

The unpalatable truth is that two arms of the state – the legislative and judicial – have ethical obligations in respect of decriminalising assisted dying which they have sidestepped for more than a quarter of a century. The Constitution (RSA, 1996) has made it possible – imperative – to re-evaluate the legal status of a range of practices in our society, and thus also our common law, and we have done so: Termination of pregnancy is legal, the death penalty and corporal punishment are illegal, same-sex marriages are legal, and unfair labour practices are illegal.

But assisted dying remains the stepchild. The 'last right' goes unrecognised, thus stripping the 'last rite' of solidarity, compassion, and dignity.

In this legal hiatus, there are nevertheless courageous medical practitioners who assist patients, in the appropriate circumstances, to commit suicide, and some even practise voluntary euthanasia when it is safe to do so. But this remains under the radar, for understandable reasons – it is extremely risky and personal and professional consequences can be dire.

---

7   Voluntary euthanasia or mercy killing has four main elements – terminal illness (see footnote 6), suffering, competence, and voluntariness. Interpretation of these elements may narrow or widen the definition of assisted dying. From the *perspective of the patient*, euthanasia can be *voluntary* (an expression of the patient's free will), *non-voluntary* (the patient's will is unknown or unknowable), or *involuntary* (contrary to the patient's will but nevertheless judged to be in the patient's interest or for the patient's own good – an option limited to highly unusual and tragic circumstances that can be disregarded in a medical setting). From the *perspective of the helper*, euthanasia can be *active* or *passive* (see footnote 2).

In sharp contrast are doctors who would do everything medically possible to extend life without informed consent by either patient or surrogate, even in the face of protest by surrogates. They do so for a variety of reasons: Beliefs about what their professional values require, personal understanding of their legal obligations and duties, avoidance of legal liability for medical malpractice, religious convictions, or the pursuit of financial gain.

What exactly is the legal position regarding assisted dying in South Africa (Landman, 2022b)?

11.5.1   Common law and assisted dying

Our common law sets the currently applicable legal norm for assisted dying.

Before the advent of democracy in 1994, Dr Alby Hartmann, a general practitioner from Ceres, was found guilty of murder because he euthanised his octogenerian father who was dying of cancer (Hartmann, 1975).[8] He was sentenced to a year's imprisonment fully suspended from the rising of the court. Clearly, the court, in the person of Judge Louis van Winsen – 47 years ago already – found criminal punishment for merciful or compassionate killing in a medical context inappropriate. Dr Hartmann was, however, punished in his professional capacity and could not practise medicine again despite impassioned pleas by his patients.

The Hartmann case implicitly raised the issue of our common law that regards merciful killing in all conceivable circumstances as murder, effectively indistinguisable from murder with evil intent (*dolus*). After the adoption of the Constitution (RSA, 1996), there was a golden opportunity to review our legal position regarding assisted dying. President Nelson Mandela requested the SALC (RSA, 1998) to investigate all end-of-life decisions. A provisional report, published in 1997, solicited public comments, which were then incorporated in the final report of 1998. The report included a draft bill on all end-of-life choices. Regarding assisted dying, the commission proposed three alternative approaches for consideration. Since 1998, there have only been incidental hints about why the ANC government shelved the SALC report (RSA, 1998).[9]

---

8   Dr Hartmann's case (he was actually "Hartman") involved non-voluntary euthanasia since his father had not expressed any wish to be assisted with dying before he lost his ability to decide for himself (see footnote 7).

9   According to unconfirmed personal communication with a journalist who interviewed her, former Minister of Health Dr Manto Tshabalala-Msimang referred to assisted dying as "medicine for the rich". One of her successors, Dr Aaron Motsoaledi, said on an eNCA television show, *Judge for yourself* (10 May 2015), moderated by Judge Dennis Davis, that doctors should not kill and that "enough palliative care can help". In short, assistance with dying is claimed to be redundant in our constitutional dispensation.

In 2015, in the North Gauteng High Court, Judge Hans Fabricius recognised the right of the applicant, Adv Robin Stransham-Ford, to be legally assisted with suicide without the helper attracting criminal or professional liability (Stransham-Ford, 2015). But Stransham-Ford died two hours before Judge Fabricius's ruling.

The Minister of Justice and Correctional Services, the Minister of Health, and others took the case on appeal to the SCA (Stransham-Ford, 2016) and the appeal was upheld in December 2016. As a result, Stransham-Ford could no longer be legally assisted with dying had he not been predeceased.

In 2019, Prof. Sean Davison (2019), co-founder of DignitySA – an NPO seeking to decriminalise assisted dying – was convicted in the Western Cape High Court on three counts of murder for assisting three individuals to commit suicide. He was sentenced to three years house arrest following a plea bargain, having faced a minimum of 14 years imprisonment.

In 2017, Mr Dieter Harck, who suffers from motor neurone disease, brought an action to the South Gauteng High Court. He requests the court to allow him to end his life, with the assistance of a willing doctor, when his disease reaches the inevitable stage where death is preferable to continued life. He argues that assisted dying should not be criminalised or regarded as professional misconduct. In addition, he approaches the court in the public interest to ensure that others would likewise be allowed to seek assistance with dying. In 2021, Harck testified and was cross-examined online due to the Covid-19 pandemic. Harck's case stalled in 2022 and may resume in 2023.

The Stransham-Ford (2016) appeal is the most informative court case on the legal status of assisted dying and related end-of-life choices. Having reaffirmed the legal position that neither suicide nor attempted suicide is an offence (Stransham-Ford, 2016:Para 30), the SCA explicitly addresses assisted dying as an end-of-life choice.

First, *voluntary euthanasia* – also referred to as "mercy killing" by the court – is murder. Informed consent is not a defence available to a person who brings about the death of the deceased (Stransham-Ford, 2016:Para 38). Neither does informed consent justify a guilty verdict on the lesser charge of culpable homicide (Stransham-Ford, 2016:Para 31). Thus, a medical practitioner who administers a lethal agent to a patient at the latter's request commits the crime of murder (Stransham-Ford, 2016:Para 40). The facts of a particular case will determine the sentence (Hartmann, 1975).

Second, *assisted suicide* raises the question of the criminal liability of the medical practitioner who provides or prescribes the means with which the patient commits suicide. In answer, the SCA argued that in the Grotjohn (1970) case

> [...] the court did not decide that a criminal offence is committed *whenever* a person encourages, helps or enables someone to commit suicide or to attempt to do so. Whether they will depend on the facts of the case and issues of intention (mens rea), unlawfulness and causation. It follows that it cannot be said that in the current state of our law PAS [physician-assisted suicide] is in *all* circumstances unlawful. (Stransham-Ford, 2016:Para 54. Emphasis added.)

Thus, it needs to be established, on the basis of the facts in the circumstances of a particular case, whether a helper or encourager is liable for the crime of murder. In particular, a court would have to determine the *causal chain* that led to the death of the patient. For the helper to be found not guilty, the patient's act of suicide (such as voluntarily ingesting a substance) must be *completely independent* of, or *separate* from, the antecedent act of the helper (supplying the substance) (Stransham-Ford, 2016:Para 49). Thus, causation, as one constituent element of a crime, given the specific circumstances of a case, *may* be absent despite the fact that the helper had supplied the means that the patient thereafter self-administered to commit suicide. For example, a medical practitioner prescribes a month's supply of a legal substance for treating an illness and the patient ingests all 30 tablets at once and dies as a consequence.

Our common law regarding assisted dying can therefore be summarised as follows: Assisting suicide (depending on the facts of each case) and voluntary euthanasia (always) are crimes of murder.

11.5.2   The Constitution and assisted dying

But our common law must harmonise with our Constitution (RSA, 1996). Our constitutional rights in all probability embed a right to assisted dying that departs from our common law. There appears to be a formidable and untenable tension that needs to be removed by developing the common law in light of the Constitution's Bill of Rights.

Constitutional rights underpinning the establishment of a right to assisted dying are the rights to (1) dignity (RSA, 1996:Sec 10); (2) freedom and security of the person (RSA, 1996:Sec 12(1)), which includes the right not to be treated or punished in a cruel, inhuman, or degrading way (RSA, 1996:Sec 12(1)(e)); and (3) bodily and psychological integrity (RSA, 1996:Sec 12(2)), which includes the right to security of and control over one's body (RSA, 1996:Sec 12(2)(b)). Personal autonomy is the thread that runs through all these constitutional rights.

In addition, assisted dying calls for an interpretation of the right to life (RSA, 1996:Sec 11) that reconciles it with the right to dignity (RSA, 1996:Sec 10). In this regard, Judge Kate O'Regan made some instructive observations in the Constitutional Court (Makwanyane, 1995):

> The right to life incorporates the right to dignity; they are intertwined; the right to life is more than a right to mere existence because it is the right to be treated as a human being and with dignity; without dignity, a human life is substantially diminished; without life, there cannot be dignity.

Thus, recognising the right to life does not entail that preserving merely biological life, irreversibly devoid of quality and dignity, is a constitutional imperative.

Our right to life does not entail a duty to live. We can waive a right. It should be no different with the right to life.

The action by Dieter Harck in the South Gauteng High Court – an initiative by a terminally ill person with *pro bono* legal representation – is currently the only attempt to reconsider our common law. So, the recognition of a constitutional right to assisted dying hinges on a lone private initiative while terminally ill people are denied their constitutional rights to, among others, dignity, freedom and security of the person, and bodily integrity, including control over one's body.

11.5.3 Decriminalising assisted dying: Harmonising the Constitution and common law

What, then, is to be done about current apathy towards constitutional recognition of a right to assisted dying? There are two routes ahead – directly via Parliament or indirectly via the courts. But whichever one we follow, Parliament holds the key to decriminalising assisted dying.

According to the SCA, the proper approach to constitutional litigation in our courts should be followed (Stransham-Ford, 2016:Para 95). A court can only consider the constitutionality of assisted dying once an appropriate case is brought before it. In the Stransham-Ford (2016) appeal case, the SCA found that the North Gauteng High Court (Stransham-Ford, 2015) had erred in respect of both the facts and the law. In future, any party – a terminally ill patient or an organisation like DignitySA – could pursue litigation in the public interest with the benefit of "*full* argument and time to reflect" (Stransham-Ford, 2016:Para 76. Emphasis added.).

Significantly, the SCA gave future initiatives – as well as the current one by Dieter Harck – a significant boost when it predicted that "[w]hen an appropriate case comes before our courts *the common law will no doubt evolve* in the light of the considerations outlined there and the developments in other countries" (Stransham-Ford, 2016:Para 101. Emphasis added).

Any court considering the decriminalisation of assisted dying will have to pay particular attention to section 39(2) of the Constitution (RSA, 1996), which requires that in the development of the common law the court must strive to give effect to the nature, purport, and objects of the Bill of Rights (Stransham-Ford, 2016:Para 55).

Significantly, the SCA considered the well-known case of Carter (2012) that resulted in decriminalising assisted dying in Canada. The court suggests, in the form of a question, that common law crimes of murder and culpable homicide should be developed, by redefining one or more of their constituent elements to exclude assisted dying, and illustrates how decriminalisation could be achieved:

> Assuming the basis for any judgment was a finding that a constitutionally protected right had been infringed, would the more appropriate remedy be that adopted by the Canadian Supreme Court of a *declaration of incompatibility* [between the common law and the Constitution] *joined with a suspension of the order* [pertaining to a possible future case before the court] *to enable parliament to remedy the deficiency?* (Stransham-Ford, 2016:Para 73. Emphasis added.)

The SCA sees this as an "extremely important possibility" (Stransham-Ford, 2016:Para 73) and it would include "a fair public hearing" (Stransham-Ford, 2016:Para 74), as with parliamentary hearings preceding termination of pregnancy legislation. Development of the common law could be premised on a different view of causation, intention (*mens rea*), or unlawfulness (Stransham-Ford, 2016:Para 56) and may involve a defence of necessity or a defence of consent (Stransham-Ford, 2016:Para 61). In some other jurisdictions, this is exactly what happened. The SCA points out that the possibility of a special defence for medical practitioners and carers would have to be explored (Stransham-Ford, 2016:Para 56).

The SCA regards "the legislature [as] the proper engine for legal development" (Stransham-Ford, 2016:Para 73). A court can only respond to an appropriate case brought before it. And should that happen, the court would probably refer the case to Parliament to enact the necessary legislation. This would respect the separation of powers of the legislature and judiciary. Parliament, not the courts, makes laws. Thus, a court can alert Parliament to inconsistencies in our law and impress upon it its duty to remove the tension between our commonm law and Constitution by decriminalising assisted dying.

So, we are at the mercy of that dysfunctional institution of ours – Parliament. There is no effective alternative to putting assisted dying on the agenda of our elected representatives other than via the courts. Civil society has negligible powers of persuasion. The prospects are dim indeed, judging by the past 26 years. Prof. Pieter Carstens (Ho, 2020), a constitutional law expert, states bluntly that our constitutional right to assisted dying faces "the hypocrisy and lack of courage to act by lawmakers and government".

Given this damning critique, could a case be made for a more activist approach by the SCA towards the recognition of a constitutional right to assisted dying? Arguably, in the Stransham-Ford appeal (2016), despite the flaws in the case brought before it from the North Gauteng High Court (Stransham-Ford, 2015), the SCA could have alerted lawmakers to pressing constitutional issues such as compromised autonomy, dignity, and bodily integrity that accompany non-recognition of a constitutional right to assisted dying. The SCA could have pointed out the significant practical obstacles unique to decriminalising assisted dying and that recognition of a constitutional right is left to chance, monetary resources, and political vicissitudes.

Arguably, an appeal to the Constitutional Court against Stransham-Ford (2016) could have yielded a different result, particularly if the Constitutional Court saw its role as more activist. But the losing party (the estate Stransham-Ford), having already received a cost order, lacked the resources to appeal.

Unfortunately, the SCA's references to medical evidence for the alleged effectiveness of treating physical pain are highly problematic, feeding into the pernicious misconception *that palliative care renders assisted dying redundant* (Stransham-Ford, 2016:Paras 35, 88).

Exerting control over and manipulating another's body, wilfully disregarding their autonomous preferences, through palliative sedation and, as a last resort, terminal sedation, means foisting upon them treatment that denies their constitutional rights, among others, to autonomy, dignity, and bodily integrity, including control over one's body. Overriding autonomous preferences in circumstances of end-of-life suffering constitutes a formidable harm. Hence, unwanted and inappropriate palliative care to ease physical suffering cannot make assisted dying redundant. On the contrary, having some control over one's physical and monetary assets after death while being denied control over one's body in life is, at the very least, an indefensible inconsistency.

It is perverse to make the recognition of a constitutional right to assisted dying dependent on the initiative of a terminally ill person who must *also* be able to access the necessary financial resources, while the state (the ministers who routinely oppose such cases) has endless access to taxpayer-generated legal resources.

It was quite different with termination of pregnancy. A cynic could point out, with some justification, that this discrepancy is attributable to women constituting more than half of all eligible voters while the dying do not constitute a useful voting block. Evidently, for our lawmakers, women's rights weigh heavier than the rights of the terminally ill. Moreover, terminally ill litigants, like Stransham-Ford who died two hours before Judge Fabricius's ruling, cannot reasonably be expected to continue living while the legal process grinds on through several courts.

Assisted dying is a subject about which we gain true understanding only when we or family members wish to opt for a final liberation from intractable and unbearable end-of-life suffering in our own chosen way and not according to the dictates of others. But then it is too late. Still, extensive anecdotal evidence suggests that assisted dying is gaining significant popular support.

11.6   CONCLUSION

End-of-life choices break down into four clusters – pain management that hastens death, refusal of and refraining from life-sustaining treatment, advance directives, and assisted dying as both assisted suicide and voluntary euthanasia. All of these should be clear, legitimate, and accessible end-of-life options for terminally ill persons.

The first three are standard-of-care medical practices that are unconscionably encumbered by legal uncertainty. No wonder that medical practitioners some-times fail to act in ways that properly recognise patient rights, and that patients and their families do not know their own rights.

And the fourth – assisted dying – constitutes the common-law crime of murder. As such, in all likelihood, it contradicts rights in the Constitution's Bill of Rights, which is an ethical document that sets out the moral values and moral rights upon which we agreed to build a good and just society. So, although assisted dying is on firm ethical ground, what matters in practice is the public-policy ethical imperative to decriminalise or legalise it.

Bibliography

Carter. 2012: *Carter v Canada (Attorney General)* 2012 BCSC 886 (CanLII).

Clarke. 1992: *Clarke v Hurst NO and Others* 1992 (4) SA 630 (D).

Davison. 2019: *The State v Peter Sean Davison* CC 38/2019.

Grotjohn. 1970: *Ex parte Die Minister van Justisie: In re S v Grotjohn* 1970 (2) SA 355 (A).

Hartmann. 1975: *S v Hartmann* 1975 (3) SA 532 (C). https://doi.org/10.1016/0346-251X(75)90017-2

Ho, Ufrieda. 2020. A law professor suvives cancer to begin a personal journey to make the right to die a legal right. *Daily Maverick*, 5 February. https://bit.ly/3UYquCi [Accessed 25 February 2022].

Landman, W.A. 1982. The moral equivalence of active and passive euthanasia. *South African Journal of Philosophy*, 1(1):5-10.

Landman, W.A. 1997. The ethics of physician-assisted suicide and euthanasia. *South African Medical Journal*, 87(7):866-869.

Landman, W.A. 1998. Physician-assisted suicide and voluntary euthanasia: a response. *South African Medical Journal*, 88:242-243.

Landman, W.A. 2000. Legalising asisistance with dying in South Africa. *South African Medical Journal*, 90(2):113-116.

Landman, W.A. 2001. A proposal for legalizing assisted suicide and euthanasia in South Africa. In: L.M. Kopelman & K.A. De Ville (eds.). *Physician-assisted suicide: What are the issues?* London: Kluwer Academic Publishers. 203-225. https://doi.org/10.1007/978-94-010-9631-7_13

Landman, W.A. 2012. *End-of-life decisions, ethics and the law: a case for statutory legal clarity and reform in South Africa*. Geneva, Switzerland: Globethics.net. https://bit.ly/3GFaj8y

Landman, W.A. 2022a. Bystanddood: 'n omstrede saak. *LitNet*. https://bit.ly/3V4AcmP [Accessed 22 February 2022].

Landman, W.A. 2022b. Bystanddood in die regswêreld. *LitNet*. https://bit.ly/3Xt9eXn [Accessed 22 February 2022].

Landman, W.A. & Henley, L.D. 2000. Legalising advance directives in South Africa. *South African Medical Journal*, 90(8):785-787.

Makwanyane. 1995. *S v Makwanyane* 1995 2 SACR 1 (CC).

NC (North Carolina). 1977. *North Carolina Right to a Natural Death Act*. North Carolina General Statutes (N.C.G.S.).

RSA (Republic of South Africa). 1996. *Constitution of the Republic of South Africa*. Pretoria: Government Printing Works.

RSA SALRC (Republic of South Africa. South African Law Reform Commission Report). 1998. *Euthanasia and the artificial preservation of life*. Project 86. November. https://bit.ly/3udREcR

RSA (Republic of South Africa). 2003. *National Health Act 61 of 2003*. Pretoria: Government Printing Works.

RSA (Republic of South Africa). 2018. National Health Amendment Bill. *Government Gazette*, No. 41789 of 24 July. https://bit.ly/3ACPbME

Stransham-Ford. 2015. *Stransham-Ford v Minister of Justice and Correctional Services and Others* 2015 ZAGPPHC 230; 2015 (4) SA 50 (GP).

Stransham-Ford. 2016. *Minister of Justice and Correctional Services v Estate Stransham-Ford* 9531/2015 2016 ZASCA 197 (6 December 2016).

Warren, Earl. 1962. Quotation. https://bit.ly/3i8NP5R [Accessed 22 February 2022].

12

How to Treat Private and Sensitive Medical and Genetic Data

Himla Soodyall & Jerome Amir Singh

Keywords: confidentiality; consent; data sharing; electronic health records; genetic ancestry testing; genetic data; incidental findings; non-paternity; privacy

12.1   INTRODUCTION

Genomics research has significantly contributed to the improvement of diagnosis, treatment, and delivery of health care. Fundamental to the success of these interventions is public trust and confidence in researchers and medical professionals, underpinned by a range of ethical challenges particularly those related to consent, privacy, ownership of samples, and data sharing.

Seeley and Parker (2020) have explored issues related to feedback on findings and the nature of the relationship between genome research and medical practice, while Fisher and Layman (2018) have addressed the roles of "genetic and environment[al] factors on the development of mental health and behavioural risk, resilience and individual responsivity to prevention" and intervention programmes. Fisher and Laymen (2018) have argued that the progress of utilising biospecimens in prevention science parallels the rise in the integration of large datasets, commonly referred to as 'big data', across all scientific disciplines. The use of big data "is marked by increased access to and use of individual-level data across administrative data systems with the potential to link genomic data to health, public benefits, child welfare, criminal and juvenile justice, and educational records and other personal information" (Fisher & Layman, 2018) educational, and other information stored in large integrated datasets. These advances have created a new frontier of ethical challenges for scientists as they collect, store, or engage in secondary use of potentially identifiable information and biospecimens. To address challenges arising from technological advances and the expanding contexts in which potentially identifiable information and biospecimens are collected and stored, the Office of Human Research Protections has revised federal regulations for the protection of human subjects. The revised regulations create a new format, content, and transparency requirements for informed consent, including a new mechanism known as broad consent. Broad consent offers participants a range of choices regarding consent for the storage and future use of their personally identifiable data. These regulations have important implications for how prevention scientists and oversight boards acquire participant consent for the collection, storage, and future use of their data by other investigators for scientific purposes significantly different from the original study. This chapter describes regulatory changes and challenges affecting traditional informed consent for prevention research, followed by a description of the rationale and requirements for obtaining broad consent, and concludes with a discussion of future challenges involving ongoing transparency and protections for participants and their communities.

Along with the many benefits genomics and big data analytical tools have provided to society, many concerns such as re-identification of previously de-identified participant information have been raised. The collection, storage, and secondary use of biospecimens are compounded by further challenges. An area of intense debate has been the "model of consent that would be appropriate for genomic and biobanking studies in low and middle-income countries, and what type of governance mechanism is required for safeguarding the interest of research participants and their communities in such studies" (Seeley & Parker, 2020).

From an ethical point of view, respect for the principles of autonomy (informed consent, confidentiality, truth telling, and communication), beneficence (do good), non-maleficence (do no harm), and justice (rights justice, legal justice, and distribution justice) need to be considered together when addressing questions related to how we treat private and sensitive medical and genetic data.

This chapter discusses some of the ethical issues related to the privacy of sensitive medical and genetic data.

12.2   HOW SENSITIVE IS GENETIC DATA?

Essentially, the challenge with genetic data is the type of information it may contain such as ethnicity and health relevant information, together with their re-identification potential (Sariyar, Shur & Schlünder, 2017). Generally, genetic data can be globally unique, but as soon as data becomes linkable to a specific person, it becomes an issue for that individual and their relatives, making the problem of privacy even more complex. These authors have reviewed the sensitivity of genetic data based on criteria such as the type of genetic markers used, its stability and distinguishability as inherent characteristics.

Based on these criteria, they conclude that single nucleotide polymorphisms (SNPs) are mostly useful when combined with other gene-related information, which when used alone are less critical than other forms of genetic data – adding support for their use and value in public-domain databases such as *dbSNP* (Sariyar et al., 2017; Sherry et al., 2001). Short tandem repeat (STR) data, which are mostly used for genetic fingerprinting purposes, especially in forensic applications, are less relevant for inferring further re-identification unless used in conjunction with other information. Also, copy number variants (CNVs) can contain many genes and are therefore useful for many purposes and may play a bigger role than SNP and STR data in disclosure issues. DNA methylation as an epigenetic phenomenon is less stable than other kinds of genetic markers and does not pose much risk in issues related to sensitivity. However, whole genome sequence (WGS) data is regarded as "exceptional" and require special protection. In their (Sariyar et al., 2017) view, "once the full genome of an individual has become public, it can be used in a variety of settings for unforeseeable and discriminatory purposes". Their main argument against genetic exceptionalism is that "the characteristics of genetic data are like other medical or health-related information (e.g., it can be used to disclose an individual's identity, disease risks, or drug response)".

12.3   CONSENT

Chapter 2 of the National Health Act (2003) deals with rights and duties of users and health care personnel. Section 7 focuses on informed consent, which is enshrined in one of the four ethical principles referred to as "respect for autonomy". As Moodley (2023) outlines, "autonomy literally means self-rule". It refers to the right of every individual to make decisions for himself or herself. In health care, this entails allowing the patient to make the final decision about his/her treatment after the relevant information was clearly explained to them. It is also suggested that this principle should not be used for persons who are incapacitated, ignorant, infants, young children, suicidal, some drug-dependent patients, and patients with severe psychiatric illness that would incapacitate them (Moodley, 2023).

Informed consent is essential for enrolment of participants for research, clinical trials, and diagnostic testing for patients. However, questions arise about ethical issues related to divulging information about deceased patients. One case that highlights some of the controversy around the sensitivity of this issue relates to the publication of the book, *Mandela's Last Years: The True Story of Nelson Mandela's Final Journey* published by Dr Ramlakan, the head of his medical team (Ramlakan, 2017). Rule 13(2)(c) of the Ethical Rules of Conduct by the Health Professionals Council of South Africa (HPCSA) state that confidential information about a deceased person should only be divulged "with the written consent of his or her next of kin or the executor of the estate" (HPCSA, 2016a). "Next of kin" is not clearly defined which leaves open the question of whether a spouse or only immediate genetic relatives qualify as next of kin. As in this case, problems arise when there is conflict among family members and the executors about giving written consent. It is recommended that "in such cases the specific order of priority for consent by relatives in the National Health Act (2003) be followed" (McQuoid-Mason, 2017).

McQuoid-Mason (2017) recommended that certain questions be considered prior to divulging medical information on deceased individuals, such as (1) when is it ethical to publish such information? (2) which family members or next of kin can consent to publication? (3) when is it legal to publish such information? (4) does it make a difference if the deceased is a public figure? and (5) whether family members have legal standing to prevent or claim damages for such publication on behalf of the deceased.

Having evaluated these questions using principles in medical ethics and the law, McQuoid-Mason (2017) noted that if a doctor has made disclosures about a deceased person's medical treatment in breach of the rule 13(2)(c), the deceased person's next of kin or the executor of the estate may file a complaint with the HPCSA, and disciplinary action can be taken against the doctor for unethical conduct. The problem arises if some family members give consent and others do not, and actively oppose the publication. Unfortunately, the rule does not define "next of kin", nor clearly indicates which next-of-kin takes precedence over others.

McQuoid-Mason argues that the National Health Act [section 7(1)(b)] specifies the order of persons who can give consent on behalf of incompetent live patients and suggests that this could be used as a guide when determining which next-of-kin relatives should have the right to give written consent for the publication of personal medical information of a deceased person. This is based on people who are authorised to give consent on behalf of a patient to access medical treatment.

In terms of the Act, "the order of precedence is a spouse or partner, a parent, a grandparent, an adult child or a brother or sister of the person" (McQuoid-Mason, 2017). However, the South African Law Reform Commission (SALRC) has noted that this precedence "could be interpreted to imply that a brother should be consulted before a sister" (SALRC, 2018). The SALRC noted that "while there is justification for consulting a spouse or partner before consulting a child and consulting a child before consulting a sibling due to marriage, an intimate partnership or degree of family relationship, there is no justification for determining that a brother should be consulted before a sister" (SALRC, 2018). The SALRC has therefore determined that the wording in the National Health Act (2003) is discriminatory based on gender and hence in breach of section 9 of the Constitution.

Regarding when it is legal to publish information about a deceased person, the constitutional and common-law right to privacy concerning their health status must be upheld. According to McQuoid-Mason (2017), "the right is not un-limited and may be infringed where the person concerned consents, where there is a statutory duty to make disclosure (e.g., in the case of child abuse), where the disclosure is true and in the public interest or where the disclosure is privileged". The defence of truth and public interest are relevant when addressing disclosures concerning health status of public figures.

Public figures are "people who have by their personality, status or conduct exposed themselves and their families to such a degree of the publicity as to justify public disclosures of certain aspects of their private lives. Such persons include politicians, actors, entertainers, sportsmen and sportswomen, war heroes, and others who are regarded as having a limited right to private lives" since they have sought or consented to publicity (McQuoid-Mason, 2017). Should such personalities fail to carry out their professional duties or make false statements, then the media has a duty to inform the public.

President Mandela was a world-famous public figure and was always at the centre of much publicity. However, he was entitled to a private life and the public needed to respect that unless his private life contradicted what he stood for as a statesman. His and his family's wish for privacy after he retired from political life should have been respected.

Conduct that is unethical under the rules of the HPCSA may not necessarily be actionable under the law. There is no general protection for the personality rights of deceased persons. Consequently, if a doctor intentionally discloses private information about a deceased patient, there would be no action for damages in law because the person is deceased (McQuoid-Mason, 2017). Even the next-of-kin have no grounds to sue the doctor under these circumstances. "This is because the right to sue for breach of confidentiality or invasion of privacy vests in deceased persons during their lifetime, and not in their next of kin or executors after their death" (McQuoid-Mason, 2017).

This situation was resolved by the publishers withdrawing the book from circulation and never went to court. Despite the legal right to sue for breach of confidentiality or invasion vesting with deceased persona during their lifetime, the sharing of confidential health details of deceased persons raises profound ethical issues and arguably constitutes a moral harm.

12.4 CONFIDENTIALITY

The National Health Act (2003) makes it an offence to disclose patients' information without their consent, except in certain circumstances. Sections 14, 15, and 16 of the Act are pertinent with regard to confidentiality. Sections 15 and 16 describe how patient information may be disclosed by a health care worker "for any legitimate purpose within the ordinary course and scope of his or her duties where such access or disclosure is in the interests of the user" (National Health Act, 2003).

Respect for confidentiality is important to safeguard the well-being of patients and to ensure the confidence of society in the doctor-patient relationship. "Health information is not only based on objective observations, diagnoses, and test results, but also subjective impressions about the patient, their life-style, habits, and recreational activities. The improper disclosure of such highly sensitive information could harm patients' reputation or result in lost opportunities, financial commitments, and even personal humiliation (Beltran-Aroca et al., 2016).

The HPCSA places confidentiality as central to the doctor-patient relationship and a core aspect of the trust that holds the relationship together. The HPCSA's official guidance, *Confidentiality: Protecting and Providing Information* (2008), emphasises these key principles:

1. Patients have a right to expect that information about them will be held in confidence by health care practitioners. Confidentiality is central to trust between practitioners and patients. Without assurances about confidentiality, patients may be reluctant to give practitioners the information they need to provide good care.

2. Where health care practitioners are asked to provide information about patients, they should:

    a. Seek the consent of patients to disclosure of information wherever possible, whether or not the patients can be identified from the disclosure; Comprehensive information must be made available to patients with regard to the potential for a breach of confidentiality with ICD10 coding.

    b. Anonymise data where unidentifiable data will serve the purpose;

    c. Keep disclosures to the minimum necessary.

3. Health care practitioners must always be prepared to justify their decisions in accordance with these guidelines.

There are two general exceptions where it is necessary to question whether it is essential to maintain confidentiality: (1) when the safety of others or (2) public health is threatened (Beltran-Aroca et al., 2016). The HPCSA advocates that the risk of harm must be serious enough to outweigh the patient's right to confidentiality and recommends that consent of the patient should be sought first before disclosure unless this is not forthcoming.

Given the emphasis on confidentiality in the National Health Act (2003) and the HPCSA guidelines, the Constitutional Court ruling on the case of *NM, SM and LH v Charlene Smith, Patricia de Lille and New Africa Books* has been criticised by Mark Heywood representing the Aids Law Project in this case (Section27, 2007).[1]

This case was taken to the Constitutional Court by three women (NM, SM, and LH) against Charlene Smith, Patricia de Lille, and New Africa Books since the defendants had published their full names and HIV status without their consent in the biography of De Lille, written by Charlene Smith and published by New Africa Books. The women had participated in clinical trials and raised concerns about the illness and fatalities among the participants. They submitted that the consent forms for the trials were not properly explained to them. De Lille was contacted to help investigate the complaints. Professor SA Strauss was appointed to conduct an inquiry into the allegations of misconduct and subsequently issued a report on the trials (the Strauss Report). This report contained the applicants' names and HIV status.

"The women argued that the disclosure of their names and HIV status in the book was an invasion of their rights to privacy, dignity, psychological integrity and mental and intellectual well-being." They asked the Court to grant them relief on the following issues: "(1) an order directing the defendants to issue a private apology to each plaintiff, (2) an order directing the defendants to cause the

---

1   https://bit.ly/3VhTTr8

offending passages to be excised or removed from all unsold copies of the book, and (3) an order directing the defendants to pay damages of R200,000 to each plaintiff" (Parker & Lucassen, 2018; Section27, 2007). In this judgment, Judge Schwartzman (Section27, 2007) referred to previous case law which confirmed that the "right to privacy entitles an individual to decide when and under what circumstances private facts may be made public". He further acknowledged that "because of the ignorance and prejudices of large sections of our population, an unauthorised disclosure [of HIV status] can result in social and economic ostracism" and "can even lead to mental and physical assault".

In summary, Mark Heywood (Aids Law Project) presented some explanation for Judge Schwarzman's decision as follows (Section27, 2007):

- De Lille and Smith have, by their long-standing involvement with people living with HIV/AIDS, demonstrated that they are unlikely to intentionally invade the privacy of a person living with HIV.

- The women's names and HIV status was contained in the report of an official inquiry, commissioned by a public body into a matter of public interest. Nothing in the report suggested that any part of it was confidential. Accordingly, the defendants were entitled "to assume" that in mentioning the plaintiffs' names and HIV status, they were acting in terms of a consent furnished by the plaintiffs to the inquiry.

- There was no legal duty on the defendants to establish the nature of the consent provided by the women for the use of their names in the report.

- Although he noted that publishing the names without informed consent had "transgressed the norms and standards of the profession" ethically, the dispute concerned legal issues and was "not a question of journalistic ethics or standards."

- The fact that the plaintiffs had not consented to the disclosure of their names and HIV status and had asserted this right through legal action after the publication of the book in March 2002, entitles the plaintiffs to damages and to an order for the removal of their names.

- In this respect, only the publishers are liable for the damages which occurred after the women asserted their rights by starting legal action in April 2002.

Judge Schwartzman nevertheless awarded limited damages and gave the following reasons (Section27, 2007):

- The women's fear that their family and community would come to learn of their HIV status through the book did not materialise. This finding is in fact incorrect since NM testified how her boyfriend had come to know of her status through his friends who read the book. Their relationship deteriorated and he subsequently burned down her house.

- ▦ The women's fears "of a likelihood that the disclosure of their status in the book will lead to this fact becoming well known is more imagined than real" because:

    - ▪ The plaintiffs have little formal education and are illiterate in English. "The English literacy level of the community in which they live was not explored in evidence. What is known is that some of the people with whom they associate read magazines and newspapers."

    - ▪ Since the publication of the book, apart from the first plaintiff's boyfriend, the plaintiffs were not confronted by anyone else who had read the book.

    - ▪ "Biographies, especially those read by politicians, are directed at, and read by a limited number of people. This limited readership is unlikely to include people with whom the plaintiffs come into regular contact."

- ▦ All three plaintiffs "in any event led stressful lives that are linked to the economically strained circumstances in which they grew up and in which they appear to continue to live, their lack of education and economic opportunity, and their HIV positive status."

- ▦ The publishers are only liable for damages caused by the book subsequent to its publication and the publisher having become aware of the fact that the plaintiffs had not consented to their names and HIV status being disclosed.

While the AIDS Law Project welcomed the recognition that their clients' rights to privacy were violated and the order that their names be deleted from the book, they

> were unhappy with other fundamental aspects of this judgment both in terms of its findings and reasoning. It remains our opinion that Patricia De Lille and Charlene Smith should have been held liable precisely because they are acutely aware of the impact of stigma and discrimination on people living with HIV. The disclosure of our clients' full names and HIV status in De Lille's book did not add anything and no harm would have been done had their initials or pseudonyms been used instead. It was, for example, not disputed that neither De Lille nor Smith approached the plaintiffs to ascertain whether or not their names could be used in the book even though they both acknowledged that the plaintiffs had the right to determine the ambit of the disclosure of their names and HIV status. (Section27, 2007)

The AIDS Law Project also expressed its disappointment with the low award of damages made in this case which seems to completely disregard large portions of the plaintiffs' testimony about the impact of the publication of the book on their lives.

This case once again highlights some discrepancies in the way ethical issues and the law are interpreted.

12.5 HOW DOES THE DUTY OF UPHOLDING CONFIDENTIALITY APPLY WHEN SHARING GENETIC INFORMATION WITH FAMILY MEMBERS?

Genetic information from family members can be important in the identification, treatment, and counselling of patients at risk of inherited disorders. Despite this, some patients are not happy to share relevant information with other family members making it difficult for medical professionals to treat other family members who may benefit from the information, fearing breaching patients' confidentiality. Parker and Lucassen (2018) discussed

> four ways in which genetic information can fail to be communicated to families; (1) where a patient explicitly refuses to share genetic information with a family member for whom it might be useful; (2) where a patient, for one reason or another, simply never gets around to telling their relatives about it; (3) where a patient is overwhelmed by their own diagnosis and does not feel able to cope with sharing just yet; or (4) where a patient is unaware of the fact that there are relatives who might benefit or has lost contact with relatives.

They contend that "a duty of confidentiality should not prevent the use of familial genetic information in the care and treatment of family members. Although a familial factor may first be identified in a single individual, this does not necessarily make it sensitive to, or identifying of, that person" (Parker & Lucassen, 2018). Finally, notwithstanding the importance of confidentiality in medicine, in situations where there is a risk of death or serious harm, they suggest sharing of relevant information.

While the default position for health care professionals to treat patient information as confidential and disclosure without consent as the exception, not the rule, Dheensa, Fenwick and Lucassen (2016) argue that this approach to confidentiality and autonomy is based on an "inaccurate conceptualisation of patients as separate from others, free from social and familial constraints". By contrast, they suggest that "relational approaches to autonomy stress that patients develop their autonomy through social embeddedness and engagements with others; that one person's choices affect other people's autonomy; and that despite wanting to protect their personal interests, people are interested in maintaining family and community relationships" (Dheensa et al., 2016).

Along the same lines is the joint account model of confidentiality, where the genetic information is conceptualised as familial and "belonging" to all the relatives it might affect, not just the individual in whom it was first identified. These authors interviewed 33 patients at large genetic centres in the United Kingdom. The interviews included questions related to hereditary conditions regarding consent, confidentiality, and information sharing in genetic medicine. They found that generally the participants had altruistic tendencies and thought of genetic information as familial, which aligns with the relational joint account model. Overall, participants supported sharing, but noted two reasons where health care professions might find it difficult to share if a patient had refused consent. First, the result had been generated from one person's blood, which might confer special rights for them over it and second, personal information (the condition and its effect on an individual) and familial information (the familial mutation) were entangled. However, they could not articulate any special rights a tested person may have over the result that would justify non-disclosure. Based on these inputs, the authors recommend that health professions inform participants about sharing information before seeking informed consent for their engagement.

Sharing of clinical and genetic data has many benefits like promoting research efficiency, expediting translational efforts of research results, ensuring traceability and transparency of published data, and maximising the utility of existing databases and lessening the burden to participants. Successful collaborations and sharing of data include genomic research for cancer (e.g., International Cancer Genome Consortium [Zhang et al., 2019]) and rare diseases (e.g., Global Alliance for Genomic Health [GA4GH, 2013] and the International Rare Diseases Research Consortium [IRDiRC, 2011]) (Takashima et al., 2018). In genomic research for cancer and rare diseases, patient family members (e.g., parents, children, siblings, aunts, or uncles) can provide important information and their genomic information is submitted to a repository or database and shared broadly. Privacy protection, security, and respecting participants' consent, however, remain ethical concerns. Takashima et al. (2018) argue that when sharing clinical and genomic data, there is a need to consider protection of the patients' own data and their family members' data. To overcome the risk of re-identification of individuals from data when sharing clinical and genomic data, the authors reported that their survey showed that the public and patients considered that familial data sharing in research should be protected more strictly. They conclude that all stakeholders – researchers, sample collectors, laboratory scientists, data analysts, database operators, institutional review boards and public and research participants, fulfil their own responsibilities to protect patients' and their families' privacy and interests while advancing genomic science and medicine.

12.6 CONFIDENTIAL GENETIC TESTING AND ELECTRONIC HEALTH RECORDS

Although paper records and human interpretation of laboratory results have sufficed in the past, the synthesis and interpretations of large amounts of complex genomic information requires electronic tools capable of delivering to patients and health care professionals the right amount and type of information at point of care (Hazin et al., 2013). Electronic health records have more recently been introduced to facilitate these processes. Many electronic medical record systems allow patients to access their results online without the presence of professional help. Electronic medical record systems allow sharing of health information and test results with other health professionals, some of whom may or may not know the patient, leading to inadvertent disclosure.

Black, Barton and Perlmutter (2021) commented on their review of 10 well-known centres that conducted presymptomatic testing for Huntington's disease and found that there were still many unresolved issues between the "virtues of a shared medical record and the goal of patient control of sensitive medical information". The authors propose that medical record systems adapt to and respect the patient's desires for confidentiality and allow people undergoing presymptomatic testing to restrict access to this sensitive information.

Huntington's disease, an autosomal dominant neurodegenerative disorder, is typically late-onset, most commonly between the ages of 30-50, but individuals of any age can present with it if the disease is diagnosed in the family. Patients present with severe progressive decline in motor control and cognitive faculties and exhibit behavioural disturbances. Due to the nearly 100% penetrance of this adult-onset condition, the decision for an individual to undergo testing, especially prior to the onset of symptoms, is difficult, as the results may affect their life and family and also produce serious psychosocial reactions and lead to future financial planning, educational, and employment complications (Eno et al., 2020)patient requests for increased confidentiality may be in conflict with the legal obligations of medical providers to document patient care activities in the electronic health record (EHR. Although some Acts (e.g., The Genetic Information Non-discrimination Act of 2008 [Code of Federal Regulations, 2012]; Genetic Information Nondiscrimination Act of 2009 [GINA, 2009] and the Affordable Care Act [ACA, 2010] in the USA) protect individuals from health insurance discrimination, other insurance products such as disability, life, and long-term care are not protected by these laws (Eno et al., 2020). Pretest counselling and confidential testing to protect the well-being of those who choose to be tested are highly recommended.

Arias and Karlawish (2014) reached similar conclusions with preclinical studies of Alzheimer's disease. They concluded that "current legal and regulatory mechanisms are not sufficient to protect against harms that could have very real consequences for subject of preclinical Alzheimer's disease trials" (Arias & Karlawish, 2014). They suggested that research institutions must address shortcomings in the design of the electronic medical recording system, revise laws to limit discrimination, and disclose details of risks associated with the loss of confidentiality.

12.7   INVOLUNTARY DISCLOSURE OF CONFIDENTIAL GENETIC INFORMATION TO RELATED THIRD PARTIES

When an individual has been diagnosed with a hereditary genetic condition, their immediate family members may wish to know the probability of themselves or their lineage developing the condition. It has been argued that an individual has a moral obligation to share their diagnosis of a hereditary condition with relevant genetically close family members so that these individuals can choose whether to be tested themselves (Singh, 2023). This moral duty to disclose is not necessarily confined to the immediate family. Some have argued that adults who have been diagnosed with a hereditable condition, or parents of a child diagnosed with a hereditable condition, have an ethical duty to inform relatives in the extended family about the condition (Andrews, 1987). This moral duty arises from kinship bonds (Wertz, Fletcher, Berg & WHO Human Genetics Programme, 2003). The moral duty to disclose to relevant parties becomes challenging when the patient diagnosed with the condition (or in the case of a minor child diagnosed, his or her parents) refuse to voluntarily disclose the diagnosis to relevant family members. Section 16 of the HPCSA's Guidelines, *Seeking Patient's Informed Consent: The Ethical Considerations* – which governs consent to genetic screening and testing – states that informed decision-making involves a health care practitioner explaining "any significant medical, social or financial implications of screening or testing for the particular condition or predisposition" (HPCSA, 2016b). 'Social implications' could be interpreted as including the need to consider the implications of the test for related third parties (Singh, 2023).

In a report, *Review of Ethical Issues in Medical Genetics*, the World Health Organization noted the stance of the US President's Commission – a multi-disciplinary body of legal experts, ethicists, and clinicians – on the issue of genetic confidentiality (Wertz et al., 2003). The Commission held that the genetics professional may, unless it is prohibited by law, override individual confidentiality provided the following conditions are met:

- All efforts to persuade the individual to disclose the information voluntarily have failed.

- There is a high probability of harm to the relatives (including future children) if the information is not disclosed, and there is evidence that the information could be used to prevent harm.

- The harm averted would be serious.

- Only genetic information directly relevant to the relatives' own medical status would be revealed. Information relevant to the individual must remain confidential.

The duty to warn blood relatives came up in the UK case of *ABC vs St Georges Healthcare NHS Trust and Others* (YIP DBE, 2020). In this case, a patient, XX, was diagnosed with Huntington's disease while serving a prison sentence. An offspring of an individual who has Huntington's disease has a 50% chance of developing the condition. XX refused to disclose his diagnosis to either of his daughters, despite learning that one of his daughters (ABC) was pregnant. The health care professionals treating XX were also aware that ABC was pregnant. However, they took the position that they should not override XX's confidentiality. The health care providers thus did not notify ABC that she was at risk of inheriting the gene for Huntington's disease timeously enough for her to terminate her pregnancy. ABC had her baby, and a few months later, a member of XX's medical team accidently disclosed XX's diagnosis to ABC. Several years later, ABC was diagnosed with the genetic mutation for Huntington's disease. She subsequently developed a psychiatric condition due to her diagnosis and became concerned about her daughter's health, as she too had a 50% chance of inheriting the gene for Huntington's disease. ABC brought a negligence claim against the three Trusts responsible for the relevant health care professionals who treated XX, arguing that the Trusts breached their duty of care to her by failing to notify her timeously that she was at risk of inheriting the gene for Huntington's disease, to enable her to terminate her pregnancy.

In deciding the case, the court had to establish: (i) whether a duty of care existed between XX's clinicians and ABC; and (ii) if so, whether the clinicians breached this duty of care (i.e., acted negligently by omitting to inform ABC), and whether this omission caused ABC to suffer loss/harm (i.e., whether the element of causation was satisfied). In determining whether a duty of care existed between XX's clinicians and ABC, the court held that while ABC was not a patient of the three defendants, there was a close proximal relationship between ABC and the second defendant (D2) as ABC was involved in the family therapy arranged by D2's clinicians and they had material information about ABC and her particular circumstances. The court held that it was foreseeable, and D2 actually foresaw that ABC was at risk of suffering harm if they withheld information about her genetic risk from her. As such, the court held that D2 owed a duty of care to ABC to "balance her interest in being informed of her genetic risk against her father's interest in preserving confidentiality in relation to his diagnosis and the public interest in maintaining medical confidentiality generally". The court underscored that this duty of care was not "a broad duty of care owed to all relatives" of the patient in relation to genetic information. Instead, this duty of care was likely to arise only in prescribed circumstances where there was a close proximal relationship between the medical professionals and the at-risk person.

Having established that a duty of care existed between D2 and ABC, the court noted that ABC's negligence claim against D2 would succeed if: (i) D2 had breached their duty of care to ABC; and (ii) ABC would have terminated her pregnancy had she been timeously informed of the risk during her pregnancy. The court held that while a duty of care existed, D2's decision not to disclose XX's condition to ABC did not amount to a breach of the duty of care as the decision was "supported by a responsible body of medical opinion and was a matter of judgment open to [D2] after balancing the competing interests". The court also held that ABC had not established that she would have tested and undergone a termination of her pregnancy had the risk been timeously disclosed to her during her pregnancy. Given these factors, the court dismissed ABC's negligence claim against D2.

While ABC was unsuccessful in her claim as she had not satisfied the court that she would have undergone testing for the Huntington's gene and terminated her pregnancy based on a positive result, this case is significant in England – and arguably other settings which have legal systems based on English common law, such as South Africa – as it established that clinicians have a duty of care to at-risk relatives of their patients who have been diagnosed with hereditary diseases.

12.8   INCIDENTAL FINDINGS: THE RIGHT TO KNOW AND THE RIGHT NOT TO KNOW

Every so often, during biomedical research, researchers obtain information on participants that are outside of the scope of the research study. These findings have been referred to in the literature as "incidental findings" and has engaged some debate among researchers as to whether these findings should be disclosed to participants. For example, researchers collecting imaging data for a particular purpose may find an abnormality that poses a health risk to the participant, or genetic screening can reveal variants that are associated with higher relative risks of certain conditions. It is also possible to detect non-paternity from some studies.

Schaefer and Savulescu (2018) hold the view that reporting of incidental findings "should be based primarily on the possibility of medial benefit, factoring in the findings' validity, clinical actionability, and significance to health or reproduction" (Schaefer & Savulescu, 2018). They direct attention to participants' autonomy, privacy, and promoting the interests of participants. To assist with dealing with such scenarios, it is suggested that researchers should anticipate the possibility of incidental findings in advance of the study and should have a plan as to how they would deal with them. This plan should be conveyed to participants during the consent process so that participants are informed of such possibilities.

While various researchers have debated what incidental findings to disclose, there are three criteria – validity, significance to health (and sometimes reproduction), and clinical actionability – which have been described as the best-mediated-interest standard as outlined by Schaefer and Savulescu (2018). According to these authors, validity refers to the accuracy and reliability of the findings. In other words, a mere suspicion of a problem would not merit reporting, but a finding informed by a number of clinical studies might. Significance to health and reproduction refers to whether the finding could have a substantial impact on someone's health or (via reproduction) that of his/her offspring. Clinical actionability refers to the potential for a clinical intervention to alleviate the health issue, e.g., treatment for breast cancer.

The best-mediated-interest standard has been viewed as problematic since it is overly narrow in its clinical focus. It is argued that participants may have an interest in receiving incidental findings that are not related to health or are health-related but not actionable (Schaefer & Savulescu, 2018). They qualify their view by stating that "misattributed paternity would be of crucial interest to a purported father paying child support. And some people will have a nonmedical interest in learning about a genetic predisposition to currently incurable conditions like Alzheimer's on grounds that the knowledge can let them better plan their lives".

Several factors have contributed towards the argument for non-disclosure of incidental findings. Some commentators have suggested that such information can sometimes by psychologically harmful – "it may induce anxiety, fear, survivor guilt, depression, or other negative mental states" (Schaefer & Savulescu, 2018). Even if there is a right to know, it may not be absolute, and the negative effects of some findings, especially those which are not actionable, may override that right.

It is suggested that the decision about disclosure should involve weighing the positive reason(s) to provide information, respecting the right to know, against uncertain negative reason(s) against it (psychological harm). Also, disclosure should be limited to circumstances, when after appropriate explanations, participants would understand the implications of such information. It is recommended that researchers respect people's rights to know about themselves (Schaefer & Savulescu, 2018).

12.9 HOW TO DEAL WITH GENETIC TESTING WHEN IT REVEALS NON-PATERNITY?

An ethical issue that may cause medical providers extreme anguish is what to do when genetic testing reveals non-paternity as an incidental finding. The rate of this misattributed parentage is estimated to be between 1% to 10% of all births (Prero et al., 2019). When this outcome is discerned and disclosed, the result can be devastating to the entire family. The child, other children, and both parents may be severely and permanently harmed. This disclosure may also jeopardise mothers' safety, result in child support being withdrawn, result in family members' losing inheritance, and cause bitter custody disputes (Howe, 2021).

The value conflicts this poses for providers are exceptionally difficult. Providers' views on what they should do when this question arises have differed. Some have favoured, for example, never telling parents this outcome. Others spell out what they will do in advance. Still others tailor their responses to families' different needs (Howe, 2021).

Mothers may also find out that they are not biological parents. This may come about when children are born because of in vitro fertilization (IVF). Mistakes in IVF procedures may be made. With IVF, it may then also benefit parents if providers anticipate these incidental findings and discuss this with parents in advance. Providers informing these parents that a mistake could occur with IVF may, on the other hand, scare them. Thus, due to the most remote chance that this could occur, it may be better here to not inform them (Howe, 2021).

Howe (2021) discusses other concerns parents may have about the effects of genetic information on their relationship with their children in other contexts. An example occurred "when a transgender parent did not want his child to know that after he had given birth to his child, he changed his gender. He feared that his child might find this out after viewing his father's medical records. Here, even if this wouldn't occur, he still may have had this underlying concern".

Providers' options may be limited in what they can do to relieve parents' concerns in some instances. Then, they refer these parents to counsellors in the hope that this might help them reduce their fear. These parents too might decide, because of this counselling, to share information about themselves with their children that they wanted to keep secret, after all.

Parents' culture may also affect what providers can and should disclose. In some cultures, for example, a woman convicted of consented infidelity may face most severe adverse consequences. Providers should keep in mind, though, that even when parents share the same culture, as when they are next door neighbours, their views may wholly differ as much as they would if they were from different cultures. Providers must initially then explore both parents' views fully and separately so that they do not inadvertently favour one parent's views over the other, by not exploring each to the degree that they could and should. If two parents have irresolvable differences, mediators or, again, counsellors may help (Howe, 2021).

Perhaps the most common approach providers take is, when possible, medically, to inform, first and only, mothers of this risk of discovering non-paternity (Howe, 2021). This can occur if these mothers initially come in alone. Providers then can leave it up to these mothers to decide whether anyone will be tested and if so, who this will be. If the mother suspects that her child's father may not be the biological father, she may choose to not ask this father to be tested. This respects her autonomy and may be most beneficial to all. Providers may be willing to do this, however, only if there are no risks of adverse medical consequences to anyone. This approach also allows the provider to sustain a more positive relationship with the mother since it allows her to decide. The mother, too, then, may not know or even ever know whether her husband – or another former partner – is their child's biological father. This may be what she would want. The provider might, then, take initiative to explore this with her before she decides. Providers may not want to offer mothers this decision-making option on the ground that the mother chose to engage in what they see as an indiscretion. They may believe that she should bear this decision's consequences. This view is for several reasons ethically problematic. Chief among these problems is that the consequences may be profoundly destructive to the child and family. This harm may far outweigh all other considerations. The provider, also, has no ethical basis for taking on this judging role (Howe, 2021).

Another approach discussed by Howe (2021), quite the opposite of the one above, may occur after providers discover non-paternity incidentally. These providers may then tell these mothers that they must tell these fathers, as, for instance, within a week. Further, they may inform the mothers that if they have not told the father by then, these providers will.

Providers may do this for several reasons. They may think that those in the medical profession should not keep secrets. They may think that fathers have an absolute right to know. They may also use these two above reasons to "justify their imposing personal view that the mother should be punished for her past indiscretion. They may do this without their knowing that they are using these reasons to rationalize their imposition of their morally unjustifiable personal bias" (Howe, 2021).

A third approach is for providers to inform both parents initially that any information they find incidentally they will not disclose unless it is medically relevant. This practice of total non-disclosure has been used to protect family members' relationships by keeping them intact in other contexts. Transplant centres, for example, may inform family members before a transplant is carried out that if for some reason the transplant is cancelled, the staff will not tell the family why. A reason for this policy is that parents and other donors may refuse to donate their kidney at the last minute. There may also be other reasons for cancelling the transplant than these parents' own interest, but the staff's policy not to inform the family will prevent the family from a possibly devastatingly effect. This transplant policy is controversial. It illustrates, however, another instance in which medical staff may agree to keep a family secret to themselves (Howe, 2021).

A fourth approach sometimes carried out is for providers not to forewarn either parent that genetic testing can produce this incidental finding. Some parents may not know this unless their provider tells them. They may not be aware that genetic testing conducted for an entirely different medical reason could also reveal non-paternity. If, though, the provider tells the parents this, such that they learn this for the first time, the alleged fathers – who almost always will be the biological fathers – may, in response, want to have a paternity test. They may seek this out even at another institution. Then, the same harmful outcomes for their family may come about (Howe, 2021).

Therapeutic privilege (also known as therapeutic exception) is an exception to the general rule of informed consent and applies in the uncommon instance where a health professional may be excused from revealing information to a patient if disclosing it could pose a serious psychological threat to the patient (Singh, 2023). The notion of therapeutic privilege allows health professionals to withhold 'psychologically sensitive information' in situations where the nature of the information to be conveyed to the patient (for example, XY genotype in a female patient) could cause 'grave psychological harm' to that patient or their family. The therapeutic privilege presumes full disclosure, but is delayed until the individual is psychologically and cognitively competent to process the information (Wertz et al., 2003).

Some experts advise obtaining a second opinion about the likelihood of psychological harm before opting to defer or delay disclosure (Wertz et al., 2003). However, in the absence of timely access to mental health professionals, and when assessment shows that emotional harm is possible, nondisclosure or delayed disclosure of the full scientific facts may be justified (Wertz et al., 2003). The notion of therapeutic privilege is recognised in South African law. Section 6(1) of the National Health Act (2003) states: "Every health care provider must inform a user (patient) of (a) the user's health status *except in circumstances where there is substantial evidence that the disclosure of the user's health status would be contrary to the best interests of the user.*" The decision to invoke therapeutic privilege and determining what is in the best interests of the patient is left to the discretion of the health profession.

As a medical scientist doing population genetic research and offering genetic ancestry tests to the public and sharing individual results with subjects, one of the authors (Soodyall) has had to withhold Y-chromosome DNA results when returning reports. In one study, when examining the transmission of Y-chromosome DNA in conjunction with genealogical information in an isolated clan community, there were a few instances when the inferred Y-chromosome lineage linked with a particular founding father and his descendants did not match and could not be explained by new mutations but could be attributed to non-paternity. With input from the Chief in the district, some cases were attributed to a scenario in which a woman conceived out of wedlock and the child was then registered with her fathers' surname to protect the family, resulting in a different Y-chromosome lineage being introduced in the family not concordant with the family surname. Due to the sensitivity of these situations, Soodyall would leave out the Y-chromosome result in the report and only discuss the mitochondrial DNA results with the individual.

Another scenario presented when she had done an ancestry test from a profiled person and presented his results to him. Years later, another male with the same surname came for a genetic ancestry test, but they did not detect a match to this individual in their database. Soodyall was subsequently informed that these individuals' father was the profiled person that they had previously tested, and when the two results were compared, the 'son' had a very different profile to the father. Soodyall did not disclose this to the son and did not mention to him that she had compared the two results. However, in her explanation of the results to him, she informed him that sometimes when these tests are done, some changes are known to occur in a stepwise fashion with STR markers during spermatogenesis. Whether the son discussed the result with his father, and they compared results, was never disclosed to Soodyall and neither came back to her for further explanations. In both examples above, non-disclosure of the test results was in the best interest of the subjects.

Acknowledgements

The authors wish to thank Ms Rajeshree Mahabeer for her assistance with editing and formatting this paper.

Bibliography

ACA. 2010. Affordable Care Act (ACA). *HealthCare.Gov.* https://bit.ly/3ExLhWq

Andrews, L.B. 1987. *Medical genetics: a legal frontier.* American Bar Foundation.

Arias, J.J. & Karlawish, J. 2014. Confidentiality in preclinical Alzheimer disease studies. *Neurology,* 82(8):725. https://doi.org/10.1212/WNL.0000000000000153

Beltran-Aroca, C.M., Girela-Lopez, E., Collazo-Chao, E., Montero-Pérez-Barquero, M. & Muñoz-Villanueva, M.C. 2016. Confidentiality breaches in clinical practice: what happens in hospitals? *BMC Medical Ethics,* 17(1):52. https://doi.org/10.1186/s12910-016-0136-y

Black, K.J., Barton, S.K. & Perlmutter, J.S. 2021. Presymptomatic testing and confidentiality in the age of the electronic medical record. *The Journal of Neuropsychiatry and Clinical Neurosciences,* 33(1):80-83. https://doi.org/10.1176/appi.neuropsych.20030068

Code of Federal Regulations. 2012. *Genetic Information Nondiscrimination Act of 2008.* https://bit.ly/3OCbwzK

Dheensa, S., Fenwick, A. & Lucassen, A. 2016. "Is this knowledge mine and nobody else's? I don't feel that." Patient views about consent, confidentiality and information-sharing in genetic medicine. *Journal of Medical Ethics,* 42(3):174-179. https://doi.org/10.1136/medethics-2015-102781

Eno, C.C., Barton, S.K., Dorrani, N., Cederbaum, S.D., Deignan, J.L. & Grody, W.W. 2020. Confidential genetic testing and electronic health records: a survey of current practices among Huntington disease testing centers. *Molecular Genetics & Genomic Medicine,* 8(1):e1026. https://doi.org/10.1002/mgg3.1026

Fisher, C.B. & Layman, D.M. 2018. Genomics, big data, and broad consent: a new ethics frontier for prevention science. *Prevention Science: The Official Journal of the Society for Prevention Research,* 19(7):871-879. https://doi.org/10.1007/s11121-018-0944-z

GA4GH. 2013. *Global Alliance for Genomics and Health.* https://www.ga4gh.org/

GINA. 2009. *Genetic Information Nondiscrimination Act: OHRP guidance (2009).* HHS.gov. https://bit.ly/3gw3RWZ

Hazin, R., Brothers, K.B., Malin, B.A., Koenig, B.A., Sanderson, S.C., Rothstein, M.A., Williams, M.S., Clayton, E.W. & Kullo, I.J. 2013. Ethical, legal, and social implications of incorporating genomic information into electronic health records. *Genetics in Medicine: Official Journal of the American College of Medical Genetics,* 15(10):810-816. https://doi.org/10.1038/gim.2013.117s

Howe, E. 2021. Ethical issues when non-paternity is an incidental finding. *International Journal of Pregnancy & Child Birth,* 7:1-4. https://doi.org/10.15406/ipcb.2021.07.00218

HPCSA (Health Professionals Council of South Africa). 2016a. *HPCSA guidelines for good practice in the health care professions. Seeking patients' informed consent: the ethical considerations.* https://bit.ly/3EWrVf0

HPCSA (Health Professionals Council of South Africa). 2016b. *HPCSA guidelines for good practice in the health care professions. Booklet 1: general ethical guidelines for health care professions.* https://bit.ly/3EAG3sT

IRDiRC. 2011. *IRDiRC: International Rare Diseases Research Consortium.* https://bit.ly/3EHZVdU

McQuoid-Mason, D. 2017. Disclosing details about the medical treatment of a deceased public figure in a book: who should have consented to the disclosures in Mandela's Last Days? *South African Medical Journal,* 107:1072-1074. https://doi.org/10.7196/SAMJ.2017.v107i12.12764

Moodley, K. 2023. Respect for autonomy. In: K. Moodley (ed.), *Medical ethics, law and human rights: a South African perspective* (3rd edition). Van Schaik (in press).

National Health Act. 2003. *National Health Act 61 of 2003.* South African Government. Pretoria: Government Printing Works. https://www.gov.za/documents/national-health-act

Parker, M. & Lucassen, A. 2018. Using a genetic test result in the care of family members: how does the duty of confidentiality apply? *European Journal of Human Genetics*, 26(7):955-959. https://doi.org/10.1038/s41431-018-0138-y

Prero, M.Y., Strenk, M., Garrett, J., Kessler, A., Fanaroff, J.M. & Lantos, J.D. 2019. Disclosure of misattributed paternity. *Pediatrics*, 143(6):e20183899. https://doi.org/10.1542/peds.2018-3899

Ramlakan, V. 2017. *Mandela's last years: the true story of Nelson Mandela's final journey by the head of his medical team*. Penguin Books.

SALRC (South African Law Reform Commission). 2018. *Project 25. Report on statutory law revision: legislation administered by Department of Health*. https://bit.ly/3Vats6P

Sariyar, M., Suhr, S. & Schlünder, I. 2017. How sensitive is genetic data? *Biopreservation and Biobanking*, 15(6): 494-501. https://doi.org/10.1089/bio.2017.0033

Schaefer, G.O. & Savulescu, J. 2018. The right to know: a revised standard for reporting incidental findings. *The Hastings Center Report*, 48(2):22-32. https://doi.org/10.1002/hast.836

Section27. 2007. *NM, SM and LH v De Lille, Smith and New Africa Books*. 4 April. https://bit.ly/3Xw5DI3

Seeley, J. & Parker, M. 2020. Editorial: ethical practice and genomic research. *Global*

Bioethics, 31(1):164-168. https://doi.org/10.1080/11287462.2020.1855712

Sherry, S.T., Ward, M.H., Kholodov, M., Baker, J., Phan, L., Smigielski, E.M. & Sirotkin, K. 2001. DbSNP: the NCBI database of genetic variation. *Nucleic Acids Research*, 29(1):308-311. https://doi.org/10.1093/nar/29.1.308

Singh, J.A. 2023. Law and the health professional in South Africa. In: K. Moodley (ed.), *Medical ethics, law and human rights: a South African perspective* (3rd edition). Van Schaik (in press).

Takashima, K., Maru, Y., Mori, S., Mano, H., Noda, T. & Muto, K. 2018. Ethical concerns on sharing genomic data including patients' family members. *BMC Medical Ethics*, 19(1):61. https://doi.org/10.1186/s12910-018-0310-5

Wertz, D.C., Fletcher, G.F., Berg, K. & WHO Human Genetics Programme. 2003. *Review of ethical issues in medical genetics: Report of consultants to WHO / D.C. Wertz, J.C. Fletcher, K. Berg. WHO / HGN/ETH/00.4.* WHO IRIS. https://bit.ly/3idulNz

YIP DBE. 2020. *ABC v St George's Healthcare NHS Trust & Ors* [2020] WHC 455 (QB). 28 February. https://bit.ly/3U9UB8C

Zhang, J., Bajari, R., Andric, D., Gerthoffert, F., Lepsa, A., Nahal-Bose, H., Stein, L.D. & Ferretti, V. 2019. The International Cancer Genome Consortium data portal. *Nature Biotechnology*, 37(4):367-369. https://doi.org/10.1038/s41587-019-0055-9

13

Cyberspace-related Risk Aspects in the Medical Ecosystem

Basie von Solms

Keywords: cybersecurity; cybersecurity governance; cybersecurity risks; cyberspace; internet of medical things (IoMT); medical ecosystems; medical ethics

13.1 INTRODUCTION

New developments in technology have, over the ages, always been core drivers in the dramatic improvement in all areas of health care. Such developments include the availability of newer and more effective drugs, the possibility to implant a stent and a pacemaker in the body to address a problem which, only a few years earlier, may have needed a massive invasive operation. Technological developments, operating in what we today experience as 'cyberspace', have already become massive new drivers in improving health care, and will continue to do so at a dizzying pace in coming years. However, as has always been the case with any new technology, there are always risks which must be managed as comprehensively as possible to prevent the new technology from causing negative consequences.

In this chapter, we will try to give an overview of how cyberspace has already impacted the medical ecosystem, and what are some of the important risks which must be identified and managed.

The chapter is structured as follows:

- Some technical background
- Risks in cyberspace and attack methods
- Examples of cyberattacks on hospitals and medical devices

- Cybersecurity measures to mediate the risks of a cyberattack

- The internet of medical things (IoMT)

- Online operations and surgical robots

- Medical ethics and cybersecurity

- A cyber-incident response plan (CIRP) in the medical ecosystem

- Cybersecurity governance in the medical ecosystem

- Conclusion

We start off by giving some technical background used in this chapter.

13.2   SOME TECHNICAL BACKGROUND

13.2.1   Defining a few concepts

As background to sections in this chapter, some concepts must be defined. While many definitions do exist, and many different definitions can be provided from existing literature, the definitions which are provided below are mostly based on the author's personal experience of the relevant concept over many years and may therefore be criticised by the 'purists'. Nevertheless, the purpose is to make concepts as understandable as possible and is specifically directed at the non-technologists.

- The internet: In its simplest form, the internet can be visualised as millions of computers and computing devices connected via millions of computer networks. Such computers include big enterprise type computers, desk top computers, laptops, tablets, smart phones, and many more. The internet can therefore be seen as purely an interconnected technical infrastructure on which more advanced applications can be built.

- The World Wide Web (WWW): On every one of the computers and devices making up the internet, there may reside databases containing data, information, and software. In its simplest form, the WWW can be seen as all these databases, and therefore the data, information, and software in these databases, connected via the internet infrastructure. The WWW is therefore built on the underlying internet infrastructure.

- Cyberspace: Again, with the risk of oversimplifying, cyberspace can be seen as the internet and the WWW together. This means that cyberspace can be seen as everywhere where there is some computing device connected to other computing devices. This *interconnectedness* is maybe the main characteristic of cyberspace. In this chapter, we will specifically investigate risks which arise because of this *interconnectivity*.

- Cybercrimes: Cybercrimes are crimes performed in and through cyberspace.

- Cyberattacks: Cyberattacks are the methods and actions used by cyber-criminals to break into (hack) computer and data systems to perform cybercrimes.

- Ransomware attack: This is an attack method used by cybercriminals in which the computer system of a company is penetrated, and all the data stored and managed by the computer system is encrypted. This makes such data inaccessible and unavailable to the authorised users. In most cases, a ransom amount is then demanded by the criminals to restore the data to useable format.

- Malicious software (Malware): Malware is unauthorised software which can be loaded onto compromised computers, phones, and intelligent devices to perform unauthorised actions.

- Cybersecurity: Cybersecurity is an encompassing term referring to all actions and measures implemented to protect computer and data systems against cyberattacks.

- The Internet of Things (IoT): Because of the interconnectivity of cyberspace, more and more (small) devices like sensors are connected to it, making it possible to monitor and manage such devices remotely. Such devices may be simple sensors measuring for example rainfall, temperature, and more. This 'extended' cyberspace is called 'the internet of things' where these 'things' refer to the connected devices and sensors.

- The Internet of Medical Things (IoMT): The IoMT can be seen as a subset of the IoT covering the collection of medical devices and applications that connect to health care IT systems through cyberspace. In this case, the 'Things' are medically related sensors, equipment, and more.

- Cyberspace-based Medical or Health Care Ecosystem: The cyberspace-based medical ecosystem can be seen as an infrastructure (people, enterprises, devices, computer systems, and more) that use cyberspace and the Yom to deliver, monitor, and manage health care services.

- The Cloud: The cloud refers to servers and databases that are used to store data, but are not on the same site where the data is provided or captured from. These servers and databases are accessible via cyberspace. This means that you store your data somewhere in cyberspace without actually knowing where the server of database is situated. Cloud service providers provide and manage such services.

As this chapter is all about the cyber risk aspects related to the medical eco-system, including the attack methods used by cybercriminals, it is good to first understand the general risk aspects in cyberspace we are exposed to every day and the attack methods used. This will help as many of such risks and attack methods are exactly the same as those experienced in the medical ecosystem. In the next paragraph, we will investigate cyber risks and attack methods. There are many such risks and attack methods, but we will concentrate on just a few.

13.3   RISKS IN CYBERSPACE AND ATTACK METHODS

Because of its interconnectedness, cyberspace provides a good platform to cybercriminals to launch cyberattacks through. They may launch an attack on a system on the other side of the world from where they are physically located, as the specific targeted system can be reached through cyberspace. As an example, image a hospital in country X having a website. The website allows anybody in the world to access the website and get information about the specific hospital. For this reason, a cybercriminal in country Y, thousands of kilometres away from country X, can access this hospital's website, and try to penetrate the rest of the hospital's medical ecosystem to perform unauthorised actions.

Cybercriminals have different reasons why they attack and hack computer systems, and we will concentrate on two such reasons – getting access to personal and other types of data and getting access to some electronic device to use as a springboard for further unauthorised actions. We will now briefly discuss these two reasons.

13.3.1   Getting access to personal and other types of data

Data has become extremely valuable, and criminals want to get access to different types of data which they then sell or use in ways to force the owners of the data to react to their demands. They can get access to such data by different means, including directly hacking into the central database or trying to get (steal) the login data from a user of the company. They then use this login data to perform an (unauthorised) login to the system, masquerading as the user.

In particular, personal health data is very high on their list, and therefore attacks on medical databases are common. Such stolen medical data can be used to blackmail a patient whose data was stolen, or even to blackmail a whole hospital through a ransomware attack. In other cases, they use personal medical data to try to get login parameters to the patients' financial systems, and even to misuse stolen electronic scripts to get illegal drugs.

As explained above, the interconnectivity of the medical ecosystem just increases this risk as personal patient data can be collected from different places, sent between different systems, shared between different doctors and medical staff, and stored in different places.

Furthermore, the Yom will have many more devices and sensors connected to the care of a patient, and all the data captured by such devices is being sent along networks and even cyberspace. There are national initiatives by countries to force health care providers to upload all patient data to a central data base managed by some central body. Such a database will be a treasure trove for cybercriminals and needs excellent security and protection.

Interconnectivity in cyberspace has massive benefits for the medical ecosystem, but also carries massive risks in terms of patient and related medical data (Green, 2018; Khalik, 2018).

We will expand on these aspects later in the chapter.

13.3.2 Getting access to electronic devices, sensors, and other components of the IoMT

With more and more people doing banking via cyberspace and online systems, cybercriminals are committed to getting access to a client's smart phone to steal the client's login details. This is done by infecting the smart phone with malicious software. This software now waits until the client logs into an online bank account, captures the login information, and sends it back to the cyber-criminal. Apart from using the stolen login information in an unauthorised way, or planting malware on the user's phone, the criminals can try to intercept the communication between the phone and the bank, for example changing the bank account number the client intended to transfer money to.

Any device, sensor, or 'thing' connected to cyberspace can potentially be misused in the way described above, and many other ways too. In the Yom, many such devices already exist and will just increase in number in the future.

Pacemakers are intelligent devices that are implanted in a person's body to help control their heart's rhythm. In many cases, such pacemakers have built-in communication facilities that can communicate back to the physician via cyberspace and provide data in real time. The physician, which may be hundreds of kilometres away, can now monitor the person's heartbeat, and in emergencies, even send a message to the device to perform a specified emergency action like increasing the rhythm.

Just like the smart phone above, such a pacemaker or the communication between the pacemaker and the doctor can be hacked. Malicious software can be loaded on the pacemaker, or the doctor's commands to the pacemaker can be changed, causing potential deadly consequences. In 2013, former US Vice President Dick Cheney's doctors disabled his pacemaker's wireless capabilities to thwart terrorists and possible assassination attempts (Vaas, 2013).

More and more people today use different forms of health and fitness monitoring devices. The main benefit of such devices is that they can be interconnected into the medical ecosystems and are therefore all components of the IoMT.

> Wearable medical devices and home health monitoring devices are becoming more prevalent among patients of all ages. These devices allow vital data to be transmitted from a patient's home directly to hospital and other health care staff, resulting in real-time monitoring of a patient's health. (Ronte, Taylor & Haughey, 2018)

Such sharing of often very sensitive medical data creates motivation and reason for cybercriminals to try to compromise such systems to get their hands on the sensitive data.

Within the IoMT, such risks will grow as more and more devices are used to monitor, control, and manage patient health care in the medical ecosystem. Cyber-attacks against such Yom components will grow and become more sophisticated.

> [...] cybersecurity issues are pervasive across medtech (medical technology), as the increasing numbers and capability of connected medical devices present additional risks for data security. (Ronte et al., 2018)

We will expand on these aspects again later in this chapter but will in the next section firstly investigate a few examples of how these risks were exploited in real life.

13.4　EXAMPLES OF CYBERATTACKS ON HOSPITALS AND MEDICAL DEVICES

In subsection 13.3.1 above, we considered the cyberattacks to steal data and, in our context, medical data. In this section, we will first look at the theft of personal medical data, and then at the compromise of medical equipment. It is claimed that medical data is up to 10 times more valuable than a credit card number (Alpine Security, 2021).

Attacks to steal personal medical data can happen on an individual level, where a specific person's sensitive medical data is compromised, and the person is blackmailed. Such an event occurred in Finland where a database of a clinic was compromised, and the data used to blackmail individual patients (Sipilä, 2020).

The attacks can, however, also be made directly on a health institution, where the medical database of the institution is hacked, and the whole database is encrypted through a ransomware attack. This makes all the data unavailable to all concerned. A ransom amount is then demanded, and if paid, the data may be decrypted to be used again, but in many cases paying the ransom does not solve the problem. Such an attack can of course have a devastating effect on the institution's medical infrastructure and the relevant patients.

> Cybercriminals have begun to target the healthcare industry with ransomware – malware that encrypts an infected device and any attached devices or network drives. After encryption, cybercriminals demand a ransom before releasing the devices from encoding. Without adequate disaster recovery and backup plans, many businesses are forced to pay the ransom. (Aver, 2021; Spence et al., 2018)

Several cases have been reported where such a ransomware attack caused the death of patients.

> German authorities are investigating the unknown perpetrators on suspicion of negligent manslaughter, the Associated Press, German news outlet NTV, and others reported. The event under investigation occurred last Friday when the unidentified woman was turned away from Düsseldorf University Hospital because a ransomware attack hampered its ability to operate normally. The woman was rushed to a hospital about 20 miles away, resulting in about a one-hour delay in treatment. She died. (Goodin, 2020)

In subsection 13.3.2 above, we considered cyberattacks on devices. Cyberattacks will of course make medical data unavailable, as discussed above, but can also compromise medical devices and equipment. Such devices and equipment are mostly intelligent devices, meaning they are computers themselves, and if their software is compromised, they cannot operate. As part of the IoMT, many devices are connected to a hospital's computer system. This interconnectivity creates risks as a cyberattack on a specific device can potentially spread to the rest of the equipment in the hospital, and make them unavailable (Miliard, 2021; Rothschild, 2020).

Many more examples of compromised medical systems have been reported, and the question now is of course how to protect oneself against such attacks. We will expand on this in the next section.

13.5   CYBERSECURITY MEASURES TO MEDIATE THE RISKS OF A CYBERATTACK

Cybersecurity is a very big and important field as cyberattacks are growing daily. A report from McAfee estimated that global losses from cybercrime topped $1 trillion in 2020, and they are expected to skyrocket to more than $6 trillion in 2021, according to a report produced by Cybersecurity Ventures, which was sponsored by Intrusion (Morgan, 2017).

Furthermore, as mentioned above, hospitals and medical institutions are becoming a growing target for cyberattacks (Weiner, 2021). "Healthcare has become the most targeted industry for cybercriminals" (Steger, 2020). Hospitals should therefore be specifically wary and ensure that their cybersecurity and cyber protection are based on internationally accepted best practices such as the ISO 27000 series of documents (Irwin, 2020).

It is not the purpose of this chapter to extend too deeply into cybersecurity practices, but institutions must understand a number of important aspects related to cybersecurity attacks. Firstly, there is no such thing as 100% cybersecurity. No enterprise, or hospital, can totally prevent cyberattacks – the best that can be done is to lower your cyber risks as much as possible, and manage the cyber risk environment constantly and as comprehensively as possible.

Secondly, no cybersecurity plan can be based on technology only. Products such as firewalls, anti-virus software, and more are essential, but is not sufficient. The human part of cybersecurity is just as important. Reports claim that more than 90% of successful hacks against a company has a human origin. Creating a cybersecurity culture in the company where every employee is cyber aware and knowledgeable on how to recognise and prevent a cyberattack is maybe the core of a good cybersecurity plan. "A holistic approach designed with people at the heart – Did you know that people are the single biggest risk factor to cyber-attacks? Many organisations overlook the human side of cybersecurity" (Deloitte, 2020).

Thirdly, it is essential to understand that cybersecurity is a corporate governance responsibility. This means that the accountability for cybersecurity resides with the board of directors of the company – the buck stops right at the top! We will expand on this aspect in section 13.10 below on cybersecurity governance in the medical ecosystem.

In the next section, we expand the concept of the internet of medical things.

13.6   THE INTERNET OF MEDICAL THINGS (IoMT)

As the concept of the IoMT is crucial to modern integrated health care, and as components of the IoMT are open to cyberattacks, we have to discuss the concept in more detail.

As briefly defined in subsection 13.2.1 above, the IoMT can be seen as a collection of medical devices, interconnected via networks (and cyberspace). These devices may be individual sensors connected to a patient. For a specific hospital, it may be medical devices on site, but also remote medical devices, all connected to a central computer and database within the hospital. These devices can collect data directly, and then send that to some central processing computer and data store. The data may also be stored in the cloud, which can cause further risks.

Examples of such medical devices may be a range of sensors connected to the patient, including devices to monitor parameters such as heart rate, respiration, blood oxygen saturation, skin temperature, blood glucose, blood chemistry, and body weight. Furthermore, parameters like behavioural parameters (e.g., motion, acceleration, mood) linked to health and well-being can also be collected (Mittelstadt, 2017).

Many of these devices may be in the physical hospital environment itself, but many may also be remotely located, for example fitness devices which patients can wear at any place and any time. Such collected data are then transmitted via cyberspace, and other network technologies, to some central computer.

Figure 13.1 below gives some idea of the IoMT (Dilawar, Rizwan, Ahmad & Akram, 2019).

It is widely reported that medical devices and components of the IoMT often do not have very good cybersecurity protection and are hackable.

> More than 60 percent of all medical devices are exposed to some degree of risk, according to a recent report from healthcare cybersecurity company CyberMDX. It's crucial, then, for healthcare systems to understand the vulnerabilities of Yom tools and how to protect them – both today and in the future. (Kawamoto, 2017; Steger, 2020)

According to Critical Insight (n.d.), the top six hackable medical IoT devices are:

- Infusion and insulin pumps
- Smart pens
- Implantable cardiac devices
- Wireless vital monitors
- Thermometers and temperature sensors
- Security cameras

The IoMT is an essential component of comprehensive health care in the future, but does have significant risks, including cyber risks attached, which will have to be managed and regulated very well.

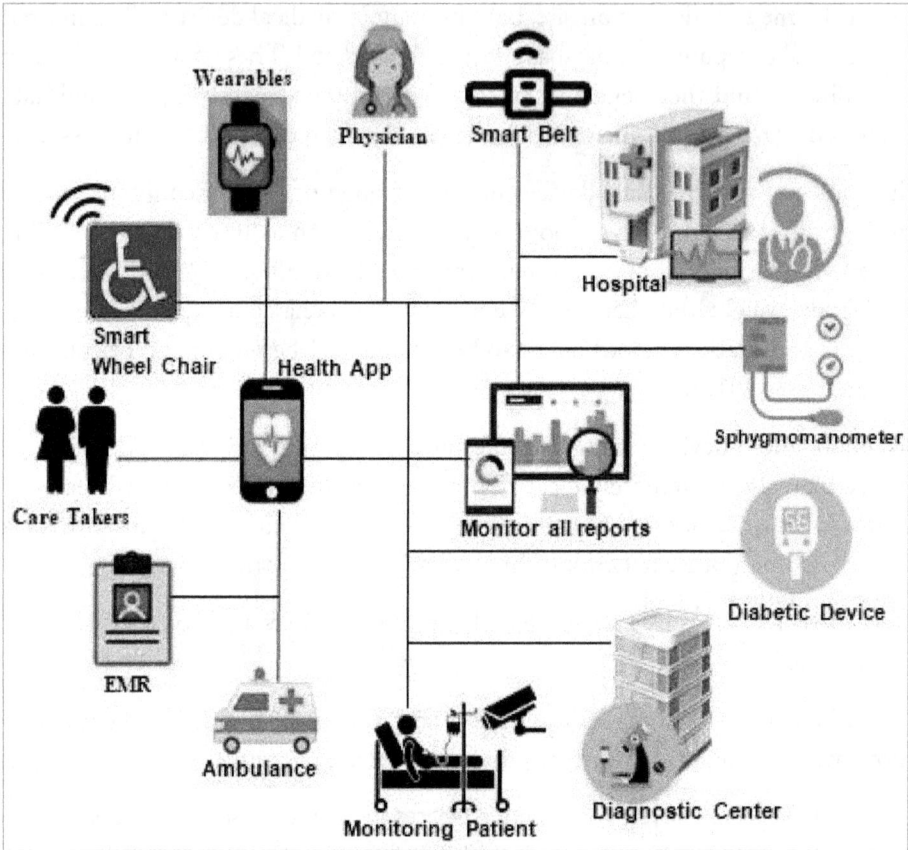

FIGURE 13.1: The internet of medical things (IoMT)

13.7 ONLINE SURGICAL OPERATIONS AND SURGICAL ROBOTS

In this day and age, robotic surgery is performed regularly. The patient is surrounded by different robots, controlled from an onsite surgeon, using controls and screens connected to the robots. This connection is via dedicated data transmission cables directly connecting the robots to the surgeon's control centre. The surgeon's instructions reach the robots nearly immediately and the surgeon always has full and direct control. The surgeon can now manipulate the robots through the controls to perform the delicate activities required for the operation. Prostate operations have been performed very successfully in this way (Intuitive, n.d.).

When the surgeon and the patient are in different locations, maybe in different cities, this approach becomes much more difficult, complex, and risky. Although the setup is identical as described above, direct dedicated transmission lines are not always possible. The surgeon's instructions are sent to the robots via cyberspace. A core requirement for this approach is of course the speed of the communication network, as any delay can cause disaster and even death. With the advancement in 5G communication systems, the required speed is theoretically possible – this makes online surgical operations possible where the surgeon and patient are in different locations.

The potential benefits of such interventions should be clear – the expertise of skilled surgeons can now be used more widely, and surgical operations can now be performed in rural hospitals where surgeons with the specific necessary skills may not be available (Madder, 2020). This approach has the promise to provide experts with specialised surgical interventions in remote areas, which would otherwise not be possible. The technologies of the 4th Industrial Revolution make such approaches viable, "delivering top-tier surgical expertise anywhere in the world" (Amerding, 2015).

Although such approaches sound exciting, using cyberspace confronts it with all the inherent risks associated with cyberspace discussed in this chapter. In many cases such online operations using surgical robots will be cases where interruptions can be life threatening, and even fatal. Multiple risks exist, of which availability and speed of the network connection between the surgeon and the hospital are crucial. The network connection can be lost at a crucial stage during the operation, or the connection may suddenly slow down – both with potentially fatal consequences (Madder, 2020).

Cybercriminals are of course aware of all these risks and implications and can launch a cyberattack on the communication network between the surgeon and the hospital and take it off the air or deliberately slow it down. Furthermore, if the communication network is not properly secured through advanced encryption, the integrity of the data flowing over the network can be compromised. The cybercriminal can hack into the network and change the instructions sent by the surgeon to the robot, causing the robot to perform incorrect and potentially dangerous actions. Reports do exist of cybersecurity researchers which successfully hacked into and hijacked a surgical robot. This stopped the robot and made it impossible for the surgeon to continue (Storm, 2015).

Therefore, although such online operations using surgical robots have immense potential, severe cybersecurity-related risks must still be addressed and resolved. In the last instance, it must also be accepted that no systems operating in cyberspace can be 100% secured – there will always be the potential that cyberattacks can be successful. There may be some ethical aspects related to this approach of online operations and surgical robots, and that will be addressed in the next section.

13.8   MEDICAL ETHICS AND CYBERSECURITY

13.8.1   Background

The normal definition of cybersecurity is that it is the people, processes, and technology needed to ensure the confidentiality, integrity, and availability of data in cyberspace. In a financial environment that may mean that a bank must ensure that clients' financial data is protected against unauthorised persons viewing it (confidentiality), their financial data must be protected against unauthorised changes (integrity), and their financial data must be available when they need it (availability) – the CIA principle. In this scenario, the bank does not really have to worry about the client's personal safety and that cyberattacks on the bank will have a direct effect and impact on the client's life and safety. The cybersecurity officer of a bank can, with little risk, decide to take the bank's whole computer system offline if a cyberattack is noticed, or to contain such an attack. Furthermore, financial institutions have developed very strong cybersecurity protection measures for lowering the risk of unauthorised access to client's data, and also have a more 'closed' environment of employees who may have access to the bank's computer systems – therefore, although the risk is never eliminated, it can be lowered significantly in such a financial environment.

However, this totally changes when we look at medical and health care data in the IoMT. Cybersecurity in medical ecosystems has potentially a much more direct impact on patients' safety and even their lives. ICU ventilators are very good examples of a type of equipment which can be seen as life supporting (Kacmarek, 2011). Many more hospital employees have access to the devices and sensors connected to the hospital's computer systems, and many of them may not be very aware of the risks and possibilities of compromising sensitive private patient data. In section 13.4 above, we gave brief examples of what such consequences can be.

The ethical dilemma when the medical ecosystem is involved, is much more complex. Three aspects will now briefly be investigated:

- the security and privacy of patient data
- the cybersecurity management of the IoMT
- the security of medical sensors.

13.8.2   Ethical decisions related to the security and privacy of patient data

As indicated in section 13.2 above, medical personal data is extremely valuable, and is a growing target for cybercriminals. Very often, personal medical data is collected from many locations, and not only in a hospital. It is therefore much more difficult to secure all this data during transmission and storage. In many cases, for example in an emergency, such data can be collected, transmitted, stored, and processed without the knowledge and approval of the patient. This can result in ethical questions and even legal consequences.

The amount of data captured through all such sensors and devices is immense and will just keep growing. New ways of storage are needed for these masses of data and using the cloud has become a very obvious choice. Cloud storage creates its own security and protection problems, many of which are not yet properly solved. This stored patient data can also be accessed by a much wider group of medical staff, increasing the risk of unauthorised access and misuse.

Some ethical questions, which do arise in such a case, include:

- Is all the data collected about a patient really necessary?
- How are patients involved in decisions to collect, store, and process their data?
- How can the patient be assured that such collected data is not misused?
- How can the number of people having access to a patient's data be limited to enforce better access control?

Surely, such questions have a strong technical implication, but in this case, ethical aspects also play a major role. As discussed in section 13.10 below, these ethical aspects must be part of the governance in the medical ecosystem and must therefore be addressed at board level.

13.8.3   Ethical decisions related to cybersecurity management of the IoMT

The cybersecurity officer of a major hospital must make much more difficult and sensitive decisions. Suppose the officer notices a cyberattack on a life-supporting system used by patients and connected to the hospital's computer system network. Suppose further this life-supporting system is at that moment supporting some patients in real time. The officer must now make some serious decisions and take action to contain the attack.

On the one hand, the officer can take the life-supporting system offline to contain the attack and prevent it from spreading to other connected systems. This may, however, risk the lives of the patients connected to the specific life-supporting system. On the other hand, the officer can leave the life-support system online but risk infecting the hospital's wider networks and computer systems. This decision is eventually not just a cybersecurity decision (as the bank's cybersecurity officer could decide), but also has serious ethical consequences. The hospital's cybersecurity officer, who is basically a technical person, must now make a decision which may have life and death implications. There is no way this officer can do that alone. The whole medical ecosystem of the hospital, interconnected to the hospital computer systems, the IoMT, and staff are now all involved in a basically technical cyberattack and cybersecurity decision. Medical ethics and cybersecurity have now become integrated as far as management and decisions are concerned.

13.8.4   The ethical decisions related to the security of medical sensors

Very often medical sensor devices themselves do not have built-in cybersecurity protection, and then they are nevertheless implemented without proper security protection, endangering the privacy and lives of patients. "Medical IoT devices have great benefits to patient care but can leave medical centers and hospitals wide open to cyber-attacks" (Archon, n.d.).

The question now should be: is it ethical to install medical sensors if it is known beforehand that they may have serious security flaws, which can impact on patients' privacy and security? To address this aspect, before implementation, it must be ensured that all such devices are robustly designed, reliable, and secured cybersecurity-wise. This is not only a technical issue but also an ethical one, which demands input and consent from top management. This is an important aspect, discussed in section 13.10 below on cybersecurity governance in the medical ecosystem (Mittelstadt, 2017).

13.8.5   Summary

Medical ethical aspects within the IoMT are growing and will keep growing as new devices are developed and implemented. The relationship between cyber-security and ethics in the IoMT must get more attention and must be accepted as a core component of the medical ecosystem. "Medical ethics can no longer be separated from cybersecurity in healthcare" (Frenz, 2021).

Taking all these risks and concerns into account, it is very important in the medical ecosystem to have a cyber-incident response plan. Quick and well-planned actions in the case of a cyberattack are essential for the safety and well-being of everyone, especially the patients. This matter is discussed in more detail in the next section.

13.9   A CYBER-INCIDENT RESPONSE PLAN IN THE MEDICAL ECOSYSTEM

As mentioned in the previous paragraph, a cyberattack on the medical ecosystem and the IoMT can potentially result in death. It is therefore irresponsible not to be properly prepared for such an eventuality, and to act with the greatest speed.

It is important for any company exposed to cyberattacks to have a cyber-incident response plan (CIRP). Such a plan provides clear guidance on what must happen if a cyber-incident occurs. For the medical ecosystem, such a CIRP is even more important. The example discussed above about decisions to be taken if a cyber-attack happens is an example of why a CIRP is essential. Of course, it is important to take preventative action to prevent any cyberattack as far as possible, but more is needed. A CIRP must clearly spell out what must be done if such an attack does happen – at that point in time, everybody should know immediately how to react. Such plans are a normal plan demanded by security good practices but is often lacking in the medical ecosystem (ECRI, 2020). This aspect is again mentioned in the following section.

13.10   CYBERSECURITY GOVERNANCE IN THE MEDICAL ECOSYSTEM

13.10.1   Background

Cybersecurity governance is a component of corporate governance, meaning the responsibility and accountability of cybersecurity governance lies squarely on the shoulder of the board of a company (Fortium, 2017; Price, 2018a; Scholtz, 2021).

The main objective of corporate governance is to provide direction and guidance in a company, including:

- Determining the strategic direction and objectives of the company;

- Ensuring that the necessary policies, procedures, and resources are in place to achieve the strategic objectives;

- Overseeing and ensuring that the strategic objectives are accomplished (WHO, 2014); and

- Understanding the relevant ethical aspects and be prepared to act properly.

International good practices for corporate governance emphasises that cyber-security governance is a core component of corporate governance. If the company operates in cyberspace in any way, the implication is therefore that the accountability and responsibility to ensure that all data, transactions, and operations are cyber-secured, resides with the board. In cyberspace, the board must understand

and accept that cybersecurity governance is not (only) a technical issue, but a business risk management issue where the buck stops in the boardroom.

Cybersecurity governance in the medical ecosystem involves all of the above but includes more – this makes it even more essential that the board of a health care institute making use of the IoMT must take on this responsibility and accountability. As already noted in section 13.8 above on medical ethics and cybersecurity, the involvement of the IoMT can cause certain situations where life and death are at stake, and where the final decisions are actually that of the board. This aspect is emphasised by stating that operating in the IoMT requires the extensions of existing governance mechanisms to ensure safety and security (Skierka, 2018).

> Cybersecurity is an essential part of maintaining the safety, privacy and trust of patients. More money and effort must be invested into ensuring the security of healthcare technologies and patient information. Security must be designed into the product from conception and not be an afterthought. Cybersecurity must become part of the patient care culture. (Coventry & Branley, 2018)

This is basically what cybersecurity governance in the medical ecosystem is all about. It, however, seems that there is "lack of appreciation among health care executives (about) the business risks of cyber breaches" (He, 2021).

Subsection 13.10.2 will provide a few steps which should be part of every medical institution's cybersecurity strategy plan.

13.10.2 A few guidelines to the board for cybersecurity governance (CSG) in the medical ecosystem

In this section, we will provide a number of guidelines for the board of a health care enterprise to ensure that the very important and strategic matter of cybersecurity governance in the medical ecosystem is properly implemented. The board must take these guidelines seriously to ensure strong oversight of the whole cybersecurity area.

The board must:

1. ensure that they understand and accept that cybersecurity governance is a corporate governance accountability, and they have an important oversight role regarding cybersecurity;

2. accept that the cybersecurity buck stops with them;

3. ensure that cybersecurity is a standing item on the board agenda;

4. ensure that regular feedback is provided to the board about the status of cybersecurity in the enterprise to be able to perform their oversight role;

5. ensure that there is at least one cybersecurity expert on the board (even an outside expert);

6. ensure that a culture of cybersecurity awareness is established and enforced;

7. create a cybersecurity risk policy, approved and signed by the board. This must include the cyber-incident response plan (CIRP), discussed in section 13.9 above, and must have representation from the legal department;

8. ensure that international good practices in cybersecurity, like encrypting data, are implemented in the enterprise;

9. create a cyber-risk governance committee as a subcommittee of the board, reporting directly to the board;

10. understand that operating the medical ecosystem has potentially very serious business risks;

11. understand that the accountability for cybersecurity governance cannot be delegated to executive management or the chief security officer – some responsibility can be delegated, but the board stays accountable; and

12. understand the ethical risks in operating in the medical ecosystem.

Price (2018b) provides more background on this matter.

13.11 CONCLUSION

The medical ecosystem will see massive growth in the coming years, primarily driven by the IoMT. This will again create a greater dependence on cyberspace, which will again provide a larger attack service for cybercriminals. To counter these cyberattacks, cybersecurity must be at the core of the medical ecosystem. This reality must be accepted by the board of an enterprise, exercising their corporate governance oversight role to ensure that the enterprise is prepared against cyberattacks as far as possible.

Bibliography

Alpine Security. 2021. *Comprehensive guide to Yom cybersecurity: risks, safeguards, and what we protect.* https://bit.ly/3GHu27G [Accessed 25 February 2022].

Archon. n.d. *Medical IoT device security risks and solutions.* https://bit.ly/3GJv7fm [Accessed 25 February 2022].

Armerding, T. 2015. *Surgical robots: smart but insecure.* https://bit.ly/3V6QSKq [Accessed 25 February 2022].

Aver, H. 2021. *Ransomware attacks on healthcare.* https://bit.ly/3VnCgWx [Accessed 25 February 2022].

Coventry, L. & Branley, D. 2018. *Cybersecurity in healthcare: a narrative review of trends, threats and ways forward.* https://doi.org/10.1016/j.maturitas.2018.04.008

Critical Insight. n.d. *Top 6 hackable medical IoT devices.* https://bit.ly/3Xnzank [Accessed 25 February 2022].

Deloitte. 2020. *Cyber transformation.* https://bit.ly/3tZ4JGy [Accessed 25 February 2022].

Dilawar, N., Rizwan, M., Ahmad, F. & Akram, S. 2019. Blockchain: securing internet of medical things (Yom). *International Journal of Advanced Computer Science and Applications,* 10(1). January. https://doi.org/10.14569/IJACSA.2019.0100110

ECRI. 2020. *Getting started with a cybersecurity incident response plan for your medical devices.* https://bit.ly/3ugzION [Accessed 25 February 2022].

Fortium. 2017. *Cyber security: the buck stops in the boardroom.* https://bit.ly/3tYxGlX [Accessed 25 February 2022].

Frenz, C. 2021. *Importance of medical ethics in cybersecurity.* https://bit.ly/3F0gFOQ [Accessed 25 February 2022].

Goodin, D. 2020. *A patient dies after a ransomware attack hits a hospital.* https://bit.ly/3ECCK4A [Accessed 25 February 2022].

Green, J. 2018. *Centralised medical records database: convenient or risky?* https://bit.ly/3V6Mvif [Accessed 25 February 2022].

He, Y. 2021. *Health care cybersecurity challenges and solutions under the climate of Covid-19: scoping review, 2021.* https://doi.org/10.2196/29877

Intuitive. n.d. *Prostate surgery.* https://bit.ly/3F1BwkS [Accessed 25 February 2022].

Irwin, L. 2020. *What is the ISO 27000 series of standards?* https://bit.ly/2JHfB4f [Accessed 25 February 2022].

Kacmarek, R. 2011. *The mechanical ventilator: past, present, and future.* https://doi.org/10.4187/respcare.01420

Kawamoto, D. 2017. *Hacked IV pumps and digital smart pens can lead to data breaches.* https://bit.ly/3VqCMDu [Accessed 25 February 2022].

Khalik, S. 2018. *Greater protection of patient data when national electronic medical records become mandatory.* https://bit.ly/3UalcSR [Accessed 25 February 2022].

Madder, R. 2020. *Robot surgery could be the future of health care in remote areas.* https://bit.ly/3OwuDeo [Accessed 25 February 2022].

Miliard, M. 2021. *Hospital ransomware attack led to infant's death, lawsuit alleges.* https://bit.ly/3VtRk5j [Accessed 25 February 2022].

Mittelstadt, B. 2017. *Ethics of the health-related internet of things: a narrative review.* https://doi.org/10.1007/s10676-017-9426-4

Morgan, S. 2017. *Cybercrime damages $6 trillion by 2021.* https://bit.ly/2K6QZnp [Accessed 25 February 2022].

Price, N. 2018a. *The relationship between cybersecurity and corporate governance.* https://bit.ly/3tVb0Dl [Accessed 25 February 2022].

Price, N. 2018b. *How to transform corporate governance for your hospital board.* https://bit.ly/3AIf6lP [Accessed 26 February 2022].

Ronte, H., Taylor, K. & Haughey, J. 2018. *Medtech and the internet of medical things.* https://bit.ly/2OafRdy [Accessed 25 February 2022].

Rothschild, F. 2020. *Medical devices are double-edged swords for hospitals: vital for patient care but vulnerable to cyberattacks.* https://bit.ly/3V5HfeW [Accessed 25 February 2022].

Scholtz, T. 2021. *Security & risk strategy.* https://bit.ly/3EYVMmT [Accessed 25 February 2022].

Sipilä, J. 2020. *Patients in Finland blackmailed after therapy records were stolen by hackers.* https://cnn.it/3U3b26M [Accessed 25 February 2022].

Skierka, I. 2018. *The governance of safety and security risks in connected healthcare.* The Institution of Engineering and Technology. https://doi.org/10.1049/cp.2018.0002

Spence, N., Bhardwaj, N., Paul, D. & Coustasse, A. 2018. *Ransomware in healthcare facilities: a harbinger of the future?* https://bit.ly/3Ukxb0B [Accessed 25 February 2022].

Steger, A. 2020. *What makes Yom devices so difficult to secure?* https://bit.ly/3V1eYGi [Accessed 26 February 2022].

Storm, D. 2015. *Researchers hijack tele operated surgical robot.* https://bit.ly/3OxavsC [Accessed 25 February 2022].

Vaas, L. 2013. *Doctors disabled wireless in Dick Cheney's pacemaker to thwart hacking.* https://bit.ly/3AHXiHy [Accessed 26 February 2022].

Weiner, S. 2021. *The growing threat of ransomware attacks on hospitals.* https://bit.ly/3U6fce6 [Accessed 25 February 2022].

WHO. 2014. *Health systems governance for universal health coverage.* https://bit.ly/3TYVukk [Accessed 25 February 2022].

14

How will Biotechnology Transform Human Health?

The peril and promise of genetic engineering

Susan Hall

Keywords: biotechnology; genetic engineering; genetic enhancement; genetic therapy; human nature; inequality; risk

---

14.1 INTRODUCTION

Technological advancement often gives rise to novel ethical problems. Technology opens up new possibilities, in that it allows us to do things which we have not been able to do before, and as a result, it inevitably raises the question as to whether these are things we *ought* to be doing, and if so, whether our prevailing moral norms and principles are adequate to deal with our new abilities. This is as true in the context of health care as elsewhere. Consider the development of life support technologies such as the medical ventilator, and the ethical questions this raised as to the extension of the concept of 'death' (Nair-Collins & Miller, 2017). More recently, the implementation of machine learning as a diagnostic and predictive tool in clinical medicine (Char, Shah & Magnus, 2018) and the use of big data analysis in biomedical contexts (Knoppers & Thorogood, 2017) have provoked ethical debate. The same is true of *biotechnological* development in medicine.

Biotechnology is defined by the Organisation for Economic Co-operation and Development (OECD) as "[t]he application of science and technology to living organisms, as well as parts, products, and models thereof, to alter living or nonliving materials for the production of knowledge, goods and services" (OECD, 2013:156). The best known and probably most contentious possible application of biotechnology in the context of health care is genetic engineering. Genetic engineering involves the modification of a biological organism's DNA. Genetic engineering in humans may be carried out in germline or somatic cells,[1] and might be carried out for therapeutic purposes (genetic therapy) or to improve upon normal human functioning (genetic enhancement). This application of biotechnology holds great promise. The development of CRISPR/Cas9 technology, for example, creates exciting possibilities for the treatment of various forms of cancer, as well as cardiovascular, metabolic, haematological, and other hereditary diseases (Li et al., 2020). Some genetic therapies have already been approved by the US Food and Drug Administration (FDA) and the European Medicines Agency (EMA) to treat devastating monogenetic diseases such as spinal muscular atrophy (Chaytow et al., 2021). To many, however, the prospect of the development and use of interventions which aim to manipulate our genetic makeup evokes discomfort or repugnance, particularly when such interventions aim not only to treat but also to enhance. Some contend that these technologies represent a threat to the human species, or fear that their potential for harm may outweigh any positive consequences.

In what follows, I will outline the bioethical debate surrounding genetic engineering.[2] I will firstly consider two groups of arguments against the development and use of gene editing technologies which focus on (1) the inherent nature of genetic modification itself and its relationship to human nature, and (2) the likely consequences of gene editing. I will explore possible lines of defence against these challenges. Finally, I will briefly put forward the case that both genetic therapy and some forms of genetic enhancement hold great potential for the transformation of human health, and, in the case of enhancement, human well-being more generally. We should therefore be cautious of rejecting these technologies out of hand.

---

1   Ormond et al. define somatic gene editing as "the alteration of cells that cannot contribute to gamete formation and thus cannot be passed on from the individual to offspring" and germline gene editing as "genome editing that occurs in a germ cell or embryo and results in changes that are theoretically present in all cells of the embryo and that could also potentially be passed from the modified individual to offspring" (2017:69).

2   This overview is partially based on research completed as part of my PhD dissertation (Hall, 2012).

14.2   GENETIC ENGINEERING AND HUMAN NATURE

Genetic engineering is aimed at the manipulation of the human genome. Many people feel uneasy about this prospect, as it seems to strike at a fundamental aspect of our common humanity. The concern is that modifying our genes will necessarily involve or lead to the modification of human nature, either because it represents a threat to our species membership, or because it will undermine values and attitudes that are regarded as foundational to our uniquely human identities. Arguments of this kind take issue with both the means (in the case of genetic engineering in general) and goals (in the case of genetic enhancement in particular) of the modification of the human genome.

14.2.1   The threat to species membership

The concern that genetic engineering will modify our genetic identities in such a way that we (or at least some of us) will no longer be members of the human species is largely focused on the possibility that this may weaken or undermine human commonality and threaten our recognition of the moral status of others. George Annas, for example, worries that "altering our nature necessarily threatens to undermine both human dignity and human rights" (2000:772) – a position also shared by Fukuyama (2002:101) – and calls for an "international treaty banning specific 'species altering' techniques and species-endangering experiments" (Annas, 2000:779). The purported link between species membership and moral status is emphasised in the Universal Declaration on the Human Genome and Human Rights in the statement that the "human genome underlies the fundamental unity of all members of the human family" (UNESCO, 1997:3). This implies that the modification of the human genome via genetic engineering could imperil this fundamental unity, and thereby our recognition of the moral status of others.

This argument also encompasses anxiety about posthumanism. Again, this concern is based upon the idea that genetic engineering will transform human nature to the extent that enhanced individuals will no longer be categorised as members of the species *Homo sapiens*. The worry is that the boundaries that currently determine membership of the human species will be eroded as two "subspecies" (Sandel, 2007:15) emerge: humans who maintain their naturally given genetic characteristics, and genetically modified posthumans. This development, some suggest, could further destabilise our "sense of moral community" based on common species membership (Buchanan et al., 2000:95) and may lead to what Agar refers to as "polarization" (2004:134) between humans and genetically engineered posthumans.

While we may accept the possibility that genetic engineering could alter the human genome in ways which ultimately alter the human species, we need not agree that this is morally problematic. The human genome is, after all, subject to evolutionary forces, and will continue to change in the future. It is therefore unclear precisely why random change exacted by evolution should be preferable to directed change exacted by human interventions if it cannot be shown that the latter is considerably riskier than the former (Buchanan, 2011:137; Caplan, 2009:202; Harris, 2007:34). In other words, if genetic engineering entails a move away from what we currently regard to be human nature, based on our genetic characteristics, this will merely constitute a hastening of a process that will occur in any case as a result of evolution.

But what of the argument that genetic modification may, in its potential to undermine species membership, also threaten the basis of our recognition of moral status, human dignity, and by extension, universal human rights? Commentators respond to this assertion by questioning whether human nature, as the basis of moral recognition and human rights, can be reduced to brute biological characteristics. Rather, "[t]here are many candidates for the qualities that serve to give us our inalienable rights … but none hinge on a taxonomic designation" (Juengst, 2009:52). Theories of human rights usually regard such rights as stemming not simply from our genetic identity as human beings, but rather from the presence of interests, in that morally relevant beings have an interest in being treated in particular ways. While we might feel intuitively that "all humans have 'human rights' precisely because they are human", an interrogation of this idea reveals that it is "problematic as a theory of moral status" (Beauchamp & Childress, 2009:68). Rather, we are inclined to grant moral status and rights to those beings which have certain capacities such as the ability to reason, to form a conception of themselves as the subject of autonomous action, and to engage in moral deliberations, and while such qualities usually correspond with human species membership, this is neither a necessary nor a sufficient condition for our recognition of such moral status (Beauchamp & Childress, 2009:68).

To deny the conception of rights outlined above and to insist instead that moral status is bestowed upon us solely as a result of our genetic identity as human beings is to indulge in what Peter Singer refers to as "speciesism" (1993:88): the belief that moral status is conferred by the brute fact of our membership of the human species, based upon a prejudice in favour of our own kind. This amounts, according to Juengst, to the "moral idolatry" of the human genome (2009:52). If such a conception of moral status is unreliable, and moral status depends instead upon the presence of morally relevant characteristics, this implies that genetic engineering, despite its potential to erode the current boundaries of species membership, need not represent a threat to our recognition of the moral status or rights of others.

14.2.2 The threat to human values

The second concern with respect to genetic engineering, and genetic enhancement in particular, is that it will undermine or come into conflict with *attitudes* or *values* that we regard as foundational to our humanity, and that this will have a dehumanising effect on genetically modified individuals and on society as a whole. The concern in this case is not the threat to the genetic basis of species membership, but to the values and attitudes that give meaning to our humanity (Fenton, 2008:3). In other words, the dehumanising effect attributed to genetic engineering is related to its posited potential to undermine those values and attitudes which are regarded as constitutive of human nature, or which give content to our notion of "what it means to be human" (Robert, 2005:28).

14.2.2.1 *Giftedness*

The first value which is thought to be threatened by the prospect of genetic engineering is the value of 'giftedness'. Both Leon Kass (2003) and Michael Sandel (2007) suggest that the goal of genetic enhancement in particular is problematic because it constitutes a striving towards mastery of the natural world, and, more importantly, of ourselves. In so doing, it undermines our appreciation of the "giftedness" of our natural human abilities and endowments (Sandel, 2007: 26-27). This 'giftedness' entails a recognition that our abilities are "not wholly our own doing, nor even fully ours": a recognition that fosters an attitude of "humility" (Sandel, 2007:27). If we develop the ability to shape our genetic capacities, these could no longer rightly be regarded as "gifts for which we are indebted" but would instead be perceived as "achievements for which we are responsible" (Sandel, 2007:86-87). Leon Kass, the onetime chairman of The President's Council on Bioethics, echoes these sentiments, regarding an attitude of "hubris" as central to the project of genetic enhancement (Kass, 2003:18).

However, as Kass notes, the difficulty which such an argument immediately encounters is that we typically do not humbly accept the "giftedness" of disease and dysfunction (Kass, 2003:19). What Kass therefore seeks to argue is that there is something morally objectionable about the drive to enhance human nature that does not apply to medical treatment in general. Kass attributes this to the attitude expressed in genetic enhancement "that seeks wilful control of our own nature" and contrasts this with medicine as "servant and aid to nature's own powers of healing" (Kass, 2003:18), a point which Sandel echoes:

> Although medical treatment intervenes in nature, it does so for the sake of health, and so does not represent a boundless bid for mastery and domination. Even strenuous attempts to treat or cure disease do not constitute a Promethean assault on the given. The reason is that medicine is governed, or at least guided, by the norm of restoring and preserving the natural human functions that constitute health. (Sandel, 2007:46-47)

One may, however, question the contention that intervening in our own natures to bring about enhancement constitutes hubris, while intervening in our own natures to cure or prevent disease or dysfunction does not. Buchanan, for example, argues that it is simply illogical to assert that it is acceptable to transform the given when it comes to curing disease and dysfunction, but not when it comes to improving normal functioning (Buchanan, 2011:3). In his view, it does not follow from the fact that "one ought to be appreciative of the good things one has and aware that many of them are unearned" that "one should refrain from ever trying to improve one's life or the lives of others" (2011:3). Harris echoes this point in his failure to be persuaded by the argument that we should accept the "gifted nature" of human talents but not the giftedness of disease and disability (Harris, 2007:112). Both Kass and Sandel argue that the distinction between treating disease and enhancing function lies in the fact that medical practice aids or restores natural human functioning. Harris, however, points out that disease and disability are themselves an aspect of natural human functioning (2007:35). Thus, the rejection of interventions that seek to manipulate nature would seem to exclude the practice of medicine altogether.

It is also important to note that it is not only through the practice of medicine that we routinely seek to exercise "wilful control over our own nature" (Kass, 2003:19). Attempts to master nature, and specifically, attempts to act upon and improve our own natures and the natures of others, are hardly novel pursuits: they are constitutive not only of the goals of medicine, but also of law, childrearing, and education, and the striving towards improvement and enhancement has always been a project which characterises human life (Buchanan, 2011:xi). In fact, the whole history of human culture and civilisation may be regarded as the history of human attempts to alter and shape the naturally occurring state of affairs, including our naturally occurring human natures: we have "long tinkered with ourselves using all manner of technologies from clothing to medicines to agriculturally produced food to telescopes to computers to airplanes" (Caplan, 2009:202), and in this sense, "Sandel's warning that one should not imperil gifted-ness comes several millennia too late" (Buchanan, 2011:79).

One may also question whether the genetic engineering of human beings is self-evidently motivated by a desire for mastery. All such interventions cannot be assumed, without further argument, to be necessarily driven by a desire for mastery or for total control over the given world, and as such, the argument against enhancement based upon this premise fails (Buchanan, 2011:79), as it involves a "vast empirical generalization ... about the psychology of those who pursue enhancement" (Buchanan, 2011:9). In other words, it is perfectly feasible that one may seek to improve upon some aspect of human genetic functioning without thereby seeking, or expecting to achieve, mastery over the natural world or over our own natures.

14.2.2.2 The structure of agency and the value of effort

Michael Sandel advances a further objection to genetic engineering which focuses on the means which this technology would employ. In his view, "[o]ne aspect of our humanity that might be threatened by ... genetic engineering is our capacity to act freely, for ourselves, by our own efforts, and to consider ourselves responsible – worthy of praise or blame – for the things we do and for the way we are" (Sandel, 2007:25). In other words, our achievements could no longer be regarded as flowing (entirely) from our own efforts but would rather be the result of technological achievement. Sandel's point here is related to the value we ascribe to the effort which we expend in achieving our goals. Genetic enhancement in particular has the potential to bypass the "substantial discipline and effort" which we currently invest in our attempts to "produce the desired feature or capability" and negates the fact that "a valued human activity is [sometimes] defined in part by the means it employs, not just by the end at which it aims" (Brock, 1998:58). We ascribe virtue to the means which are employed when our advantages are acquired through effort and hard work, and therefore regard the resulting advantages as honourable and deserved. The advantages that could be acquired through genetic enhancement, however, could be regarded as unmerited, as they are not acquired through such virtuous means (Mehlman, 2003:112).

However, one may object to this account of the value of effort, and the extent to which this value is likely to be compromised by genetic engineering. As Harris points out, many enhancing technologies "leave plenty of room for effort, skill training [and] hard work" (2007:133). The causal relationship between genetically modified genotypes and phenotypes (the eventual characteristics or traits of an organism) will vary, and will depend upon environmental influences, including one's own actions and efforts, a point which Sandel concedes in his assertion that "the roles of effort and enhancement will be a matter of degree" (2007:25). While enhanced individuals may be engineered for high levels of intelligence, for example, this genetic disposition is worthless without education, with all the associated effort in terms of study and discipline which that implies.

Allhoff (2005) also makes two points in opposition to the argument against genetic engineering from the value of effort. Firstly, he points out that "successive generations have always had more resources available to them than previous generations", and that we routinely expend less effort in the achievement of our goals than our ancestors. Motorised transport, technological study aids, and domestic appliances, among other technologies, have greatly reduced the effort and transformed the means by which we realise our ends. We do not regard this as problematic, or the ultimate achievement of our goals as any less laudable as a result. Secondly, he points out that some people, due to their genetic advantages as provided by the genetic lottery, do not need to expend as much effort to achieve their objectives as others. We do not regard their accomplishments as any less valuable, or any less their own, despite this (2005:46). Genetic engineering therefore does not seem to represent an unprecedented departure from the existing state of affairs. Taken together, these counter arguments suggest that such technologies would not represent the kind of novel disruption to human agency that critics of enhancement suggest it would.

14.2.2.3   The goodness of fragility

A further objection to genetic engineering which focuses on its purported threat to human values concerns the value of fragility. Human beings are by nature vulnerable creatures, and are susceptible to misfortune, adversity, disease, and disability. Some have expressed the concern that the revolutionary potential of genetic engineering to reduce or nullify this human fragility is morally problematic. The reasoning behind this position is that the physical and mental frailties of human beings, which will be the targets of such technologies, are in fact valuable aspects of the human condition, or, in other words, that "the limitations" which our bodies impose upon us with regard to the achievement of our goals "might have ethical significance that [will be] imperilled by efforts … to overcome all such limitations" (McKenny, 1998:223). Winkler argues in this regard that the "power over uncertainty or contingency" (1998:242) which enhancement technologies offer us could lead to a sacrifice of our "full humanity" (1998:248), as this humanity is partially constituted by a tendency to "love and honour the body in all its fragility, imperfection and finitude" (1998:249).

Why should we feel that the fragility of the body is something to be valued, taking into account that much of the history of civilisation represents an attempt to overcome it? One of the principal answers offered in reply to this question is that the experience of our frailty and vulnerability makes possible important modes of "self-formation" in our responses to adversity (McKenny, 1998:235). Our failure to recognise "the goodness of fragility" (Parens, 1995:141), then, will actually impoverish rather than improve human beings by, for example, oblite-rating the experience of caring for others who are more vulnerable than ourselves, or by removing the opportunity to develop capacities of perseverance and forbear-ance in response to our own finitude.

There are several problems with this objection to genetic engineering. Firstly, the modification of the human genome will not lead to heaven on earth. Genetic engineering will not make us invulnerable, and nor will it remove all adversity or contingency from our lives (Buchanan, 2011:81; Savulescu, 2007:287). Is it nonetheless problematic that genetic engineering is at least *directed towards* the eradication of human fragility, even if this is a goal which can never be completely accomplished?

The difficulty here is that the insistence upon the value of human fragility is based upon a particular world view which is not universally shared. Some insist, for example that it is not "intuitively obvious that there is necessarily ... anything good about aging, or death, or human fragility" (Allhoff, 2005:45). This is borne out by the fact that the use of multiple technologies to counteract such frailty has been regarded as morally laudable over the course of history, and it is unclear why genetic interventions should be an exception to this. Savulescu characterises positions which reject genetic modifications on the basis that they would reduce human frailty as expressing the warped argument that "because life is unpredictable, and good can come out of bad, we should choose the bad or be indifferent to it, or allow it to occur ... when we can easily and foreseeably avoid it" (Savulescu, 2007:286). On this account, the restriction of genetic engineering based on a particular world view which values fragility would be "tyrannical" in the face of competing conceptions of the good life which do not regard it as something which ought to be preserved (Harris, 2007:137). In addition, there is something deeply worrying about any position which seeks to maintain the fragility of *others* in order to preserve the self-formation that accompanies the experience of caring for them.

Thus far it appears that the transformation of human nature via genetic engi-neering, either in terms of our genetic species identity or the values which are central to our humanity, is either exaggerated or less ethically concerning than it first appears. It is worth emphasising again that attempts to alter human nature are hardly new. Human nature has not only been subject to change through evolutionary processes, but also through our own environmental interventions (Daniels, 2009:33). Compared to human beings of the not-too distant past, today "we are taller, we live longer, we have more inclusive ethical codes" (Lewens, 2009:354). These are changes that are at least partially the result of human action, including the use of technological interventions. By this token, genetic engineering is not necessarily a radical departure from what has come before, but rather the latest phase on a continuum of interventions that seek to improve upon human functioning. However, there is a further set of arguments against genetic engineering which I have not yet considered. What if the consequences of genetic engineering are not improvement, but disaster, or what if its benefits are outweighed by far greater costs? It is to these possibilities that I now turn.

14.3   CONSEQUENTIALIST ARGUMENTS AGAINST GENETIC ENGINEERING

Consequentialist arguments against genetic engineering hold that there are negative consequences which are likely to follow from genetic modification, and as these consequences are ethically undesirable, we should avoid them by refraining from developing and utilising such technologies. There are two possibilities that are frequently identified in this regard. On the one hand, genetic engineering, despite the benefits that it might appear to offer, may also have negative consequences for the person who is targeted by the intervention. Here the primary concern is that these technologies may not be safe, and that the inherent risks of genetic engineering are greater than conventional forms of medical treatment due to the nature of genetic functioning. On the other hand, one may accept that genetic engineering may benefit the targeted individual, but still hold that its use would be bad for society as a whole. Here, the most commonly stated worry is that inequitable access to such technologies will exacerbate social and global inequalities, and lead to injustice.

14.3.1   Genetic engineering is medically hazardous

The worry that genetic engineering may be medically hazardous is frequently expressed (Anderson, 1989:686; Borenstein, 2009:524; Kamm, 2009:127; Kass, 2003:14; Mehlman, 2003:71; The President's Council on Bioethics, 2003:48), and ought to be taken seriously. While the possibility of dangerous and unforeseen side effects is always a relevant concern with respect to new medical procedures, genetic engineering may be particularly vulnerable to such concerns. The pleiotropic nature of genes, in that most genes appear to have more than one function and to affect more than one body system (Coors & Hunter, 2005:21), implies that it may be difficult for researchers to predict the effect of a given genetic intervention. Coors and Hunter draw our attention to an incidence of genetic intervention in mice, which caused over-expression of the p53 gene. This intervention reduced the incidence of cancer in the affected mice, but also significantly lessened their life expectancy (2005:21). This example illustrates the danger that "even modest alterations in the best studied genes ... can have completely unexpected consequences for aspects of the organism that were not at all suspected to be related to the function of the gene" (Coors & Hunter, 2005:22). This risk is amplified by the polygenic nature of most complex human traits and disorders which would likely be the targets of enhancement interventions and many therapeutic interventions respectively.

A second point which is raised in support of the particularly hazardous nature of genetic engineering has to do with the inheritability of germline genetic interventions. Genetic interventions are usually classified as somatic cell or germline interventions. Somatic cell genetic interventions (whether therapeutic or enhancing) entail "the insertion of a ... gene into somatic, or body, cells of a patient", while germline interventions, often viewed as more controversial, aim at genetic alterations at the level of the "gametic cells" in such a way that "children of the patient would receive the [altered] gene" (Anderson, 1989:682). Germline genetic interventions, even in their therapeutic manifestations, are unique technological interventions in that their effects would not be limited to the treated patient, but would be passed onto their offspring (Brock, 1998:62). Where the safety of a particular intervention has not been established, or, more pertinently, where unforeseen negative effects of an intervention are delayed, the future person may be harmed by a genetic intervention which affects them but which they have not consented to. This may be a good reason to avoid at least germline genetic interventions until safety can be definitively established.

However, the fact that a procedure is risky does not necessarily give us reason to disavow it entirely, particularly if its potential benefits would be very great, and for this reason, medical risk may not be a knock-down argument against the practice of genetic engineering. While safety concerns, particularly with regard to new and revolutionary interventions, should always be at the forefront of researchers' minds, this suggests the need for the utmost caution, but does not necessarily imply that an outright ban on genetic engineering is justified (Baylis & Robert, 2004:14). If genetic interventions are inherently more risky than other novel medical interventions, they ought to be approached with greater caution. However, if it can be shown, through extended and careful research, and controlled clinical testing, that genetic interventions can overcome the difficulties identified above, and could be practiced in a relatively safe and effective manner, this objection simply disappears.

In addition, the possible effect of germline genetic engineering on future generations is not unique to such interventions. As Moseley points out, "[h]umans alive today do many things which may have unforeseeable and negative consequences for future generations but which appear ethically acceptable" and that normal procreation in general is subject to this very same complaint (Moseley, 1991:643). If we assume that rational persons will not choose interventions that run clear risks of bringing about obviously negative consequences for their offspring and descendants, we cannot reject genetic interventions purely on the basis of remote risks which have not been proven without calling into question many other human practices, especially in the realm of scientific interventions, which we currently consider to be not only ethically acceptable, but desirable. As Harris points out, "insistence on rigorous risk assessment and on only proceeding if in all the circumstances of the case the risks are acceptable is a feature not only of all medical and scientific advance but of all human decision making whatsoever" (2007:33). Thus, while the risks of genetic engineering must be taken very seriously, the presence of such risks does not constitute a definitive argument against this practice.

14.4   GENETIC ENGINEERING AND INJUSTICE

The concern that genetic engineering may lead to or exacerbate injustice is situated within the framing assumption that the benefits of genetic engineering primarily accrue to the individual, and that this benefit should be balanced against the likelihood of its "social or collective harms" (Buchanan, 2011:36). The worry here is that genetic engineering, and particularly genetic enhancement, will bring about or widen inequalities between individuals and groups in society in a way which will be unjust. If, as is likely, genetic engineering is at least initially an expensive intervention which is not covered by national health schemes or health insurance, only those who are already financially advantaged will be able to make use of it. If these genetic interventions confer "advantages in competitions for social goods such as wealth, status or power" (Gardner, 1995:69), this improved ability to compete will therefore increase the variance of the distribution of social goods (Gardner, 1995:74), contributing to "the widening gap between the well-off and the less-so" (Baylis & Robert, 2004:12).

The purported connection between genetic enhancement and injustice is not only relevant with regard to inequality within societies, but also inequality between societies (Mehlman, 2003:127). Concerns have already been expressed that the benefits of new biotechnological advances may not be made available in many African countries as a result of their prohibitive cost (Benatar, 1998:169). In countries where greater provision is made for access to health care beyond the primary level, it is likely that access to genetic engineering will be distributed more equitably among the population than in countries where only the wealthy will be able to fund it. The ethical issues at stake here are therefore not confined to the sphere of personal morality but are significant with respect to global bioethics. This is particularly relevant in the African context, where the distribution of health care resources, and particularly the just distribution of global health care resources, is already of major ethical concern. Research into genetic modification may represent a misallocation of resources in a context where the basic health needs of millions of people remain unfulfilled. We do not need genetic engineering to provide all children with mosquito netting or to vaccinate everyone against measles (Davis, 2009:149).

It may certainly be the case that access to genetic engineering technologies may be inequitably distributed, at least initially, and probably for some time. However, brute inequality does not necessarily imply injustice. For the inequality created by genetic engineering to be morally concerning, it must also be unjust. This raises some difficult questions, as the notion of justice itself is extremely difficult to define or to reduce to a single theory (Harris, 1992:192). However, some general remarks on this matter may suffice.

Firstly, we should note that rather than being born into equality, we are all already subject to the natural inequality imposed by the genetic lottery (Holtug, 1999:138). Some of us are naturally genetically advantaged competitors, and some are less fortunate (Brock, 1998:67). However, one may counter that this naturally given inequality is not the result of human action, and therefore not within the sphere of behaviour that can be morally censured. The situation with respect to genetic engineering is different. Here, what specifically concerns many is the possibility that sophisticated genetic therapies and enhancements would only be available to those in society who are already wealthy and powerful. The competitive advantages accompanying access to these technologies could therefore be bought in a way that natural genetic advantages cannot be.

Once again, however, we may question whether this really represents such a radical departure from the status quo. It is already the case that the financially advantaged can purchase competitive advantages. We are not only already subject to naturally occurring inequality as a result of the genetic lottery, but also to inequality brought about by expensive environmental enhancements available only to the wealthy. For example, private school education indisputably exacerbates social inequalities between the rich and the poor, as does inequitable access to the most sophisticated medical treatments. While we ought to be concerned by the possible inequality which may be caused by the future use of genetic engineering, we ought to be equally concerned with the vast inequalities that are already present in and between our societies, and that may clearly be deepened by the ability of the wealthy to purchase environmental enhancements and other competitive advantages. In addition, it is not necessarily the case that "[f]airness ... require[s] that benefits should not be provided to any" until they are widely accessible (Harris, 2007:28).

Harris sums up this position as follows:

> So when enhancements make life or lives better they are justified if they do just that [even] if they also confer positional advantage that is no part of their justification and will in fact always constitute a moral disadvantage of their use, although whether this disadvantage constitutes a decisive argument against either the use or the permissibility of the enhancement will depend upon many other factors, among which are the degree of advantage, the degree of unfairness it creates, and the likelihood of the unfairness being minimized over time or by other factors such as compensation. (2007:30)

Another somewhat idealistic possibility is that modification of the human genome could be employed to diminish, rather than exacerbate, inequalities (Savulescu, 2006:321). How might this be so? Firstly, while genetic interventions may initially only be available to the wealthy, this may ultimately give way to a situation in which their distribution will be more equitable. Moore points out that the vast majority of new medical technologies are initially only available to the rich, but as they are further developed and refined, costs are lowered, and eventually "procedures that were once cost prohibitive are ... available to everyone" (Moore, 2000:117).

Secondly, it has been suggested that genetic enhancement could be used to improve our ethical sensibilities through genetic means, in other words, that "genetic moral enhancement" (Faust, 2008:397) could be used to improve our sense of responsibility towards others, thus heightening our feelings of solidarity and our moral intuitions as to the demands of justice, rather than merely being used as a tool to gain a competitive edge over others.

Finally, some suggest that active use could be made of genetic modifications to counter or diminish the natural inequality that is the result of the genetic lottery, the results of which are "arbitrary from a moral perspective" (Rawls, 1971:64). If our natural genetic advantages and disadvantages are not something which we can be said to deserve (Rawls, 1971:86), an argument can be made for the redistribution of genetic goods by the means of both genetic therapy and enhancement, favouring not the wealthy and powerful, but those who are worse off, genetically or otherwise. While this suggestion may be somewhat idealistic in terms of the current financially driven medical market, it does indicate that the obligation to reduce inequality can at least in principle be called upon as a motivating factor for the development and use of genetic engineering, rather than a factor militating against it. Holtug suggests in this regard that "people who are badly off through no fault of their own" (1999:42), for example, because of genetic disease, should be compensated via the provision of genetic therapy to satisfy the principle of justice.

This raises an interesting possibility. If the successful development of genetic engineering technologies results in a situation in which the "natural distribution" of abilities would no longer be "simply [a] natural fact" (Rawls, 1971:87) their distribution would rightly fall within the province of a theory of justice. Savulescu highlights various alternatives in this regard: "We can allow our lives to be determined by the natural lottery, or by wealth. Both of these lead to injustice." In contrast to this, he suggests that "[j]udicious use of enhancement, based on a rational policy" can, in fact, operate to reduce inequality and injustice (Savulescu, 2006:336).

Consequentialist arguments against genetic engineering rightly draw our attention to the possible negative outcomes of these technologies, including medical risks and the exacerbation of inequality and injustice. While we ought to take these concerns into account in making decisions about when and how to make these interventions available, it is also clear that the worries raised here do not apply only to genetic engineering, but also to other interventions such as environmental enhancements and novel medical treatments in general. Caution is appropriate, but the possibilities identified above are not sufficient to justify the outright rejection of genetic engineering. This is especially the case if we consider not only the possible negative consequences of genetic modification, but also its transformational promise.

14.5   THE PROMISE OF GENETIC ENGINEERING

Genetic therapies are already available for several disease conditions. For example, while they do not yet amount to a cure, three therapies designed to enhance SMN (survival motor neuron protein) production have recently been approved for the treatment of SMA (spinal muscular atrophy), a disease which causes muscles to become weak and waste away, and which predominantly affects children. In its most severe form, and left untreated, it leads to death before the age of two (Chaytow et al., 2021). The FDA has also approved genetic therapies for the treatment of cancers such as acute lymphoblastic leukaemia and lymphoma. Clinical trials are currently underway for the treatment of rare neurological diseases such as ALS (amyotrophic lateral sclerosis), a disease that affects the nerve cells responsible for controlling voluntary muscle movement, and for which there is currently no cure; for treatments to restore vision; and for treatments to combat sickle cell disease, among others. The potential of genetic therapy for reducing suffering and for restoring function in a way that expands opportunity is not something that we should dismiss based on misplaced repugnance.

What of genetic enhancement? While we should certainly take into consideration the moral concerns with enhancement discussed thus far, we should also consider the "cost of not making use of enhancement technologies" (Buchanan, 2011:37). While most would acknowledge the moral desirability of combatting disease and disability to restore normal functioning, we need not accept that this is as far as morality requires us to go. Normal functioning, as Buchanan notes "is simply functioning that is typical of the organism as it happens to be now", without reference to what we value (2011:3-4) and a tendency to prize normal functioning above all else is to "confuse human good with what evolution delivers" (Buchanan, 2011:4). Harris, too, fails to see why the achievement of normality should represent the limit of our moral ambitions. Rather, he argues that "the most usual motive for using technology to intervene in the natural lottery of life is for the sake of the harms this will prevent or the goods that this will bring about" (Harris, 2007:54). If particular forms of general-purpose genetic enhancements can be shown to increase the likelihood of leading a good life, contribute towards well-being, and reduce the disadvantages imposed upon us by the genetic lottery, such technologies may very well be compatible with these goals.

Bibliography

Agar, N. 2004. *Liberal eugenics: in defence of human enhancement*. Oxford: Blackwell. https://doi.org/10.1002/9780470775004

Allhoff, F. 2005. Germ-line genetic enhancement and Rawlsian primary goods. *Kennedy Institute of Ethics Journal*, 15(1):39-56. https://doi.org/10.1353/ken.2005.0007

Anderson, W.F. 1989. Human gene therapy: why draw a line? *Bioethics*, 14(6):681-693. https://doi.org/10.1093/jmp/14.6.681

Annas, G.J. 2000. The man on the moon, immortality, and other millennial myths: the prospects and perils of human genetic engineering. *Emory Law Journal*, 49(3):753-782.

Baylis, F. & Robert, J.S. 2004. The inevitability of genetic enhancement technologies. *Bioethics*, 18(1):1-26. https://doi.org/10.1111/j.1467-8519.2004.00376.x

Beauchamp, T.L. & Childress, J.F. 2009. *Principles of biomedical ethics*. Oxford: Oxford University Press.

Benatar, S.R. 1998. A perspective from Africa on human rights and genetic engineering. In: J. Burley, (ed.). *The genetic revolution and human rights: the Oxford amnesty lectures 1998*. Oxford: Oxford University Press. 159-189.

Borenstein, J. 2009. The wisdom of caution: genetic enhancement and future children. *Science and Engineering Ethics*, 15(4):517-530. https://doi.org/10.1007/s11948-009-9183-9

Brock, D.W. 1998. Enhancements of human function: some distinctions for policymakers. In: E. Parens (ed.). *Enhancing human traits: ethical and social implications*. Washington, DC: Georgetown University Press. 48-69.

Buchanan, A. 2011. *Beyond humanity? The ethics of biomedical enhancement*. Oxford: Oxford University Press.

Buchanan, A., Brock, D., Daniels, N. & Wikler, D. (eds.). 2000. *From chance to choice: genetics and justice*. Cambridge:

Cambridge University Press. https://doi.org/10.1017/CBO9780511806940

Caplan, A.L. 2009. Good, better, or best? In: J. Savulescu & N. Bostrom (eds.). *Human enhancement*. Oxford: Oxford University Press. 199-209.

Char, D.S., Shah, N.H. & Magnus, D. 2018. Implementing machine learning in health care: addressing ethical challenges. *The New England Journal of Medicine*, 378(11):981-983. https://doi.org/10.1056/NEJMp1714229

Chaytow, H., Faller, K., Huang, Y.T. & Gillingwater, T.H. 2021. Spinal muscular atrophy: from approved therapies to future therapeutic targets for personalized medicine. Cell reports. *Medicine*, 2(7):100346. https://doi.org/10.1016/j.xcrm.2021.100346

Coors, M.E. & Hunter, L. 2005. Evaluation of genetic enhancement: will human wisdom properly acknowledge the value of evolution? *The American Journal of Bioethics*, 5(3):21-22. https://doi.org/10.1080/15265160591002683

Daley, J. 2021. Four success stories in gene therapy. *Nature*. [Online]. https://doi.org/10.1038/d41586-021-02737-7

Daniels, N. 2009. Can anyone really be talking about ethically modifying human nature? In: J. Savulescu & N. Bostrom (eds.). *Human enhancement*. Oxford: Oxford University Press. 25-42.

Davis, D.S. 2009. From YUCK to WOW and back again. *Religious Studies Review*, 35(3):147-150. https://doi.org/10.1111/j.1748-0922.2009.01354.x

DeGrazia, D. 2005. Enhancement technologies and human identity. *Journal of Medicine and Philosophy*, 30(3):261-283. https://doi.org/10.1080/03605310590960166

Faust, H.S. 2008. Should we select for genetic moral enhancement? A thought experiment using the MoralKinder (MK+) Haplotype. *Theoretical Medicine and Bioethics*, 29(6):397-416. https://doi.org/10.1007/s11017-008-9089-6

Fenton, E. 2008. Genetic enhancement: a threat to human rights? *Bioethics*, 22(2):1-7.

Fukuyama, F. 2002. *Our posthuman future: consequences of the biotechnology revolution.* New York: Farrar, Straus and Giroux.

Gardner, W. 1995. Can human genetic enhancement be prohibited? *The Journal of Medicine and Philosophy*, 20(1):65-84. https://doi.org/10.1093/jmp/20.1.65

Hall, S. 2012. Harm and enhancement: philosophical and ethical perspectives. Unpublished doctoral dissertation. Stellenbosch: Stellenbosch University.

Harris, J. 1992. *Wonderwoman and Superman: the ethics of human biotechnology.* Oxford: Oxford University Press.

Harris, J. 2007. *Enhancing evolution: the ethical case for making better people.* Princeton: Princeton University Press.

Holtug, N. 1999. Does justice require genetic enhancements? *Journal of Medical Ethics*, 25(2):137-143. https://doi.org/10.1136/jme.25.2.137

Juengst, E. 2009. What's taxonomy got to do with it? "Species integrity", human rights, and science policy. In: J. Savulescu & N. Bostrom (eds.). *Human enhancement.* Oxford: Oxford University Press. 43-58.

Kamm, F. 2009. What is and is not wrong with enhancement? In: J. Savulescu & N. Bostrom (eds.). *Human enhancement.* Oxford: Oxford University Press. 91-130.

Kass, L.R. 2003. Ageless bodies, happy souls: biotechnology and the pursuit of perfection. *The New Atlantis*, 1:9-28.

Knoppers, B. & Thorogood, A. 2017. Ethics and big data in health. *Current Opinion in Systems Biology*, 4:53-57. https://doi.org/10.1016/j.coisb.2017.07.001

Lewens, T. 2009. Enhancement and human nature: the case of Sandel. *Journal of Medical Ethics*, 35(6):354-356.

Li, H., Yang, Y., Hong, W., Huang, M., Wu, M. & Zhao, X. 2020. Applications of genome editing technology in the targeted therapy of human diseases: mechanisms, advances and prospects. *Signal Transduction and Targeted Therapy*, 5(1):1-23. https://doi.org/10.1038/s41392-019-0089-y

McKenny, G.P. 1998. Enhancements and the ethical significance of vulnerability. In: E. Parens (ed.). *Enhancing human traits: ethical and social implications.* Washington, DC: Georgetown University Press. 222-237.

Mehlman, M. 2003. *Wondergenes: genetic enhancement and the future of society.* Bloomington, IN: Indiana University Press.

Moore, A.D. 2000. Owning genetic information and gene enhancement techniques: why privacy and property rights may undermine social control of the human genome. *Bioethics*, 14(2):97-119. https://doi.org/10.1111/1467-8519.00184

Moseley, R. 1991. Maintaining the somatic/germ-line distinction: some ethical drawbacks. *The Journal of Medicine and Philosophy*, 16(6):641-647. https://doi.org/10.1093/jmp/16.6.641

Nair-Collins, M. & Miller, F.G. 2017. Do the 'brain dead' merely appear to be alive? *Journal of Medical Ethics*, 43(11:):747-753. https://doi.org/10.1136/medethics-2016-103867

OECD. 2013. Biotechnology. In: *OECD Factbook 2013: economic, environmental and social statistics.* Paris: OECD Publishing.

Ormond, K.E., Mortlock, D.P., Scholes, D.T., Bombard, Y., Brody, L.C., Faucett, W.A., Garrison, N.A., Hercher, L., Isasi, R., Middleton, A., Musunuru, K., Shriner, D., Virani, A. & Young, C.E. 2017. Human germline genome editing. *American Journal of Human Genetics*, 101(2):167-176. https://doi.org/10.1016/j.ajhg.2017.06.012

Rawls, J. 1971. *A theory of justice.* Oxford: Oxford University Press. https://doi.org/10.4159/9780674042605

Parens, E. 1995. The goodness of fragility: on the prospect of genetic technologies aimed at the enhancement of human capacities. *Kennedy Institute of Ethics Journal*, 5(2): 141-153. https://doi.org/10.1353/ken.0.0149

Robert, J.S. 2005. Human dispossession and human enhancement. *The American Journal of Bioethics*, 5(3):27-29. https://doi.org/10.1080/15265160591002728

Sandel, M. 2007. *The case against perfection.* Cambridge & London: The Belknap Press of Harvard University Press.

Savulescu, J. 2006. Justice, fairness, and enhancement. *Annals of the New York Academy of Sciences*, 1093:321-338. https://doi.org/10.1196/annals.1382.021

Savulescu, J. 2007. In defence of procreative beneficence. *Journal of Medical Ethics*, 33(5):284-288. https://doi.org/10.1136/jme.2006.018184

Singer, P. 1993. *Practical ethics.* Cambridge: Cambridge University Press.

The President's Council on Bioethics. 2003. *Beyond therapy: biotechnology and the pursuit of happiness.* Washington, DC: The President's Council on Bioethics.

UNESCO. 1997. *Universal declaration on the human genome and human rights.* Paris: 29th Session of the General Conference.

Winkler, M.G. 1998. Devices and desires of our own hearts. In: E. Parens (ed.). *Enhancing human traits: ethical and social implications.* Washington, DC: Georgetown University Press. 95-123.

Contributing Authors

Susan Hall

Department of Philosophy
Stellenbosch University
Stellenbosch
South Africa

Email: shall@sun.ac.za
https://orcid.org/0000-0002-1668-5185

Chris Jones

Unit for Moral Leadership
Faculty of Theology
Stellenbosch University
Stellenbosch, South Africa

Email: chrisjones@sun.ac.za
https://orcid.org/0000-0002-9483-5337

Anita Kleinsmidt

Faculty of Law
University of the Western Cape
Bellville, Cape Town, South Africa

Email: kleinsmidt@gmail.com
https://orcid.org/0000-0003-0125-7804

Willie Koen

Cardiothoracic surgeon
Life Vincent Pallotti Hospital
Pinelands, Cape Town, South Africa

Email: wkoen@iafrica.com
https://orcid.org/0000-0002-2950-4961

Mariana Kruger

Department of Paediatrics and
Child Health
Faculty of Medicine and Health
Sciences
Stellenbosch University and Tygerberg
Hospital, Stellenbosch, South Africa

Email: marianakruger@sun.ac.za
https://orcid.org/0000-0002-6838-0180

Rosaan Krüger

Faculty of Law
Rhodes University
Grahamstown/Makhanda, South Africa

Email: r.kruger@ru.ac.za
https://orcid.org/0000-0002-8894-502X

Willem Landman

Extraordinary Professor
Department of Philosophy
Stellenbosch University Stellenbosch,
South Africa

Email: willemlandman1948@gmail.com
https://orcid.org/0000-0003-0071-7426

Elmi Muller

Dean of the Faculty of Medicine and
Health Sciences
Stellenbosch University
Stellenbosch, South Africa

Email: elmimuller@sun.ac.za
https://orcid.org/0000-0003-4891-5296

Johannes R (Hanru) Niemand

Clinical psychologist in private practice
Durbanville, Cape Town, South Africa

Email: hanruniemand@gmail.com
https://orcid.org/0000-0001-7045-2924

Carike Noeth

Research Associate
Systematic Theology and Ecclesiology
Faculty of Theology
Stellenbosch University
Stellenbosch, South Africa

Email: carike@sun.ac.za
https://orcid.org/0000-0002-0787-3109

Andrea Palk

Department of Philosophy
Stellenbosch University
Stellenbosch, South Africa

Email: apalk@sun.ac.za
https://orcid.org/0000-0002-6798-0985

Jerome Amir Singh

Howard College School of Law
University of Kwazulu-Natal
Durban, South Africa

Dalla Lana School of Public Health
University of Toronto, Toronto, Canada

Email: singhj9@ukzn.ac.za
https://orcid.org/0000-0002-6275-6853

Himla Soodyall

Academy of Science of South Africa &
Division of Human Genetics
School of Pathology
Faculty of Health Sciences
University of the Witwatersrand and
National Health Laboratory Service
Johannesburg, South Africa

Email: himla@assaf.org.za
https://orcid.org/0000-0003-2488-9185

Juri van den Heever

Faculty of Science
Department of Botany and Zoology
Stellenbosch University
Stellenbosch, South Africa

Email: jurivdh@gmail.com
https://orcid.org/0000-0002-4858-4485

Anton van Niekerk

Department of Philosophy and Director
of the Centre for Applied Ethics
Stellenbosch University
Stellenbosch, South Africa

Email: aavn@sun.ac.za
https://orcid.org/0000-0003-3362-3434

Basie von Solms

Centre for Cyber Security
University of Johannesburg
Johannesburg, South Africa

Email: basievs@uj.ac.za
https://orcid.org/0000-0003-3586-6632

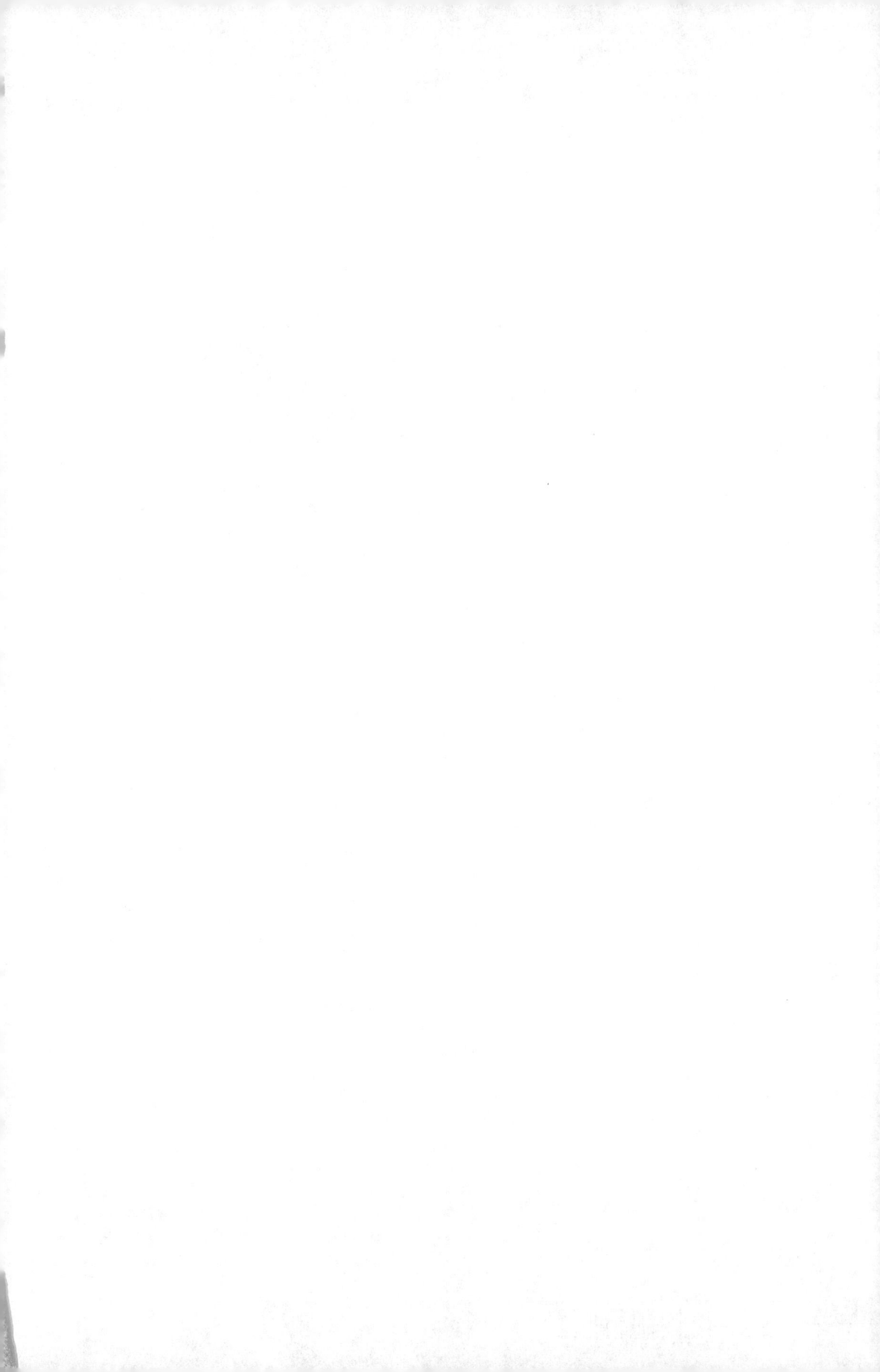